Imaging in Oncology

Editor

VIJAY P. KHATRI

SURGICAL ONCOLOGY CLINICS OF NORTH AMERICA

www.surgonc.theclinics.com

Consulting Editor
NICHOLAS J. PETRELLI

October 2014 • Volume 23 • Number 4

ELSEVIER

1600 John F. Kennedy Boulevard ● Suite 1800 ● Philadelphia, Pennsylvania, 19103-2899

http://www.theclinics.com

SURGICAL ONCOLOGY CLINICS OF NORTH AMERICA Volume 23, Number 4
October 2014 ISSN 1055-3207, ISBN-13: 978-0-323-32634-6

Editor: Jessica McCool
Developmental Editor: Stephanie Carter

Surgical Oncology Clinics of North America (ISSN 1055-3207) is published quarterly by Elsevier Inc., 360 Park Avenue South, New York, NY 10010-1710. Months of publication are January, April, July, and October. Business and Editorial Offices: 1600 John F. Kennedy Blvd., Ste. 1800, Philadelphia, PA 19103-2899. Customer Service Office: 3251 Riverport Lane, Maryland Heights, MO 63043. Periodicals postage paid at New York, NY and additional mailing offices. Subscription prices are $290.00 per year (US individuals), $421.00 (US institutions) $140.00 (US student/resident), $330.00 (Canadian individuals), $533.00 (Canadian institutions), $205.00 (Canadian student/resident), $410.00 (foreign individuals), $533.00 (foreign institutions), and $205.00 (foreign student/resident). Foreign air speed delivery is included in all Clinics subscription prices. All prices are subject to change without notice. **POSTMASTER**: Send address changes to Surgical Oncology Clinics of North America, Elsevier Health Science Division, Subscription Customer Service, 3251 Riverport Lane, Maryland Heights, MO 63043. **Customer Service: 1-800-654-2452 (US and Canada). 314-447-8871 (outside US and Canada). Fax: 314-447-8029. E-mail: journalscustomerservice-usa@elsevier.com** (for print support); **journalsonline support-usa@elsevier.com** (for online support).

Reprints. For copies of 100 or more, of articles in this publication, please contact the Commercial Reprints Department, Elsevier Inc., 360 Park Avenue South, New York, New York 10010-1710. Tel. 212-633-3874; Fax: 212-633-3820; E-mail: reprints@elsevier.com.

Surgical Oncology Clinics of North America is covered in MEDLINE/PubMed (Index Medicus) and EMBASE/ Excerpta Medica, Current Contents/Clinical Medicine, and ISI/BIOMED.

Contributors

CONSULTING EDITOR

NICHOLAS J. PETRELLI, MD, FACS
Bank of America Endowed Medical Director, Helen F. Graham Cancer Center at Christiana
Care, Newark, Delaware; Professor of Surgery, Thomas Jefferson University, Philadelphia,
Pennsylvania

EDITOR

VIJAY P. KHATRI, MBChB, FACS, MBA
Division of Surgical Oncology, Professor of Surgery, Department of Surgery; Medical
Director, Clinical Resource Utilization Management, University California, Davis
Comprehensive Cancer Center, University California, Davis Health System, Sacramento,
California

AUTHORS

SHADI AMINOLOLAMA-SHAKERI, MD
Department of Radiology, University California, Davis Health System, Sacramento,
California

ALEXANDER J. ANTONIOU, MD, MA
Russell H Morgan Department of Radiology and Radiological Sciences, Johns Hopkins
School of Medicine, Baltimore, Maryland

APARNA BALACHANDRAN, MD
Associate Professor, Abdominal Imaging, The University of Texas MD Anderson Cancer
Center, Houston, Texas

PRIYA R. BHOSALE, MD
Associate Professor, Abdominal Imaging, The University of Texas MD Anderson Cancer
Center, Houston, Texas

CHUSLIP CHARNSANGAVEJ, MD
Professor, Abdominal Imaging, The University of Texas MD Anderson Cancer Center,
Houston, Texas

HONG CHOU, MBBS
Radiology Department, Vancouver General Hospital, University of British Columbia,
Vancouver, British Columbia, Canada

DANAI CHOURMOUZI, MD, PhD
Diagnostic Radiology Department, Interbalcan Medical Centre, Thessaloniki, Greece

MICHAEL T. CORWIN, MD
Department of Radiology, University California, Davis Health System, Sacramento,
California

ANTONIOS DREVELEGAS, MD, PhD
Professor of Radiology, Diagnostic Radiology Department, Interbalcan Medical Centre,
Thessaloniki, Greece

GHANEH FANANAZAPIR, MD
Department of Radiology, University California, Davis Health System, Sacramento,
California

BRUCE B. FORSTER, MD
Radiology Department, Vancouver General Hospital, University of British Columbia,
Vancouver, British Columbia, Canada

MICHELLE S. GINSBERG, MD
Director, Cardiothoracic Imaging; Member, Department of Radiology, Memorial Sloan
Kettering Cancer Center; Professor of Radiology, Weill Cornell Medical College,
New York, New York

SARA A. HAYES, MD
Assistant Attending Radiologist, Department of Radiology; Assistant Member, Memorial
Sloan Kettering Cancer Center; Assistant Professor, Weill Cornell Medical College,
New York, New York

SUSAN HILTON, MD
Clinical Professor of Radiology, Perelman School of Medicine, University of Pennsylvania;
Chief, CT Section, Department of Radiology, Hospital of the University of Pennsylvania,
Philadelphia, Pennsylvania

J. LOUIS HINSHAW, MD
Associate Professor, Department of Radiology, University of Wisconsin School of
Medicine and Public Health, Madison, Wisconsin

LISA P. JONES, MD, PhD
Clinical Associate Professor of Radiology, Perelman School of Medicine, University of
Pennsylvania, Philadelphia, Pennsylvania

VIJAY P. KHATRI, MBChB, FACS, MBA
Division of Surgical Oncology, Professor of Surgery, Department of Surgery; Medical
Director, Clinical Resource Utilization Management, University California, Davis
Comprehensive Cancer Center, University California, Davis Health System, Sacramento,
California

RAMIT LAMBA, MBBS, MD
Department of Radiology, University California, Davis Health System, Sacramento,
California

MEGHAN G. LUBNER, MD
Assistant Professor, Department of Radiology, University of Wisconsin School of
Medicine and Public Health, Madison, Wisconsin

PAUL I. MALLINSON, MBChB
Clinical Fellow, Radiology Department, Vancouver General Hospital, University of British
Columbia, Vancouver, British Columbia, Canada

CHARLES MARCUS, MD
Russell H Morgan Department of Radiology and Radiological Sciences, Johns Hopkins
School of Medicine, Baltimore, Maryland

KOSTANTINOS MARIAS, PhD
Computational Medicine Laboratory, Institute of Computer Science, FORTH, Heraklion, Greece

WILLIAM W. MAYO-SMITH, MD
Professor, Department of Diagnostic Imaging, Rhode Island Hospital, Alpert School of Medicine, Brown University, Providence, Rhode Island

PETER L. MUNK, MD
Radiology Department, Vancouver General Hospital, University of British Columbia, Vancouver, British Columbia, Canada

BRUNO C. ODISIO, MD
Assistant Professor, Division of Diagnostic Imaging, Department of Interventional Radiology, The University of Texas MD Anderson Cancer Center, Houston, Texas

ELISSABET PAPADOPOULOU, MD, PhD
Diagnostic Radiology Department, Interbalcan Medical Centre, Thessaloniki, Greece

PERRY J. PICKHARDT, MD
Professor, Department of Radiology, University of Wisconsin School of Medicine and Public Health, Madison, Wisconsin

ANDREW J. PLODKOWSKI, MD
Assistant Attending Radiologist, Department of Radiology; Assistant Member, Memorial Sloan Kettering Cancer Center; Assistant Professor, Weill Cornell Medical College, New York, New York

JULIE H. SONG, MD
Associate Professor, Department of Diagnostic Imaging (Clinical), Rhode Island Hospital, Alpert School of Medicine, Brown University, Providence, Rhode Island

RATHAN M. SUBRAMANIAM, MD, PhD, MPH
Russell H Morgan Department of Radiology and Radiological Sciences; Department of Oncology; Department of Otolaryngology-Head and Neck Surgery, Johns Hopkins School of Medicine; Department of Health Policy and Management, Johns Hopkins Bloomberg School of Public Health, Baltimore, Maryland

ERIC P. TAMM, MD
Professor, Abdominal Imaging, The University of Texas MD Anderson Cancer Center, Houston, Texas

MICHAEL J. WALLACE, MD
Department Chair ad interim, Division of Diagnostic Imaging, Department of Interventional Radiology, The University of Texas MD Anderson Cancer Center, Houston, Texas

Contents

Neuroimaging plays a crucial role in diagnosis of brain tumors and in the
decision-making process for therapy. Functional imaging techniques can
reflect cellular density (diffusion imaging), capillary density (perfusion techniques), and tissue biochemistry (magnetic resonance [MR] spectroscopy).
In addition, cortical activation imaging (functional MR imaging) can identify
various loci of eloquent cerebral cortical function. Combining these new
tools can increase diagnostic specificity and confidence. Familiarity with
conventional and advanced imaging findings facilitates accurate diagnosis, differentiation from other processes, and optimal patient treatment.
This article is a practical synopsis of pathologic, clinical, and imaging
spectra of most common brain tumors.

In this review, the value of imaging in the management of head and neck
tumors is summarized. The many diverse tumors of the head and neck
are grouped for purposes of staging and treatment. The groupings of
malignancies consist of sinonasal, nasopharynx, salivary gland, oral cavity, oropharynx, hypopharynx, larynx, and thyroid tumors. The anatomy,
rationale for choice of imaging modality, interpretation of acquired images,
staging, treatment options, and posttherapy assessment are discussed.

Computed tomography (CT) is the primary imaging modality for the diagnosis, staging, and follow-up of most thoracic cavity tumors. Fluorine-18
fluorodeoxyglucose positron emission tomography/CT has established
itself as a supplementary tool to CT in lung cancer staging and in the
assessment for distant metastases of many thoracic tumors. Magnetic
resonance imaging is an important adjunctive imaging modality in thoracic
oncologic imaging and is used as a problem-solving tool to assess for
chest wall invasion, intraspinal extension, and cardiac/vascular invasion.
Imaging can facilitate minimally invasive biopsy of most thoracic tumors
and is vital in the pretreatment planning of radiation therapy.

comprise the ligaments, mesenteries, and connective tissues of the peritoneal and retroperitoneal spaces.

Adrenal glands are common sites of disease involved in a wide spectrum
of pathology. Several imaging studies allow accurate diagnosis of adrenal
masses, separating inconsequential benign masses from the lesions that
require treatment. This article discusses contemporary adrenal imaging
techniques, imaging appearance, and the optimal imaging algorithm for
the workup of common adrenal masses.

Modern radiologic imaging is an aid to treatment planning for localized
renal cancer, enabling characterization of mass lesions. For patients who
present with advanced renal cancer, new imaging techniques enable a
functional assessment of treatment response not possible using anatomic
measurements alone. Multidetector CT urography permits simultaneous
assessment of the kidneys and urinary tract for patients with unexplained
hematuria. Both CT and MRI play a significant role in staging and follow
up of patients treated for urothelial cancer. Newer imaging methods such
as diffusion-weighted MRI have shown promising results for improving
accuracy of staging and follow up of urothelial cancer.

Magnetic resonance imaging is the mainstay of diagnostic imaging for soft
tissue masses, but plain film, ultrasound, and computed tomography all
have roles. A subset of lesions has specific imaging features that enable
a confident radiological diagnosis with appropriate clinical correlation.
Many soft tissue masses have nonspecific appearances and should be
considered for biopsy in a specialist center. When a biopsy is required
for definitive diagnosis, careful multidisciplinary planning is essential to
avoid contamination of unaffected tissue, leading to recurrence and
unnecessary amputations. This article discusses radiological diagnosis,
biopsy, and management of the soft tissue mass.

Interventional oncology, a term commonly used to indicate the minimally
invasive procedures performed by interventional radiologists to diagnose
and manage cancer, encompasses a broad spectrum of techniques
unique to interventional radiology that have been established as a vital
part of the multidisciplinary oncologic cancer care team. This article provides an updated overview of the variety of applications of image-guided
procedures to distinct clinical scenarios, such as the diagnosis, treatment,
and management of complications of malignancies.

Imaging in Oncology

SURGICAL ONCOLOGY CLINICS OF NORTH AMERICA

Foreword

Imaging in Oncology

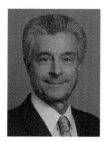

Nicholas J. Petrelli, MD, FACS
Consulting Editor

This issue of the *Surgical Oncology Clinics of North America* deals with imaging technology in cancer care. The guest editor is Vijay P. Khatri, MBChB, FACS, MBA, Professor of Surgery, from the University of California Davis School of Medicine. Dr Khatri manages a variety of cancers, with clinical interests in rectal carcinoma and primary/metastatic liver cancers. He also has experience in the management of extremity soft tissue sarcomas. Dr Khatri's research is geared toward the implementation of clinical research and conducting clinical trials.

This issue of the *Surgical Oncology Clinics of North America* runs the gamut of imaging from adrenal gland tumors, thoracic cavity tumors, soft tissue tumors, head and neck tumors, to imaging of pancreatic neoplasms, among others. The article entitled, "Diagnostic Imaging of Hepatic Lesions in Adults," by Dr Khatri and his colleagues is especially interesting and informative. Dr Khatri is also an author on the article entitled, "Emerging Modalities in Breast Cancer Imaging," with his colleague Dr Shakeri.

The last issue of *Surgical Oncology Clinics of North America* devoted to cancer imaging was guest edited by Scott Kurtzman, MD, from the Department of Surgery at Waterbury Hospital and the University of Connecticut School of Medicine, in April 2007. That edition dealt with preoperative and postoperative cancer imaging and hence it was long overdue to update imaging status in cancer care to the present day. I'd like to thank Dr Khatri and his colleagues for this edition of the *Surgical Oncology Clinics of North America* and hope that readers will share this information with all of their trainees in surgery.

Nicholas J. Petrelli, MD, FACS
Helen F. Graham Cancer Center at Christiana Care
4701 Ogletown-Stanton Road, Suite 1233
Newark, DE 19713, USA

E-mail address:
npetrelli@christianacare.org

http://dx.doi.org/10.1016/j.soc.2014.07.006
surgonc.theclinics.com

Preface

Imaging in Oncology

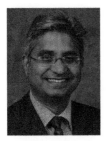

Vijay P. Khatri, MBChB, FACS, MBA
Editor

The source and center of all man's creative power…is his power of making images, or the power of imagination.

—*Robert Collier*

Imaging plays an important role along the entire trajectory of cancer management; hence, this issue of *Surgical Oncology Clinics of North America* is devoted to this topic. Leading authorities in this field have been recruited to contribute their expertise and provide a unique insight in the application of established and emerging radiological techniques. The comprehensive reviews by the authors are further enhanced by an abundance of radiographs to clarify the concepts. The issue addresses the topic in a system and disease site–based approach. I am grateful to Dr Nicholas Petrelli, Consulting Editor, for this opportunity and moreover for his unrelenting mentorship that remains unsurpassed. Dr Petrelli's consummate leadership in the educational, clinical, research, and executive aspect of surgical oncology is incomparable.

I am deeply indebted to the efforts of all the contributors and their timely submissions. Special gratitude is extended to Jessica McCool and Stephanie Carter for their tireless efforts to drive this issue to the finish line. I am confident that the audience will appreciate the depth of the knowledge imparted by the contributors and ultimately benefit our patients, who deserve our best.

Vijay P. Khatri, MBChB, FACS, MBA
Clinical Resource Utilization Management
University of California
Davis Health System
Sacramento, CA 95817, USA

E-mail address:
vijay.khatri@ucdmc.ucdavis.edu

Surg Oncol Clin N Am 23 (2014) xiii
http://dx.doi.org/10.1016/j.soc.2014.07.007
1055-3207/14/$ – see front matter © 2014 Elsevier Inc. All rights reserved.

surgonc.theclinics.com

Erratum

An error was made in the July 2014 issue of *Surgical Oncology Clinics of North America,* Vol. 23, No. 3, on page 569. The first sentence of the second paragraph included incorrect percentages. The corrected sentence should read "Compared with other breast cancer patterns, TNBC are more likely to be occult on mammography and ultrasonography imaging (19.5% vs 36%)."

Surg Oncol Clin N Am 23 (2014) xv
http://dx.doi.org/10.1016/j.soc.2014.08.001
1055-3207/14/$ – see front matter © 2014 Elsevier Inc. All rights reserved.

surgonc.theclinics.com

Imaging of Brain Tumors

Danai Chourmouzi, MD, PhD[a],*, Elissabet Papadopoulou, MD, PhD[a],
Kostantinos Marias, PhD[b], Antonios Drevelegas, MD, PhD[a]

KEYWORDS

- Brain tumors • Magnetic resonance imaging • Diffusion imaging
- Perfusion techniques • Magnetic resonance spectroscopy
- Functional magnetic resonance imaging

KEY POINTS

- A prerequisite for the diagnosis of brain tumors is knowledge of their incidence and prevalence, histopathological classification, and clinical course.
- Different tumors occur in different age groups, and the likelihood of malignancy is influenced by the age of the patient. The location of a lesion is critical to narrowing the differential diagnosis.
- Neuroimaging plays a crucial role in establishing a diagnosis and is involved in the decision-making process for therapy.
- On computed tomography and magnetic resonance imaging (MRI), findings such as calcifications, cystic components, contrast enhancement, and signal intensity on T1-weighted images and T2-weighted images allow characterization of the tumors. However, the introduction of advanced imaging techniques into clinical practice places new tools into the hands of neuroscientists.
- Functional imaging techniques can reflect cellular density (diffusion imaging), capillary density (perfusion techniques), and tissue biochemistry (MR spectroscopy). In addition, cortical activation imaging (functional MRI) can identify various loci of eloquent cerebral cortical function. Combining these new tools can increase diagnostic specificity and confidence.
- Familiarity with conventional and advanced imaging findings facilitates accurate diagnosis, differentiation from other processes, and optimal patient treatment.

CONVENTIONAL IMAGING TECHNIQUES IN BRAIN TUMORS

Intracranial tumors are a significant health problem. The annual incidence of primary and secondary central nervous system (CNS) neoplasms ranges from 10 to 17 per 100,000 persons.[1]

The authors have nothing to disclose.
[a] Diagnostic Radiology Department, Interbalcan Medical Centre, Asklipiou 10, Thessaloniki 57001, Greece; [b] Computational Medicine Laboratory, Institute of Computer Science, Plastira 100 Vasilika Vouton, FORTH, Heraklion, Greece
* Corresponding author.
E-mail address: dchourm@hol.gr

Surg Oncol Clin N Am 23 (2014) 629–684
http://dx.doi.org/10.1016/j.soc.2014.07.004
1055-3207/14/$ – see front matter © 2014 Elsevier Inc. All rights reserved.

Brain tumors include a variety of subtypes with a broad range of histopathological characteristics, molecular and genetic profiles, clinical spectra, treatment possibilities, and patient prognoses and outcomes.[2]

The diagnosis and grading of brain tumors follows the World Health Organization (WHO) classification.[3] Also, neuroimaging plays a critical role in the diagnosis of brain tumors and pre-operative planning.

Unenhanced computed tomography (CT) of the brain is considered the first line of imaging for patients with suspected brain tumor who present with acute symptoms. Contrast-enhanced CT can be helpful in detecting areas of blood-brain barrier (BBB) breakdown and defining the contrast-enhancing tumor border. However, even multidetector CT using intravenous contrast agent is inferior to magnetic resonance imaging (MRI) in terms of soft tissue resolution. Yet, the presence and distribution of calcifications in a mass and bone remodeling adjacent to a tumor are better shown on CT than MRI.

MRI is the most useful imaging technique and the imaging test of choice for patients with brain tumor. In clinical practice, numerous different MRI protocols exist for imaging brain tumors. The most widely accepted imaging protocol includes at least the following sequences: T2-weighted imaging (T2WI), fluid-attenuated inversion recovery (FLAIR), T1-weighted imaging (T1WI), and contrast-enhanced T1WI. However, conventional MRI suffers from nonspecificity with respect to different pathological processes that appear to be similar on imaging.

Discrimination of extra-axial from intra-axial brain tumors is easy with only conventional anatomic imaging; however, the major diagnostic challenge is to reliably, noninvasively, and promptly differentiate intra-axial tumors to avoid biopsy and follow-up imaging studies.

Conventional MRI provides information about peritumoral edema/mass effect, cystic/necrotic changes, the presence of hemorrhage, and distant tumor foci. These findings are often associated with aggressive tumors. However, the absence of or minimal peritumoral edema, absence of necrotic or hemorrhagic foci, lack of a mass effect, and no contrast enhancement is sometimes observed in high-grade tumors.[4] Therefore, novel functional imaging techniques are being increasingly applied to patients with brain tumors.

The implementation of echo planar imaging (EPI) allowed the development of advanced imaging techniques, providing physiological information that complements the anatomical information available with conventional MRI. Neuroimaging in neuro-oncology is no longer a tool simply evaluating structural abnormalities and identifying tumor-related complications but it has evolved into a science that incorporates functional, hemodynamic, metabolic, cellular, and cytoarchitectural alterations.[5] Functional imaging techniques can reflect cellular density/tissue microarchitecture (diffusion imaging), capillary density (susceptibility perfusion techniques), and tissue biochemistry (MR spectroscopy [MRS]). In addition, cortical activation imaging (functional MRI [fMRI]) using techniques that are dependent on blood oxygen levels can identify various loci of eloquent cerebral cortical function.[6–8]

ADVANCED MRI TECHNIQUES IN BRAIN TUMORS
Diffusion-Weighted Imaging and Diffusion Tensor Imaging

Diffusion-weighted MRI is based on a unique contrast mechanism reflecting the differences in the diffusion of water molecules within the brain tissue.[9] The technique uses ultrafast pulse sequences similar to EPI, to freeze macroscopic patient motion, and makes use of strong gradient pulses to diphase and subsequently rephase water protons. The apparent diffusion coefficient (ADC) is a physical property of the tissue, reflecting water mobility, primarily in the extracellular space. The ADC value is regulated by the size of the extracellular space; therefore, hypercellularity may lead to a significant reduction in the ADC value and significant increase in tumor necrosis. In tissues with unrestricted water diffusion, the MR signal is depressed (low intensity, or dark, on diffusion-weighted imaging [DWI], high ADC values). In contrast, restricted water diffusion increases the signal intensity on DWI (ie, bright on DWI, low ADC values).

Clinical applications of DWI in neuro-oncology include:

- Differentiating cerebral abscesses from necrotic tumors; the high cellularity and viscosity in the purulent abscess fluid restricts water diffusion (**Fig. 1**).[10]
- Assessing tumor grade; increased cellularity, decreased extracellular space, and high nuclear/cytoplasmic ratio are the factors responsible for water diffusion the restriction of water diffusion in high-grade tumors. ADC values are inversely correlated with tumor grade (ie, low-grade tumors have higher ADCs than high-grade tumors, although some degree of overlap exists between certain tumor types).[11]
- Definition of the true extent of gliomas, as restriction of diffusion may extend outside the contrast-enhancing component of a tumor (**Fig. 2**).
- Differentiating vasogenic from neoplastic infiltrative edema; ADC values tend to be lower for infiltrative edema in high-grade tumors than for edema secondary to metastatic disease.[12]

Molecular mobility in tissues may not be the same in all directions (diffusion anisotropy) because of the presence of obstacles that may limit molecular movement in some directions.[13] Highly organized tissues, such as white matter exhibit anisotropic diffusion because of the presence of physical barriers (myelin sheaths), whereas isotropic diffusion is present when molecular motion is not spatially restricted. DWI sequences have been adapted to perform diffusion tensor imaging (DTI). DTI measures water mobility based on the data obtained from 6 or more gradient directions, as opposed to three directions in DWI. Diffusion tensor–based fiber tracking is a novel method that can be used to reconstruct the major fiber bundles of the white matter.[14] The technique is based on the fact that water mobility is facilitated across the direction of fibers rather than perpendicular to their long axis.

Current established clinical applications of DTI in neuro-oncology include:

- Identifying patterns of the relationship between tumor and white matter tracts (deviation, edema, infiltration, and destruction) (**Fig. 3**).
- Revealing peritumoral abnormalities that are not apparent on conventional MRI, allowing identification of tumor margins.[15]

Perfusion-Weighted Imaging

The development and maintenance of an adequate blood supply are essential for tumor growth and invasion. In high-grade gliomas, new formation of dense vascular beds produces an extremely high local tissue blood volume. These neocapillaries are abnormal and produce markedly increased capillary permeability. Tumor angiogenesis and capillary permeability are the focus of the 2 types of microvascular imaging methods: dynamic susceptibility contrast (DSC) T2*-weighted perfusion (DSC-MRI) techniques are used to estimate the volume of the neovascular capillary bed during the first pass of a contrast bolus,[16] and dynamic contrast enhancement (DCE) T1-weighted permeability (DCE-MRI) techniques used to estimate impairment

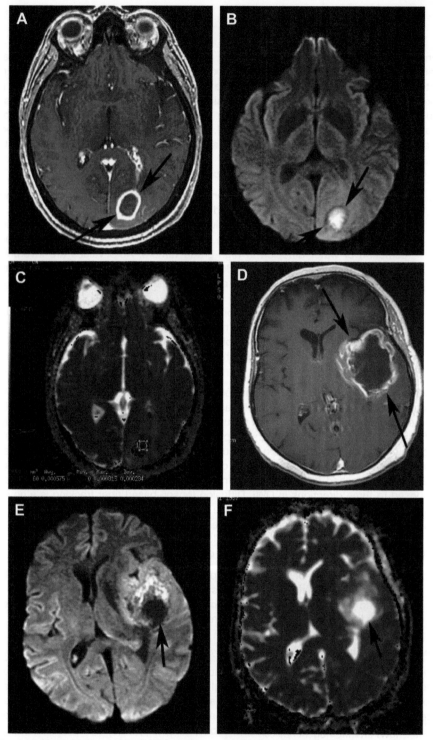

Fig. 1. Differentiating cerebral abscess from necrotic tumor based on DWI. The abscess in left occipital lobe shows ringlike enhancement (*arrows*) on postcontrast T1WI (*A*), high signal on DWI (*arrows*) (*B*), and low signal on ADC map (*C*). The glioblastoma in the left insula shows irregular ringlike enhancement on postcontrast T1WI (*arrows*) (*D*), low signal centrally on DWI (*arrow*) (*E*), and high on ADC map (*arrow*) (*F*).

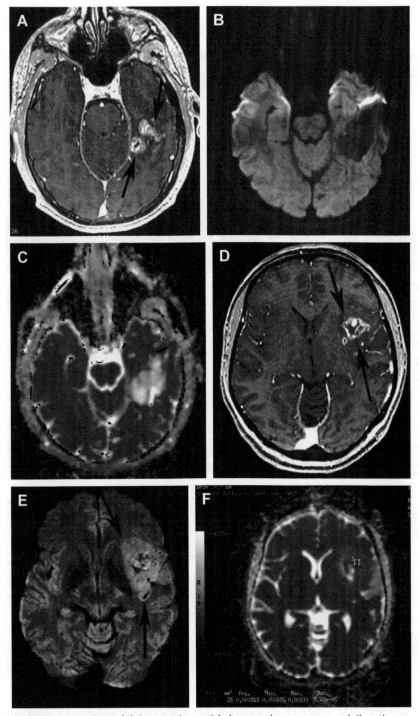

Fig. 2. Postcontrast T1WI (*A*) in a patient with low-grade astrocytoma (pilocytic astrocytoma) shows an inhomogeneous contrast-enhanced left temporal mass (*arrows*), with low signal intensity on DWI (*B*) and high ADC values (*C*), reflecting the free diffusion pattern. On the contrary, restricted diffusion pattern is identified in a patient with a left insular glioblastoma with inhomogeneous enhancement on postcontrast T1WI (*arrows*) (*D*), where the hypercellular part shows high signal intensity on DWI (*arrows*) (*E*), low ADC values (*F*), and extends outside the contrast-enhancing component of the tumor.

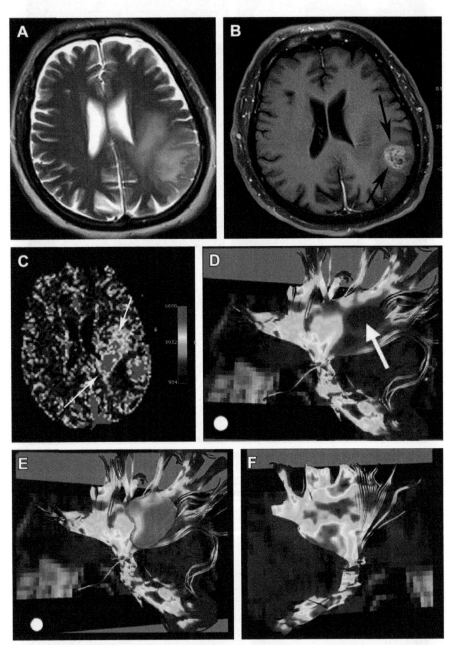

Fig. 3. Patient with glioblastoma. Axial T2WI (*A*) and postcontrast T1WI (*B*) show a left parietal enhancing tumor with peritumoral edema (*arrows*). Perfusion color map (*C*) shows the true extent of GBM, since high rCBV extends outside the contrast-enhancing component of the tumor (*arrows*). Fiber tracking of the corona radiata and fractional anisotropy color encoding (*D–F*). Red shows high fractional anisotropy, whereas blue shows low fractional anisotropy (*arrow*). The tumor is infiltrating adjacent tracts (*D, E*), because the fractional anisotropy is significantly reduced, compared with the normal contralateral corona radiata (*F*).

of the BBB by monitoring passage of the contrast into the extravascular space during the first pass and early recirculation phases.[17]

DSC-MRI of brain tumors relies on a high-pressure injection of a large contrast dose to produce a dynamic decrease in signal intensity on susceptibility T2*- weighted images acquired serially throughout the whole brain every 1 to 2 seconds during the injection. The signal change in each voxel is used to compute the relative cerebral blood volume (rCBV) of that voxel, which can then be shown as a color map or as a graph of the change in signal intensity in a given area over time (time-intensity curve). It has been shown that rCBV correlates positively with tumor vascularity.

The most important established clinical applications of DSC-MRI in diagnosis of brain tumors include:

- Tumor grading, because the average rCBV of high-grade lesions is significantly higher than that of low-grade neoplasms (**Fig. 4**).[18]
- rCBV maps can be used to select biopsy sites of likely higher grade that can be identified as areas of higher rCBV (hot area).[19]
- Sensitive definition of the true extent of gliomas, because high rCBV may extend outside the contrast-enhancing portion of a tumor (see **Fig. 3C**).[20]
- Differentiating tumor recurrence from radiation necrosis. Unlike tumors, which have increased rCBV, radiation necrosis has been shown to have diminished rCBV.[21]

Spectroscopy

MR spectroscopy (MRS) is a noninvasive method to study in vivo biochemical molecules known as metabolites. The fundamental observation, that each individual biochemical molecule resonates in a unique frequency (chemical fingerprint of the molecule), is the basic principle of MRS. Each molecule, because of its different shape and size, alters slightly the local magnetic field, introducing slight changes in the resonance frequency, the so-called chemical shift effect. The differences in proton resonance frequency are shown on the x-axis of a spectrum in units of parts per million of the resonance frequency of a standard reference compound, rather than in hertz, to produce spectra that are comparable across different field strengths. Because clinical MRS is not directly quantifiable, the y-axis of the graph represents arbitrary units of signal intensity scaled relative to the highest peak.[22,23] Principal metabolite peaks are seen in **Table 1**.

- N-Acetylaspartate (NAA) is a marker of neuronal number and function
- Creatine (Cr) is a marker of energy metabolism
- Choline (Cho) is a marker of membrane synthesis and degradation (membrane turnover)

All processes that injure neurons decrease NAA levels; all processes that injure glia or stimulate glial division increase Cho levels; all processes that disrupt aerobic glycolysis result in lactate formation; and all processes that produce necrosis release lipid and decrease Cr levels.[24,25]

The clinical usefulness of MRS is controversial. This controversy can be explained partly by the technical complexity of the method and low reproducibility, especially in the setting of a problematic magnetic field in terms of homogeneity.

The most important established clinical applications of MRS in diagnosis of brain tumors include:

- Tumor grading: qualitative or quantitative detection of high choline/NAA peak height ratios has been shown in several studies to be predictive of the presence

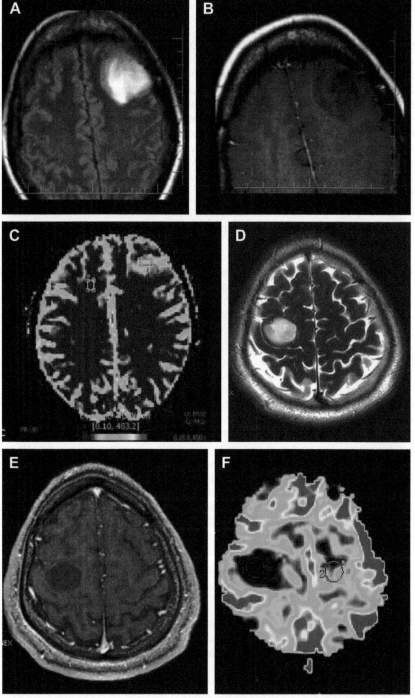

Fig. 4. Tumor grading based on DSC-MRI. Axial FLAIR image (*A*) in a patient with anaplastic astrocytoma grade III shows a hyperintense left frontal lobe tumor. On postcontrast T1WI (*B*), the lesion is unenhanced because of intact BBB. The DSC-MRI rCBV map (*C*) shows an area within the tumor with 5.7 times greater CBV value compared with normal contralateral frontal lobe, indicating tumor with high microvascular density. Axial T2WI (*D*) in a patient with fibrillary astrocytoma grade II shows a hyperintense right frontal lobe mass. The lesion does not enhance on postcontrast T1WI (*E*). Color perfusion map (*F*) shows no foci of increased rCBV.

Table 1
Principal peaks seen in MRS in brain tumors

Metabolite	Peaks (ppm)
Amino acids	0.9–1.0
Lipid	0.9–1.5
Lactate	1.3
Alanine	1.5
N-Acetylaspartate	2.0
Choline	3.2
Creatine	3.0 and 3.9
Myoinositol	3.6

of high-grade tumor (**Fig. 5**).[26] The presence of lipid/lactate in untreated glioma suggests the presence of necrotic grade IV tumor.[27,28]

- Differentiating nonenhancing tumor component from edema to better define the true extent and morphology of gliomas.
- Target biopsies to areas with high Cho/NAA ratios have been reported to increase the accuracy of tumor biopsy by targeting areas of metabolically active tumor within areas of heterogeneous glioma, thus reducing the false-negative rate.[29]
- Differentiating solitary metastasis from high-grade gliomas. Increased levels of Cho surrounding a peripherally enhancing mass reflect tumor infiltration in a high-grade glioma.

fMRI

fMRI comprises one of the recent developments in neuroimaging and has opened new horizons for the in vivo study of brain function. The method is based on the regional alteration of vascular supply in the functioning cortex, which can be detected by using EPI T2*-weighted sequences. Usually, there are 2 study phases: the rest phase and the active phase, in which the patient is asked to perform a specific task (paradigm), such as finger tapping or word production. Subsequently, the signal intensity of the rest period and activation period images are compared, and the regions that show a difference of about 2% to 3% are identified. These regions are considered as the regions of the activated cortex corresponding to the specific performed task (paradigm). With the appropriate paradigm planning, it is possible to study brain cortex functions, including motion (finger tapping), sensation (pain), language receptive and perceptive areas, as well as language motor cortex, memory centers (pictures, words), and vision (checkerboard, moving dots).[30]

Presurgical localization of eloquent cortical areas
One of the main clinical applications of fMRI is the presurgical study of the eloquent cortical areas and their localization, as well as their relation and distance to a known brain tumor. This goal is achieved by using specific targeted tasks (paradigms), depending on the location of the lesion and the findings of a thorough neurologic or neuropsychological evaluation of the patient. This presurgical study provides invaluable information for presurgical planning of the tumors (**Fig. 6**).

Lateralization (dominant hemisphere)
In the presurgical study of brain tumors, it is useful to determine the lateralization of the language and memory functions at least. This process is feasible by using language

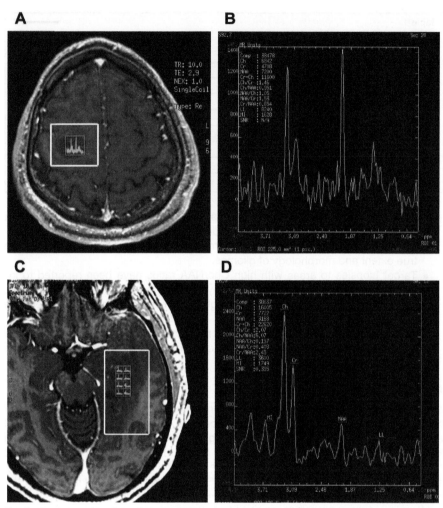

Fig. 5. Tumor grading based on MRS. MRS (*A, B*) of a nonenhancing fibrillary astrocytoma grade II in the right frontal lobe (same patient as **Fig. 4**D–F) shows mild increase of choline (choline/creatine: 1.46; choline/N-acetylaspartate: 0.95). MRS (*C, D*) of a left temporal non-enhancing glioma grade III shows increase of choline and decreased N-acetylaspartate (choline/creatine: 2.07; choline/N-acetylaspartate: 5.07).

paradigms, which show the language motor areas (Broca area) and the language receptive and perceptive areas (Wernicke-Geschwind areas).[31]

Functional neuronavigation

Functional neuronavigation refers to the transfer of the postprocessed data mainly of fMRI and DTI: tractography studies into the neuronavigational system, available as a brain mapping orientation tool during the neurosurgical procedure and to perform image-guided excision of the tumor. The objects of functional neuronavigation are:

- Presurgical risk determination of any procedure (biopsy, ablative, or gross total excision of the tumor)
- Intraoperative mapping (**Fig. 7**)[32]

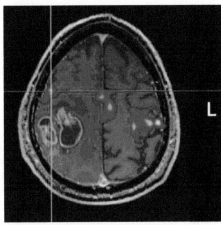

Fig. 6. Presurgical fMRI in a patient with right parietal glioblastoma. Areas of activation are superimposed on axial postcontrast T1WI. Activation foci corresponding to the hand (*red*) are displaced anteriorly.

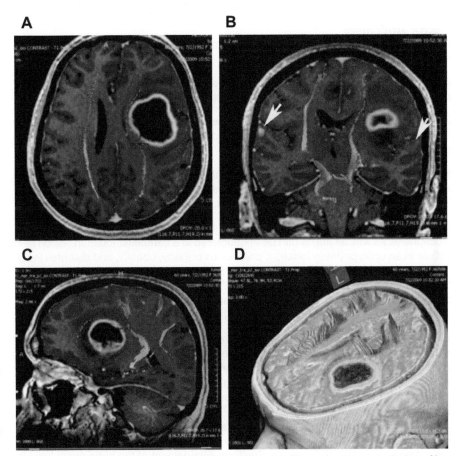

Fig. 7. Preoperative assessment of a patient with a high-grade tumor, including fiber tracking and fMRI studies. Corona radiata on tumor side is partially infiltrated, as shown on both two-dimensional multiplanar reformations (*A–C*) and on the three-dimensional object (*D*), whereas auditory cortex areas from the side of the tumor are showing lower statistical power compared with the contralateral side (*arrows* in *B*).

In this article, the most common brain tumors and their clinical presentation are examined; both conventional and advanced MRI sequences and their relative values in diagnosis are reviewed.

BRAIN TUMORS
Cerebral Gliomas

Cerebral gliomas are the most common and devastating primary brain tumors. The grading of gliomas mainly relies on histologic features, including cellularity, nuclear atypia, mitotic activity, vascularity, and necrosis, observed on light microscopy with the aid of immunohistochemistry. Among gliomas, astrocytic tumors are the most common and are usually divided into circumscribed and diffuse tumors. The circumscribed tumors are generally low grade, occurring in young patients, whereas the diffuse tumors are the most common cerebral tumors in adults with WHO grades, II, III, and IV. Circumscribed tumors, such as pilocytic astrocytoma (PA) (WHO grade I), are localized with distinct margin, and diffuse tumors are notorious in their propensity to infiltrate surrounding parenchyma, irrespective of their grade.

Pilocytic astrocytoma
Terminology PA is a WHO grade I, well-circumscribed tumor, with an indolent biological behavior.

Epidemiology PA accounts for 5% to 10% of all gliomas. Most commonly (75%) seen in the first 2 decades of life.[33] There is no recognized gender predisposition.

Location The cerebellum, hypothalamic-chiasmatic region, and the optic nerve are the most common brain locations, followed by the brainstem and the cerebral hemispheres.

Pathology A combination of compact (elongated cells) and loose (stellate astrocytes and microcysts) areas is characteristic. Hyalinization, microvascular proliferation, Rosenthal fibers, eosinophilic granular bodies, and ganglion cells can also be seen.[34]

Clinical presentation Features of increased intracranial pressure, mass effect, or hydrocephalus as well as ataxia can be encountered in a cerebellar location; vision field deficits in an optic pathway location; precocious puberty, obesity, and diabetes insipidus in a hypothalamic location; palsies of the sixth and seventh cranial nerves in the brainstem; and seizure and hemiparesis in a cerebral hemispheric location. Optic pathway PA is commonly associated with neurofibromatosis (NF) type 1, and bilateral presentation is almost pathognomonic for NF type 1.[35]

Imaging Four predominant imaging patterns of PA have been described: a mass with a nonenhancing cyst and an intensely enhancing mural nodule (**Fig. 8**); a mass with an enhancing cyst wall and an intensely enhancing mural nodule; a necrotic mass with a central nonenhancing zone; and a predominantly solid mass with minimal cystlike component. Solid, nonnecrotic tumors are less common and account for approximately 10% of cases.[36,37] Brainstem PAs usually expand the brainstem, have sharp margins with cystlike areas, and tend to grow exophytically (**Fig. 9**).[38] Chiasmatic/hypothalamic PAs are mainly solid, with cystic areas and trapped cerebrospinal fluid (CSF) pools. Fusiform enlargement of the optic nerve, usually with kinking and tortuosity, is seen in isolated optic nerve involvement. In a diffusion-weighted technique, PAs do not restrict. High ADC values can be used in the clinical setting as a reliable factor indicating low-grade tumor. Metabolite ratios of MRS and rCBV measurements on perfusion show inferior diagnostic performance, because

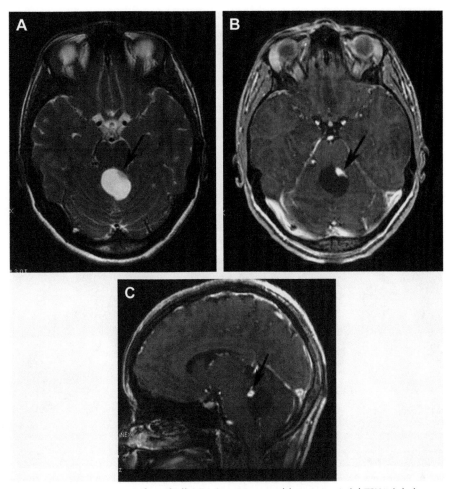

Fig. 8. Typical appearance of cerebellar PA in a 21-year old woman. Axial T2WI (*A*) shows a hyperintense cystic mass with an isointense mural nodule (*arrow*), which enhances strongly on postcontrast axial (*B*) and sagittal (*C*) T1WI (*arrow*), whereas the cyst wall remains unenhanced.

PA sometimes may have high Cho and lactate peaks and high rCBV, thus mimicking high-grade tumor.

Differential diagnosis In children, differential diagnosis should include ependymoma (EPs) and medulloblastoma (MB) in a cerebellar location. ADC values greater than 1.20×10^{-3} mm^2/s indicate PA, whereas an ADC between 1 and 1.20×10^{-3} mm^2/s is characteristic of EP. MB usually shows strong restriction, with ADC less than 0.8×10^{-3} mm^2/s.[39,40] Differential diagnosis in a chiasmatic/hypothalamic location should include craniopharyngioma (Crn), germinoma, Langerhans cell histiocytosis, and in a hemispheric location, primitive neuroectodermal tumor (PNET). In adults, differential diagnosis should include metastasis, as well as hemangioblastoma (in a cerebellar location). Marked increase of rCBV in cases of hemangioblastoma and mild increase in cases of PA with statistically significant differences have been reported.[41]

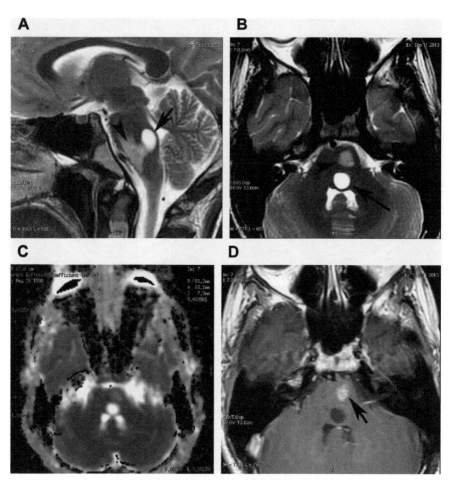

Fig. 9. Brainstem PA in a 13-year-old boy. On sagittal (*A*) and axial (*B*) T2WI, the tumor shows a bright cystic well-delineated component (*arrow*) and a mildly hyperintense solid component (*arrowheads*). ADC map (*C*) shows no evidence of restricted diffusion. Postcontrast T1WI (*D*) shows enhancement of the solid component of the mass (*arrow*).

Gangliogliomas and pleomorphic xanthoastrocytoma should be included in cases of a hemispheric location.

Therapy and prognosis Gross total resection of the tumor is usually curative. Tumors in critical or deep areas are managed conservatively, or with radiation therapy (for children >5 years old) or chemotherapy. Prognosis is excellent, with a 20-year survival rate of 79%.[33]

Low-grade infiltrative astrocytoma
Terminology Low-grade infiltrative (diffuse) astrocytoma (LGIA) is a WHO grade II neoplasm, which typically presents as a slow-growing tumor, with a tendency toward malignant transformation.

Epidemiology LGIA is usually diagnosed in children and young adults (mean 35 years of age), with a slight male predilection (male/female: 1.5:1).

Location Adult LGIA is mainly located in cerebral hemispheres, whereas its pediatric counterpart is more commonly located in the brainstem.

Clinical presentation Seizures, headache, and focal neurologic deficits depending on tumor location are the most common clinical features.

Pathology The most frequently encountered subtypes are fibrillary, protoplasmic, and gemistocytic, with gemistocytic more often associated with malignant transformation. Histopathology shows an uncapsulated, ill-defined tumor composed of astrocytes with low cellular density and mild nuclear atypia. Microcystic spaces can be encountered. Mitoses are rare.

Imaging On CT, LGIA appear as isodense or hypodense mass, which usually do not enhance after the administration of contrast medium. Calcifications and cystic spaces are rarely seen. On MRI, LGIA appear isointense to hypointense on T1WI and hyperintense on T2WI and FLAIR images, usually with subtle or no enhancement after gadolinium injection. DWI shows no restriction. MR perfusion shows relatively low rCBV. On MRS, increased Cho and low NAA levels are usually seen. However, Cho/Cr and Cho/NAA ratios are significantly lower than in high-grade gliomas (**Figs. 10** and **11**).[42]

Differential diagnosis Differential diagnosis should include high-grade glioma, cortical-based tumors (oligodendroglioma [OD], ganglion cell tumors), and nonneoplastic lesions, such as ischemic lesions and encephalitis.

Therapy and prognosis Benefit from tumor resection is reported to be controversial. Tumors in eloquent locations in neurologically intact patients are usually managed conservatively, whereas aggressive therapy is recommended at the time of malignant transformation.[43]

Anaplastic astrocytoma

Terminology Anaplastic astrocytoma (AA) is a diffusely infiltrating grade III glioma, usually arising from malignant transformation of grade II glioma and uncommonly de novo.

Epidemiology They represent one-third of all fibrillary astrocytomas and can occur at any age, but more usually in the fifth to sixth decade of life.[44]

Location Hemispheric location is the most common site of origin (65%), whereas thalamic and hypothalamic AAs are less common (20%).

Pathology Hypercellularity, nuclear pleomorphism, and mitoses are the most frequent histopathologic findings. Hemorrhage can be present, but necrosis (a hallmark of glioblastoma [GBM]) is absent.

Clinical presentation Headache, seizures, and focal neurologic deficits depending on tumor location are commonly presenting symptoms.

Imaging On CT, a hypodense ill-defined mass is seen. On postcontrast CT, focal enhancement is rarely seen. On MRI, tumors appear isointense to hypointense on T1WI and hyperintense on T2WI and FLAIR images. Fifty percent to 70% of AAs show focal, nodular, or patchy enhancement. AAs usually show areas with restriction on DWI. MRS shows increased Cho and decreased NAA levels. Perfusion MR shows foci of increased rCBV (**Figs. 12** and **13**). Surgical biopsies should be directed toward more aggressive areas of the tumor using MRS or rCBV maps.

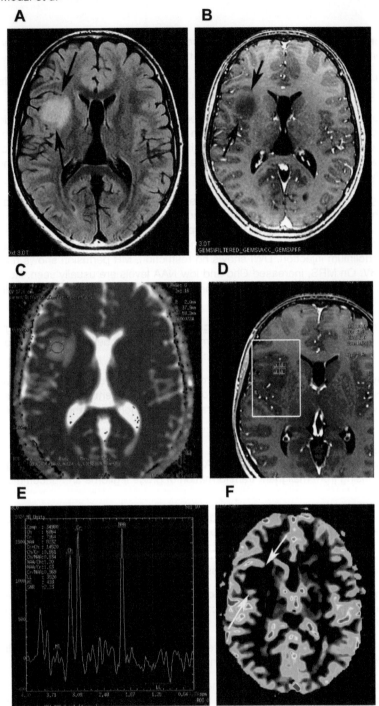

Fig. 10. Fibrillary astrocytoma grade II in a 17-year-old girl. Axial FLAIR image (*A*) shows a sharply demarcated hyperintense right insular mass (*arrows*). On axial postcontrast T1WI (*B*), the tumor remains unenhanced (*arrows*). The mass shows no evidence of restricted diffusion on ADC map (*C*) (ADC: 1.41×10^{-3} mm²/s). MRS (*D, E*) shows mild increase of Cho levels (Cho/Cr: 0.861, Cho/NAA: 0.834). Color perfusion map (*F*) shows that the mass has low rCBV (*arrows*).

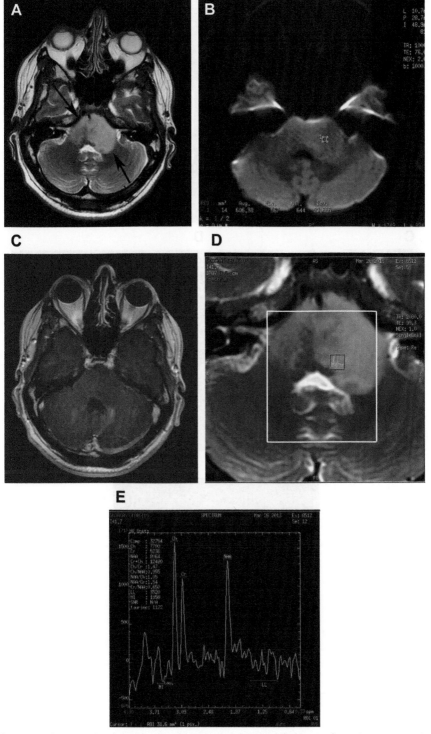

Fig. 11. Brainstem LGIA in a 26-year-old man. Axial T2WI (*A*) shows a hyperintense pontine mass displacing the fourth ventricle posteriorly (*arrows*). On DWI (*B*), there is no evidence of restricted diffusion. On postcontrast T1WI (*C*), the mass does not enhance. MRS (*D, E*) shows mild increase of Cho levels.

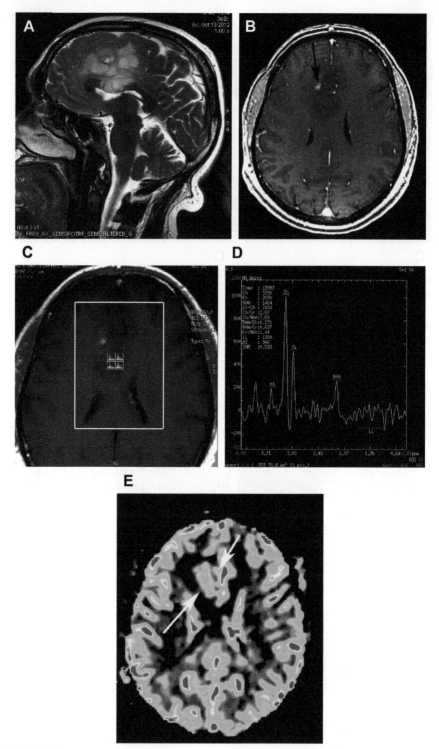

Fig. 12. Malignant transformation of grade II glioma into grade III glioma in a 45-year-old patient. Sagittal T2WI (*A*) shows a large heterogeneous right frontal mass involving the corpus callosum. On axial postcontrast T1WI (*B*), focal nodular enhancement is seen (*arrow*). MRS (*C, D*) in nonenhancing tumor component shows markedly increased Cho and decreased NAA levels. Color perfusion map (*E*) shows area of high rCBV (*arrows*), suggesting high-grade glioma.

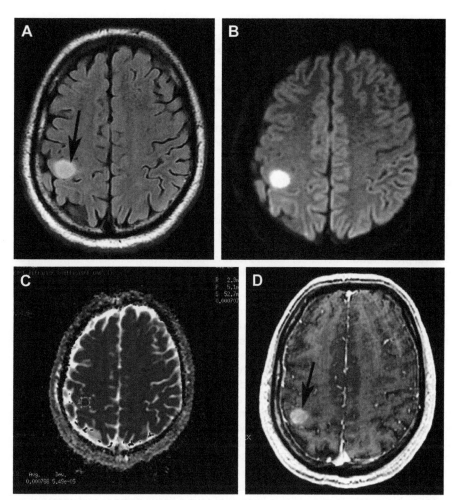

Fig. 13. De novo pathologically proven AA in a 45-year-old man presenting with seizure. Axial FLAIR image (*A*) shows a right parietal well-demarcated hyperintense lesion (*arrow*). On DWI (*B*) and ADC map (*C*), strong restriction is depicted (ADC: 0.768 × 10^{-3} mm²/s). On axial postcontrast T1WI (*D*), the lesion shows homogeneous enhancement (*arrow*).

Differential diagnosis Differential diagnosis should be made mainly from grade II gliomas. Imaging findings of AA are often indistinguishable from those of LGIA based on conventional MRI. Although there is a substantial overlap between different grades, a threshold minimum ADC tumor value of 1.07 and rCBV 1.75 provide high sensitivity and specificity in determining high-grade gliomas.[45–47] On MRS, different threshold values for Cho/Cr and Cho/NAA have been proposed in determining glioma grade. However, low-grade gliomas are generally characterized by a high concentration of NAA, low level of Cho, and absence of lactate and lipids. Progression in grade of a glioma is reflected in the progressive decrease in the NAA and myoinositol levels on the one hand and increase in Cho on the other.[48]

Therapy and prognosis Maximal surgical debulking of tumor, radiation therapy, and chemotherapy comprise the standard management of the tumor, but prognosis is poor, with a mean reported survival rate of less than 2 years.[49]

Glioblastoma

Terminology Glioblastoma (GBM) is an aggressive WHO grade IV tumor, arising either de novo or from malignant transformation of lower-grade gliomas.

Epidemiology GBMs can occur at any age but are most commonly seen in late adulthood (seventh decade of life). A slight male predilection (1.6/1) is reported. GBM represents 50% of astrocytomas.[50]

Location The supratentorial white matter of cerebral hemispheres is the most usual location of GBM. Infratentorial tumors are less commonly seen.

Pathology A high degree of cellularity, neovascularity, nuclear pleomorphism, as well as increased mitotic index, hemorrhage, and necrosis characterize most GBMs.

Clinical presentation Seizures, headache, and focal neurologic deficits depending on tumor location are the most common clinical features.

Imaging On CT, a centrally hypodense mass with peripheral hyperdense rim is usually seen. Calcifications are rare. After the administration of contrast material, GBMs usually show marked heterogeneous irregular rim enhancement. On MRI, GBMs show low signal intensity on T1WI and high heterogeneous signal intensity on T2WI/FLAIR images. Intratumoral hemorrhage at various stages of evolution and necrosis, which is the hallmark of GBM, are commonly seen. Flow voids from extensive neovascularity may be seen as well. On contrast-enhanced images, solid components show marked, usually irregular, ringlike enhancement. Distant tumor foci can also be seen. Dissemination by direct extension is usual (most characteristic is the butterfly glioma extending through the corpus callosum), whereas spread via the CSF pathway and subependymal spread are uncommon. On DWI, the solid component of GBM shows high signal (restriction) caused by high cellularity. The mean minimum ADC (0.834×10^{-3} mm^2/s) of GBM is significantly lower than that of AA (1.06×10^{-3} mm^2/s).[51] The central necrotic area shows low signal on DWI. MRS shows marked increase of Cho and decreased NAA levels. Lactate (marker of anaerobic metabolism) and lipids (marker of severe tissue damage and necrosis) are usually seen in GBM. Perfusion MR shows increased rCBV (**Figs. 14** and **15**).

Differential diagnosis The differential diagnosis should include abscess; in contrast to GBM, the central area shows marked hyperintensity on DWI and diminished ADC. The key to distinguishing GBM from solitary brain metastasis lies in the peritumoral area. The peritumoral edema of high-grade gliomas is a mixture of vasogenic edema and infiltration of neoplastic cells along the perivascular spaces, whereas metastatic peritumoral edema is purely vasogenic. Minimum ADC values of peritumoral edema in GBMs are significantly lower than those in metastases.[52] On perfusion images, peritumoral rCBV and on MRS, peritumoral metabolite ratios (Cho/Cr and Cho/NAA) are significantly higher in GBMs compared with solitary brain metastases (**Fig. 16**).[53–56] Tumefactive demyelinating lesions have little mass effect, incomplete ring enhancement, and lower Cho/Cr and rCBV than GBM.

Therapy and prognosis The tumor should be debulked as much as possible. Combination of radiation therapy and chemotherapy with alkylating agent temozolomide can be used for tumor management.[57] However, the prognosis is still poor, with a mean survival rate of 16 to 18 months after the initial diagnosis.

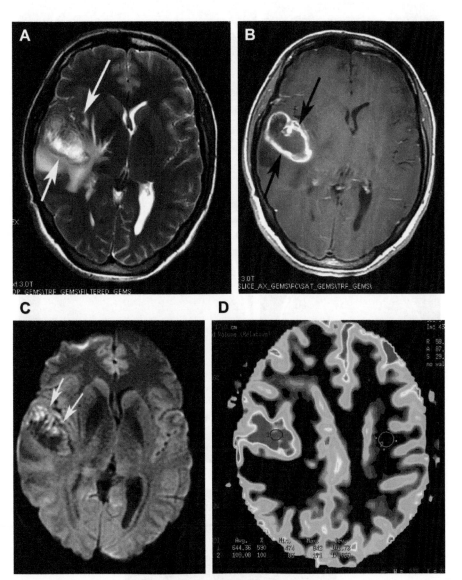

Fig. 14. GBM in a 32-year-old woman. Axial T2WI (*A*) shows a heterogeneous right temporal high signal mass with edema (*arrows*). Postcontrast T1WI (*B*) shows irregular ringlike enhancement (*arrows*). On DWI (*C*), the peripheral solid component shows high signal (*arrows*). Perfusion color map (*D*) shows marked increased rCBV.

Oligodendroglioma

Terminology Oligodendroglioma (OD) is a glial tumor arising from oligodendrocytes.

Epidemiology OD is the third most common glial neoplasm (5%–18% of glial neoplasms) usually occurring in adults (peak age for low-grade, fifth to sixth decade and for anaplastic, sixth to seventh decade), whereas in the pediatric population, it is uncommon.[58]

650

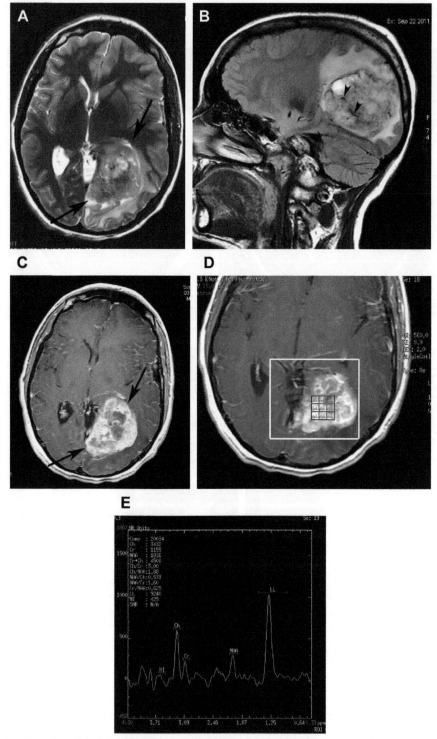

Fig. 15. Left occipital GBM in a 29-year-old woman. Axial T2WI (*A*) and sagittal FLAIR images (*B*) show a large heterogeneous mass with peritumoral edema (*arrows*). Flow voids from extensive neovascularity are seen (*arrowheads* on *B*). Axial postcontrast T1WI (*C*) shows heterogeneous enhancement of the tumour (*arrows*). MRS (*D, E*) shows increase of Cho levels and lipid/lactate peak.

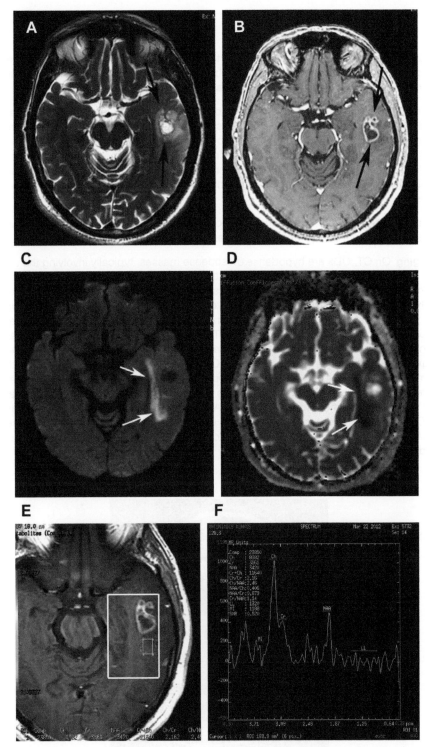

Fig. 16. Peritumoral edema in GBM. Axial T2WI (*A*) shows a left temporal hyperintense hetero-geneous mass with ringlike enhancement on postcontrast T1WI (*arrows*) (*B*). On DWI (*C*), peritumoral edema shows high signal intensity and low signal on ADC map (*arrows*) (*D*). On MRS (*E, F*), metabolite ratios in peritumoral edema (Cho/Cr and Cho/NAA) are significantly high.

Location A supratentorial location with cortical gray matter involvement is a characteristic feature of OD (frontal and temporal lobes are the most common sites). Rare sites of involvement include the cerebellum, brainstem, and the ventricular system.

Pathology OD has 2 main types: the well-differentiated low-grade OD (WHO grade II) and the anaplastic OD (WHO grade III). Histopathologic features of low-grade OD are moderate cellularity and little or no mitotic activity. Uniform round nuclei surrounded by a perinuclear halo of clear cytoplasm create a fried egg appearance. Microcalcifications, microcyst formation, and mucin production are common features. Increased cellularity and mitotic activity, pleomorphism, and necrosis are seen in anaplastic ODs.[58]

Clinical presentation Seizures and headache are the most common symptoms, and neurologic deficits can be encountered depending on tumor location.

Imaging On CT, ODs are hypodense or isodense masses, typically involving the cortex and subcortical white matter. Calcifications are seen in 34% to 80% of tumors.[59] Hemorrhagic components and areas of cystic degeneration can sometimes be seen. Calvaria scalloping/erosion can result from chronic pressure by long-standing tumors. On postcontrast CT, enhancement can sometimes be seen (**Fig. 17**). On MRI, ODs are hypointense on T1WI and hyperintense on T2WI (**Fig. 18**). Imaging features at conventional MRI cannot differentiate low-grade from high-grade OD.[60] Higher median maximum rCBV values are reported for ODs compared with astrocytomas of the same grade, leading to the exclusion of ODs from glioma grading based on rCBV measurements.[61,62] On DWI, lower ADC values do not correlate with cellularity, and there are no significant differences in minimum ADC values between subtypes and grades of ODs.[63] MRS shows increased Cho and Cr, increased myoinositol, and decreased NAA levels. High-grade tumors are characterized by significantly higher Cho levels and presence of lipid/lactate.

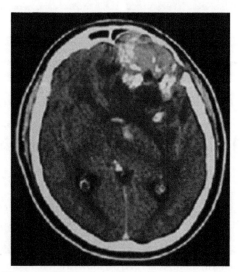

Fig. 17. Anaplastic OD in a 40-year-old man with a history of psychiatric symptoms. Contrast-enhanced CT scan shows a large heterogeneous left frontal mass with dense calcifications and erosion of the overlying calvaria.

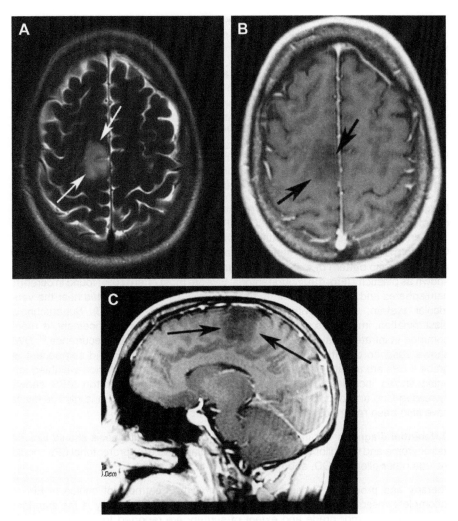

Fig. 18. OD grade II in a 38-year-old woman. Axial T2WI (*A*) shows a well-delineated high signal cortical mass (*arrows*). On postcontrast axial (*B*) and sagittal (*C*) T1WI, the lesion does not enhance (*arrows*).

Differential diagnosis Differential diagnosis should include other gliomas and DNET.

Therapy and prognosis Low-grade ODs are usually managed with surgery alone, whereas high-grade tumors are treated aggressively with surgery, radiation therapy, and chemotherapy. Ten-year survival rate is 85% for low-grade OD, 42% for tumors having undergone malignant transformation, and 15% for de novo anaplastic ODs.[64]

Ependymoma
Terminology Ependymoma (EP) is a glial tumor arising from differentiated ependymal cells of the ventricular system.

Epidemiology EPs account for 2% of all intracranial tumors in adults[65] and 6% to 12% of all pediatric brain tumors.[66] They can be found at any age.

Location Sixty percent of EPs are infratentorial (more often intraventricular in the fourth ventricle), whereas 40% are supratentorial (usually extraventricular in the cerebral hemispheres).[67]

Pathology EPs are subdivided in grade II and grade III (anaplastic). Moderate cellularity and rare mitotic activity are seen in low-grade EPs. The most characteristic microscopic pattern of EPs is the arrangement of tumor cells radially around blood vessels, known as pseudorosettes. Increased cellularity and mitotic activity, atypia, and necrosis characterize anaplastic EPs.[34]

Clinical presentation Increased intracranial pressure and hydrocephalus are usually seen in infratentorial intraventricular location, whereas supratentorial EPs usually present with seizures and focal neurologic deficits.

Imaging On CT, EPs are usually heterogeneous tumors, isodense or hypodense. Calcifications are common (40%–80%). On MRI, EPs show isointense to hypointense on T1WI and hyperintense on T2WI with moderate enhancement on postcontrast images. Cystic formation (especially in supratentorial EPs) is common. Infratentorial EPs show a characteristic pattern of extension through the foramen of Luschka and Magendie, known as plasticity (**Fig. 19**). Supratentorial EPs are most often (70%) found in cerebral hemispheres and usually present as large masses, commonly located near the ventricular system, with potential intraventricular extension (**Fig. 20**). Subarachnoid dissemination, imaged as nodular or smooth leptomeningeal enhancement, is more common in infratentorial EPs, usually of high grade, or in disease recurrence.[68] DWI shows absence of diffusion restriction, and ADC values in the solid component of grade II EPs are usually between 1 and 1.3×10^{-3} mm^2/s.[39] Perfusion-weighted imaging shows increased rCBV and poor return to baseline. Proton MRS shows increased Cho and decreased NAA levels. Increased myoinositol and glycine levels have also been reported.[69]

Differential diagnosis For infratentorial tumors, differential diagnosis should include astrocytoma and medulloblastoma. Differential diagnosis of supratentorial EPs should include other gliomas, OD, and PNET.

Therapy and prognosis Gross total resection is the treatment of choice of EP. In incomplete resected and high-grade tumors, adjuvant radiotherapy is the standard management. Tumor grade and extent of surgery are reported to be the strongest prognostic factors in EP. Infratentorial location and patient age younger than 55 years for adults and older than 3 years for children is reported to be associated with better prognosis. The 5-year survival rate for children overall is about 50%, whereas in adults 65% to 70%.[70]

Choroid plexus tumors
Terminology Choroid plexus tumors (CPT) arise from the epithelial cells of the choroid plexus. Most (80%) of these tumors are benign, slow-growing choroid plexus papillomas (CPPs), WHO grade I, whereas 20% are aggressive choroid plexus carcinomas (CPCs), WHO grade III.[71]

Epidemiology CPTs account for 2% to 4% of intracranial neoplasms in children (10%–20% of infant brain tumors, 42% of neonatal brain tumors) and 0.6% in adults.[72]

Location In children, 80% of CPPs arise in the lateral ventricles, 16% in the fourth ventricle and 4% in the third ventricle, whereas in adults, 70% of CPPs are found in the fourth ventricle, 24% in the lateral ventricles, and uncommonly, in the third

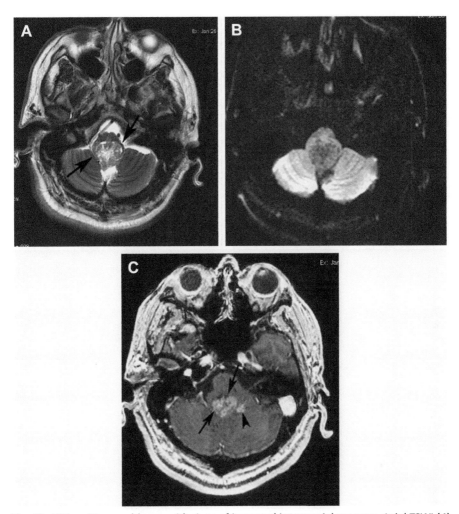

Fig. 19. EP in a 56-year-old man with signs of increased intracranial pressure. Axial T2WI (*A*) shows a heterogeneous mass filling the inferior fourth ventricle (*arrows*), with no evidence of restriction on DWI (*B*). On postcontrast T1WI (*C*), the mass shows strong enhancement (*arrows*). Note the extension of the tumor laterally to the left foramen of Luschka (*arrowhead*).

ventricle or extraventricularly.[73] Primary extraventricular location is more frequent in the cerebellopontine angle (CPA).

Pathology CPP shows cuboidal epithelial cells, with minimum mitotic activity, surrounding a fibrovascular tissue. CPC is characterized by increased mitotic activity, nuclear pleomorphism, invasion of adjacent brain parenchyma, and necrosis.

Clinical presentation Symptoms are associated with the presence of hydrocephalus and increased intracranial pressure; focal neurologic deficits, seizures, or cranial nerve palsies occur less often.

Imaging CPPs on CT appear isodense to hyperdense with irregular, lobulated or smooth margins. Calcifications (punctuate or dense) are reported in 24% of PCPs.

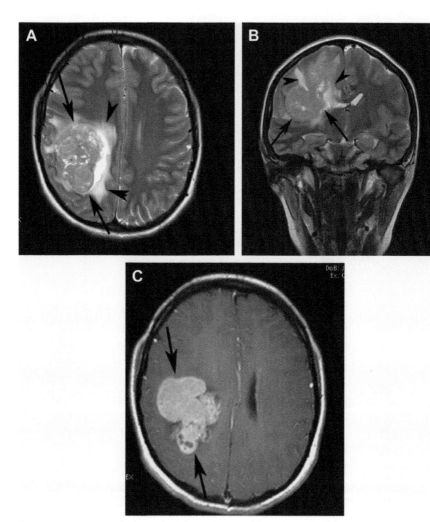

Fig. 20. Supratentorial EP grade II in a 26-year-old woman. Axial (*A*) and coronal (*B*) T2WI show a large parietal isointense mass (*arrows*) with scattered foci of high signal intensity. Note peritumoral high signal edema (*arrowheads*). Postcontrast T1WI (*C*) shows strong enhancement of the lesion (*arrows*).

On MRI, they appear isointense to hypointense on T1WI and isointense to slightly hyperintense on T2WI, with intense enhancement on contrast-enhanced images. Engulfment of the choroid plexus glomus can help differentiation of CPP from other intraventricular tumors. Areas of CSF entrapment are common. CPCs are usually more heterogeneous, with areas of hemorrhage, necrosis and flow voids, as well as subependymal and parenchymal invasion. Edema in the adjacent brain parenchyma is reported in 73% of CPCs and leptomeningeal dissemination in 45% to 62%.[74] Enlargement of the supplying choroidal artery can be seen on angiographic images. MRS of CPP shows a prominent ml peak, low to hardly detectable Cr and reduction of Cho. CPC shows a prominent Cho peak, absence of increase of ml, and low Cr and NAA levels (**Fig. 21**).[75]

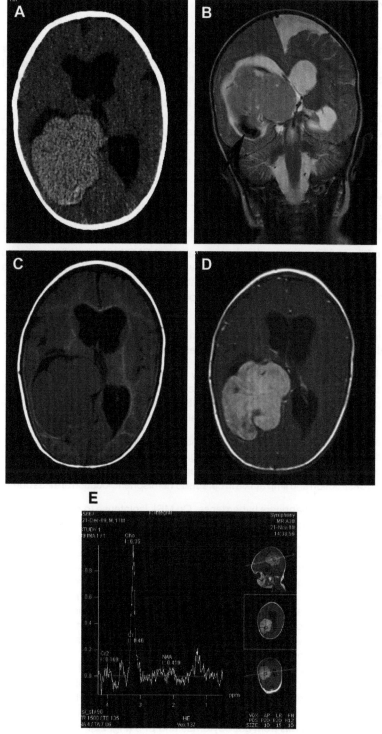

Fig. 21. CPC in a 1-year-old boy. CT scan (*A*) shows a large lobulated hyperdense intraventricular mass expanding the lateral ventricle. On coronal T2WI (*B*), the mass is isointense, with low signal area of hemorrhage in the inferior aspect (*arrow*). On axial T1WI (*C*), the mass is isointense. Postcontrast T1WI (*D*) shows strong enhancement of the tumor. On MRS (*E*), prominent Cho peak and low Cr and NAA levels are seen.

Differential diagnosis Differential diagnosis should include other intraventricular tumors, EP, subependymoma, OD, and meningioma. Perfusion MRI of CPP shows lower rcBVs compared with intraventricular meningiomas, which show high rcBVs.[76]

Therapy and prognosis Tumor resection is the treatment of choice for CPP, with shunting of the hydrocephalus when needed. CPCs are managed with surgery and occasionally, chemotherapy and craniospinal radiotherapy. CPPs have an excellent prognosis, with 100% survival at 5 years. The prognosis of CPC remains poor, with 1-year and 5-year survival 55% and 45%, respectively.[77]

Embryonal Tumors

Medulloblastoma
Terminology Medulloblastoma (MB) is a highly malignant PNET, WHO grade IV.

Epidemiology MB is the most common malignant CNS tumor in children, accounting for 12% to 25% of pediatric CNS tumors, whereas in adults, MBs represent less than 1% of brain tumors. Mean age at presentation for the pediatric population is 7 years, whereas in the adult population, it usually occurs between 20 and 40 years. Male predominance (63%) has been reported.[78]

Location Most MBs arise in the cerebellum, typically (>75%) in the vermis, whereas a lateral cerebellar hemispheric location is less common.

Pathology The classic type shows densely packed cells, with increased mitotic activity and nuclear pleomorphism. Neuroblastic rosettes, calcification, hemorrhage, apoptosis, and necrosis can be found. MB variants include desmoplastic type, MB with extensive nodularity, and the large cell anaplastic type.[79]

Clinical Presentation Duration of symptoms until diagnosis in most cases (76%) is reported to be less than 3 months. Clinical signs and symptoms are usually caused by increased intracranial pressure and hydrocephalus, whereas truncal ataxia caused by vermian destruction and limp ataxia in cerebellar hemispheric location are less common.[80]

Imaging On CT, MB appears hyperdense. On MRI, isointense to hypointense on T1WI and isointense to hyperintense on T2WI. Most MBs show marked enhancement on postcontrast images, whereas one-third show only subtle marginal or linear enhancement. Cystic/necrotic components are commonly seen,[81] whereas calcifications are less common. Spontaneous intratumoral hemorrhage is rare. Brainstem infiltration is encountered in approximately 30% of MBs. Tumor extension through the Luschka or Magendie foramina and supratentorial, spinal, or systemic metastases are less commonly seen. Local infiltration of the overlying meninges is common in desmoplastic type.[82] Adult MBs show some differences from pediatric MB in tumor location (which is more often in the cerebellar hemispheres), in tumor type (desmoplastic type more usual in adults), enhancement (which might be absent in adult MB), and in presence of necrotic/cystic areas (higher frequency in adult MBs).[83] On DWI, MBs appear hyperintense, with decreased ADC values ($<0.90 \times 10^{-3}$ mm^2/s). MRS of MB typically shows increased Cho and reduced NAA levels and occasionally, a lipid/lactate peak, but the most characteristic metabolic marker in MBs is reported to be the increase of taurine levels, differentiating MB from astrocytomas and EPs (**Fig. 22**).[84]

Differential diagnosis For pediatric MB, differential diagnosis should include EP and astrocytoma, whereas in adults, metastasis, hemangioblastoma, astrocytoma, lymphoma, and Lhermitte-Duclos disease should also be included.

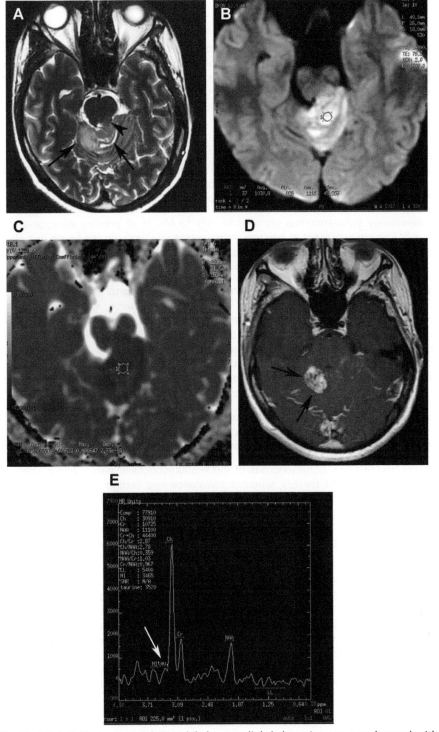

Fig. 22. Medulloblastoma. Axial T2WI (*A*) shows a slightly hyperintense mass (*arrows*) with effacement of vermian sulci extending in both cerebellar hemispheres and involving the pons (*arrowhead*). On DWI (*B*) and ADC map (*C*), restriction is noted. On postcontrast T1WI (*D*), partial enhancement is seen (*arrows*). MRS (*E*) shows increased Cho and reduced NAA levels. Taurine peak is seen at 3.4 ppm.

Treatment and prognosis Surgical resection, radiation therapy (whole brain and spine), and chemotherapy are used for tumor management. MBs are highly radiosensitive tumors, but radiotherapy should be avoided in children younger than 2 years. Recurrence in childhood MB is usually seen in the first 2 years. The overall 5-year survival rate is reported between 50% and 80%.

Tumors of Cranial Nerves

Schwannoma

Terminology Intracranial schwannomas are slow-growing tumors that arise from the perineural Schwann cells surrounding the cranial nerves. Most of them are benign, although malignant tumors have also been reported.

Epidemiology Schwannomas account for 6% to 8% of all primary intracranial tumors.[85] They may present at any age, more commonly between the fourth and sixth decades. Earlier presentation can be associated with the presence of NF type 2.[86] A slight female predominance (1.5–2:1) is reported.

Location Most schwannomas arise in the internal auditory canal (IAC) and CPA, usually from the vestibular division of the vestibulocochlear nerve, less often from the facial nerve.[87] Schwannomas of the trigeminal nerve are rare, accounting for 0.2% to 0.4% of intracranial tumors,[88] whereas schwannomas of the jugular foramen (usually from the ninth cranial nerve) are even more rarely encountered. Intraparenchymal schwannomas are extremely rare, accounting for 1% to 2% of intracranial schwannomas,[89] and are believed to originate from Schwann cells around arteries in the subarachnoid space or along the perivascular nerve plexus.[90]

Pathology Schwannomas are well-circumscribed encapsuled masses, with 2 characteristic areas: Antony type A area from compact neoplastic Schwann cells in interlacing bundles and Antony type B area, more hypocellular, with looser textured stroma.[91]

Clinical presentation Schwannomas of the vestibulocochlear nerve usually present with hearing loss and tinnitus, whereas imbalance and vertigo are less commonly encountered. Facial nerve schwannomas also present with hearing loss, but facial nerve paresis is also common.[92] Tumors of the trigeminal nerve most often present with facial pain and sensory paresthesias and less often with motor dysfunction of muscles of mastication.[87] Jugular foramen schwannomas present with a variety of symptoms, including hearing loss, nystagmus, and dysphagia-tongue atrophy.[93]

Imaging A well-circumscribed fusiform mass along the course of a cranial nerve, hypointense on T2WI, and enhancement on postcontrast images are the typical imaging findings of small schwannomas. Large lesions are characterized by isointensity to hypointensity on T1WI, hyperintensity on T2WI, and homogenous enhancement, whereas presence of cystic degeneration, calcification, hemorrhage, or fibrosis can provide heterogeneous appearance. Schwannomas of the IAC can appear as dumbbell lesions, with an isthmus connecting 2 bulbous segments, one in the IAC fundus and another in the membranous labyrinth of the inner ear or the geniculate ganglion (**Figs. 23** and **24**).

Differential diagnosis The main differential diagnosis of a schwannoma in the CPA-IAC is meningioma. The presence of IAC dilatation is suggestive of vestibular schwannoma (VS), whereas hyperostic changes of petrous bone and the dural tail sign favor a diagnosis of meningioma. Most VS show microhemorrhages on T2*-weighted gradient echo sequence.[94]

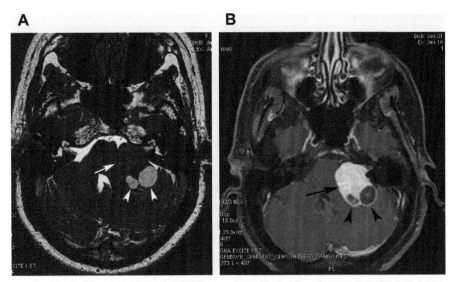

Fig. 23. Vestibular schwannoma. Thin-section constructive interference steady state image (*A*) shows an isointense left CPA angle mass (*arrow*) with cystic components (*arrowheads*) extending to the IAC. On postcontrast T1WI (*B*), strong enhancement of solid component is seen, whereas the cystic areas remain unenhanced.

Therapy and prognosis There are a variety of treatment options for the management of schwannomas, including microsurgical resection, radiotherapy, and observation.[95] Conservative management of small VS is frequently proposed in patients with small tumors, because most tumors do not grow.[96] Radiosurgery could control tumor growth and preserve hearing function and facial weakness in patients with VS.[97]

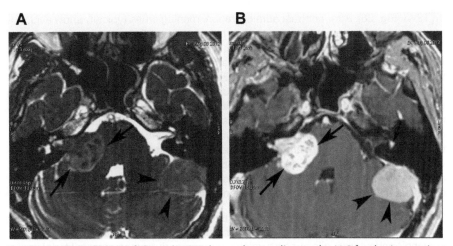

Fig. 24. (*A, B*) Typical VS of the right CPA (*arrows*) extending to the IAC fundus in a patient with NF type 2. Note meningioma (*arrowheads*) in the convexity of the left cerebellar hemisphere. Small left intracanalicular vestibular schwannoma is seen (*small arrow* in *B*).

Meningeal Tumors

Meningioma

Terminology Meningiomas are extra-axial, typically slow-growing tumors that arise from the meningothelial cells of the arachnoid.[98]

Epidemiology Peak occurrence is in the sixth and seventh decades. The female/male ratio varies with age, peaking at 4:1 in middle-aged patients. Meningiomas account for between 16% and 20% of all intracranial tumors.[99]

Location Meningiomas may be found along any of the external surfaces of the brain as well as within the ventricular system, where they arise from the stromal arachnoid cells of the choroid plexus. The most common locations include the parasagittal aspect of the cerebral convexity, the lateral hemisphere convexity, the sphenoid wing, middle cranial fossa, and the olfactory groove.[100]

Pathology Most (90%) are benign WHO grade I lesions. The most common histologic subtypes of grade I meningiomas include meningothelial, fibrous, and transitional. The more aggressive WHO grade II (atypical) meningioma shows an increased number of mitoses, cellularity, and nuclear/cytoplasmic ratio. WHO grade III (anaplastic) meningioma is characterized by the presence of malignant features, such as overt cell anaplasia, high mitotic rate, areas of necrosis, or brain invasion.[99]

Clinical presentation Symptoms relate to size and tumor location. Less than 10% of meningiomas become symptomatic.

Imaging Characteristic imaging signs suggesting an extra-axial location of meningiomas include a fluid cleft surrounding the mass, the presence of signal void pseudocapsule produced by displaced vessels or dura itself, and gray-white interface displacement. Broad dural base, linear enhancement along the dura matter on either side of meningioma (dural tail sign), and hyperostosis are often seen in extra-axial lesions as well (**Fig. 25**). Meningiomas typically appear as lobular, extra-axial masses, with well-circumscribed margins. On CT, meningiomas are typically hyperdense. The MRI signal intensity characteristics consist of isointensity to slight hypointensity relative to gray matter on T1WI and isointensity to hyperintensity relative to gray matter on T2WI (**Fig. 26**). After contrast administration, meningiomas typically show avid, homogeneous enhancement; however, they may occasionally have areas of cystic necrosis or calcification that do not enhance (**Fig. 27**). Calcifications are typically best shown on CT. Atypical imaging characteristics of meningiomas include hemorrhage, bone destruction, and extensive edema (**Figs. 28 and 29**). The distinction between benign and atypical or malignant meningiomas is not reliably made when assessing the imaging features on conventional MRI. Diffusion-weighted MRI is not found to have any additional value in determining histologic behavior or in differentiating histopathologic subtypes of meningiomas.[101] On perfusion, the differences in rCBV values between benign and malignant meningiomas are not significant. However, high rCBV values in peritumoral edema suggest a more aggressive tumor grade.[102,103] On MRS, alanine level at 1.48 ppm is often increased in meningiomas, although glutamate-glutamine and glutathione may be more specific potential markers (**Fig. 30**).[104]

Differential diagnosis There are multiple neoplastic and nonneoplastic entities that clinically and radiographically mimic meningiomas, including solitary fibrous tumors, hemangiopericytoma, gliosarcoma, leiomyosarcoma, dural metastases, Hodgkin disease, plasmocytoma, Rosai-Dorfman disease, neurosarcoidosis, melanocytic neoplasms, and plasma cell granuloma.[105]

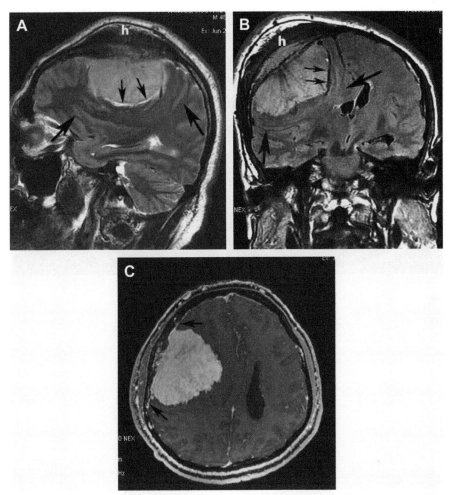

Fig. 25. Meningioma with typical imaging signs. Sagittal T2WI (*A*) and coronal FLAIR (*B*) images show fluid cleft surrounding the mass (*small arrows*), gray-white matter interface displacement (*arrows*), broad dural base, and hyperostosis (h). On axial postcontrast T1WI (*C*), linear enhancement along the dura matter (dural tail sign) is seen (*arrows*).

Treatment and prognosis The treatment of choice is complete resection, but in 50% of cases, it is not achieved, because of tumor location or surgical morbidities. The usefulness of preoperative embolization during the management of meningiomas remains controversial.[106] Radiotherapy is an established therapy in patients requiring treatment of surgically inaccessible disease and postoperatively for grade III tumors.[107] Chemotherapeutic intervention in patients with nonresectable, aggressive, and malignant meningiomas includes cytotoxic and hormonal agents, immunomodulators, and targeted agents toward a variety of growth factors.[108]

Primary CNS Lymphoma

Terminology
Primary CNS lymphoma (PCNSL) is a rare variant of extranodal non-Hodgkin lymphoma restricted to the brain, spinal cord, eye, and meninges.

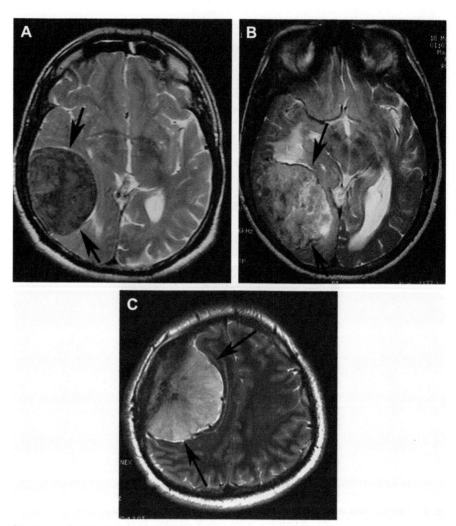

Fig. 26. Axial T2WI (*A–C*) of meningiomas (*arrows*) in different patients show low signal intensity on (*A*), heterogeneous intermediate on (*B*) and high signal on (*C*).

Epidemiology The mean age of presentation is the sixth or seventh decade. It represents up to 3.1% of all primary CNS malignancies. Twenty percent to 25% of post-transplant immunosuppressed patients and 2% to 12% of patients with human immunodeficiency virus develop CNS lymphomas.[109]

Location Locations are the cerebral hemispheres (20% to 43%), thalamus, and basal ganglia (13%–20%), corpus callosum (14%), ventricular wall and choroid plexus (12%), and cerebellum (9% to 13%).[110,111] Posterior fossa involvement is seen in 10% to 24% of cases.[112] Symmetric lesions involving the genu or splenium of the corpus callosum are referred to as a mirror pattern or butterfly pattern and tend to show subependymal and leptomeningeal spread.

Pathology Nearly all PCNSLs are diffuse large B-cell lymphomas, with T-cell lymphomas being rare.

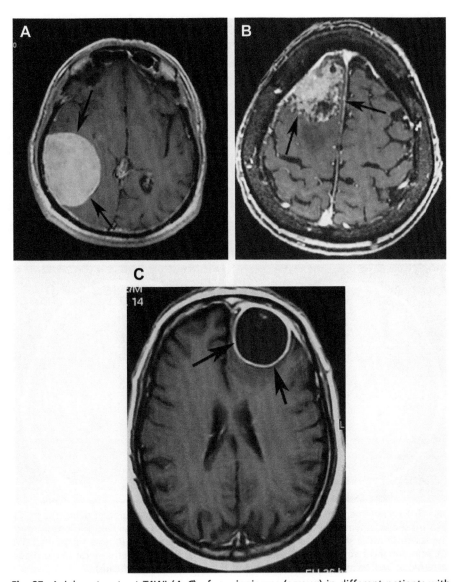

Fig. 27. Axial postcontrast T1WI (*A–C*) of meningiomas (*arrows*) in different patients with typical avid, homogeneous enhancement (*A*) cystic foci that do not enhance (*B*) and completely cystic meningioma (*C*).

Clinical presentation The clinical presentation includes focal neurologic deficits, altered mental status, and neuropsychiatric disturbances.

Imaging In most cases, lesions are solitary and tend to be large. Multiple lesions are not uncommon but tend to be small. On CT, PCNSL is typically isodense to hyperdense. Densely packed abnormal cells are believed to be responsible for the hyperdensity.[113] On T2WI, PCNSLs show low to intermediate signal intensity, which is attributed to high cellular density of the tumor. Peritumoral edema is usually present but is less prominent than in malignant gliomas or metastases. On precontrast T1WI, lesions

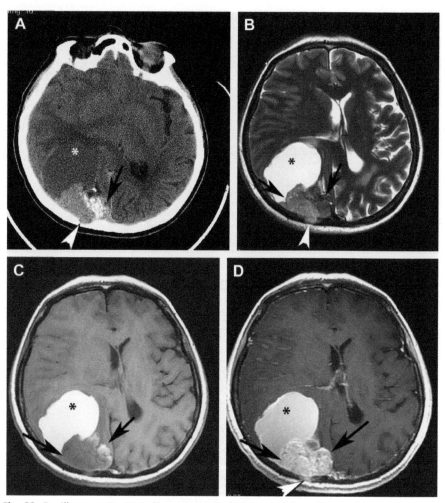

Fig. 28. Papillary meningioma in a 55-year-old woman with peritumoral hemorrhage. CT scan (*A*) shows a hyperdense occipital broad-based mass with dense calcifications (*arrow*). The lesion (*arrows*) shows intermediate signal intensity on T2WI (*B*), low signal on T1WI (*C*), and enhances strongly on postcontrast T1WI (*D*). Note the peritumoral hemorrhage (*asterisk*) as well as invasion of inner table of the calvarium (*arrowheads*).

are usually isointense or hypointense. Strong homogeneous enhancement is often present on postcontrast images. Irregular ring enhancement is rare.[114,115] PCNSL lesions often have lower ADC values ($0.51–0.63 \times 10^{-3}$ mm^2/s) than do high-grade gliomas ($0.75–0.96 \times 10^{-3}$ mm^2/s) or metastases (0.68×10^{-3} mm^2/s).[116,117] On perfusion-weighted images, rCBV is typically lower in lymphomas (1.10–2.33) than in high-grade gliomas (5.76–6.33) or metastases (4.55–5.27) (**Figs. 31** and **32**).[118,119]

Differential diagnosis Differential diagnosis includes GBM, metastasis, and toxoplasmosis in immunocompromised patients.

Treatment and prognosis Surgical resection does not improve prognosis. Stereotactic biopsy for diagnostic confirmation is recommended. Treatment options include

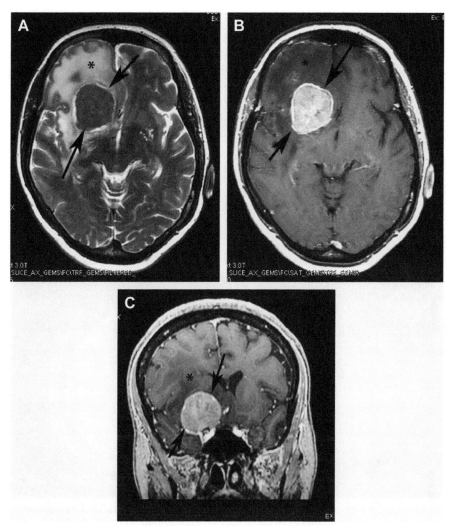

Fig. 29. Middle cranial fossa meningioma (*arrows*) with extensive peritumoral edema (*asterisks*). On axial T2WI (*A*), meningioma shows intermediate signal intensity and enhances strongly on postcontrast T1WI (*B, C*).

corticosteroids, chemotherapy, and radiation therapy. Prognosis is general poor. The 5-year survival rate is less than 10%.

Germ Cell Tumors

Intracranial germ cell tumors (GCT) are morphologic and immunophenotypic homologues of similar neoplasms, which arise in the gonads and extragonadal sites, including germinoma, teratoma, embryonal carcinoma, endodermal sinus-yolk sac tumor, choriocarcinoma, and mixed germ tumors.[120]

Germinoma
Terminology Germinoma is identical to testicular seminoma and ovarian dysgerminoma.

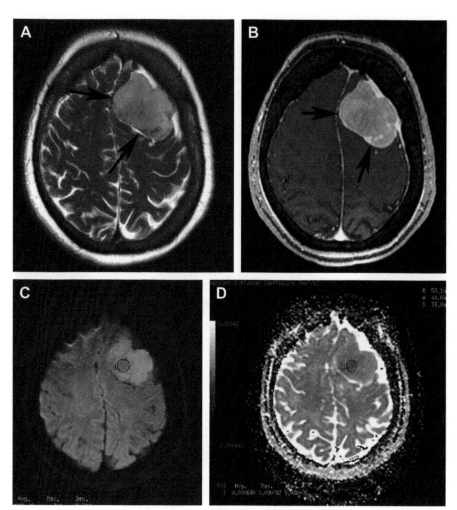

Fig. 30. Atypical meningioma. Axial T2WI (*A*) shows left frontal extra-axial homogeneous mass (*arrows*), which enhance homogeneously on postcontrast T1WI (*B*). On DWI (*C*) and corresponded ADC map (*D*), restriction of diffusion is noted. On perfusion color map (*E*), the mass is hyperperfused. MRS (*F, G*) shows a prominent Cho peak as well an alanine peak at 1.4 ppm.

Epidemiology They occur most commonly during the second decade. Pineal germinomas have a male/female ratio of 3:1, whereas suprasellar germinomas 1:1. Intracranial germinomas account for 0.5% to 2.0% of all intracranial tumors and 50% to 60% of CNS GCT.[121]

Location Germinomas have a predilection for midline structures: pineal region (>50%), suprasellar region, and anterior third ventricle. The basal ganglia are the most common off middle line site. Germinomas grow slowly and spread either to the adjacent tissue or via the subependymal or subarachnoid space.

Pathology These tumors have 2 cells pattern and they consist from lobules of primitive germ cells embedded in a matrix of lymphocytes or lymphocytelike cells.

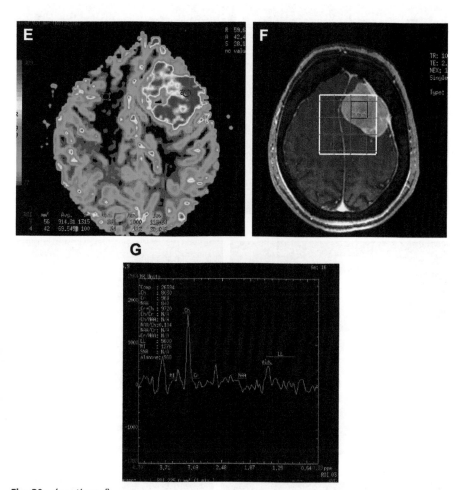

Fig. 30. (*continued*)

Clinical presentation Pineal germinoma presents with headache and Parinaud syndrome and suprasellar germinoma with diabetes insipidus and visual disturbances.

Imaging On CT, a slightly hyperdense homogeneous mass appears in most germinomas, with homogeneous enhancement after contrast medium administration. On MRI, the mass is slightly hypointense to isointense on T1WI and isointense to hyperintense on T2WI. Variably sized intratumoral cysts are common (**Fig. 33**). ADC values of 6.98 ± 0.35 and Cho/NAA ratios of 2.09 ± 0.39 in pineal germinoma have been reported.[122] In reported series,[123] germinomas showed higher ADC values than the pineal cell tumors.

Treatment and prognosis Radiation therapy is the backbone in the management of intracranial germinoma. In localized disease, chemotherapy followed by whole brain irradiation is the standard, providing cure rates in excess of 90%.[124]

Craniopharyngioma

Terminology
Craniopharyngioma (Crn) is a benign cystic sellar/suprasellar WHO grade I tumor formed from ectodermal remnants of the Rathke pouch.

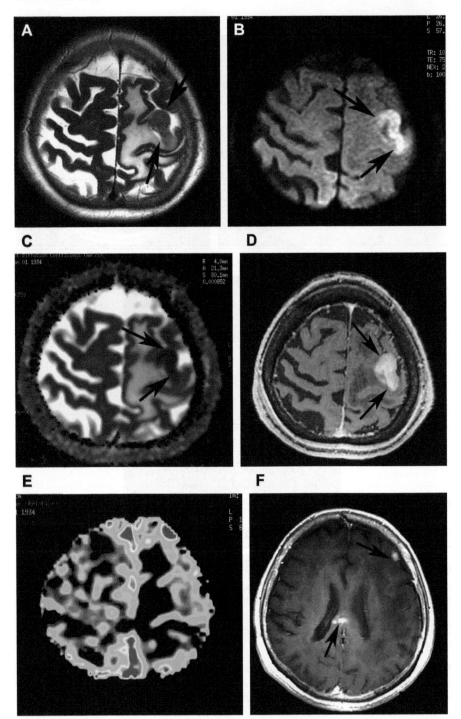

Fig. 31. Pathologically proven PCNSL in a 74-year-old woman. Axial T2WI (*A*) shows a cortical isointense lesion (*arrows*) with high signal on DWI (*B*) and low on ADC map (*C*). On postcontrast T1WI (*D*), marked homogeneous enhancement is seen (*arrows*). On perfusion color map (*E*), low rCBV is depicted. Axial postcontrast T1WI (*F*) in lower level shows foci of enhancement in the corpus callosum and left frontal lobe (*arrows*).

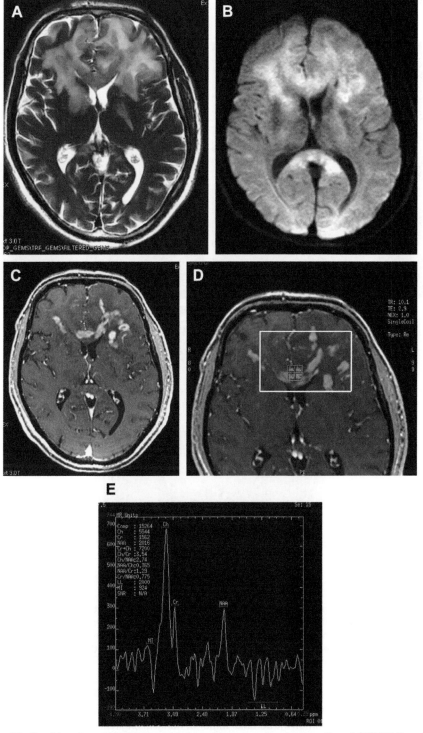

Fig. 32. B-cell lymphoma in a 65-year-old man with personality changes. On axial T2WI (*A*), multiple high signal abnormalities are seen in white matter of frontal lobes, basal ganglia, and corpus callosum. On DWI (*B*), the lesions show high signal intensity. Postcontrast T1WI (*C*) shows patchy enhancement. MRS (*D, E*) shows low NAA levels and high Cho levels and lactate peak.

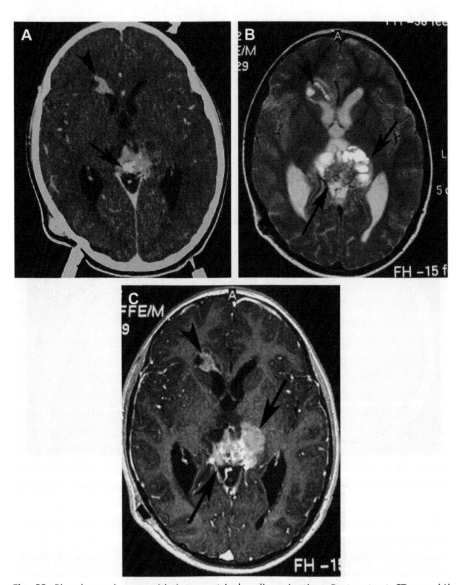

Fig. 33. Pineal germinoma with intraventricular dissemination. Postcontrast CT scan (*A*) shows an enhanced pineal lesion with characteristic calcifications (*arrow*). On axial T2WI (*B*), the lesion is isointense with foci of high signal intensity (*arrows*). On postcontrast T1WI, strong heterogeneous enhancement is seen (*arrows*) (*C*). Note the nodular enhancement in the right frontal horn (*arrowheads*).

Epidemiology Crn has a bimodal incidence, with peaks in the first and fourth decades. Crns are the most common intracranial tumor of nonglial origin in children, comprising up to 10% of pediatric brain tumors.

Location Crns can occur anywhere from the floor of the third ventricle (hypothalamus) to the pharyngeal tonsils, with more than 60% being found in the suprasellar region.[125]

Pathology The adamantinomatous type (90%) appears as a multilobulated partially solid but mostly cystic mass adhering to adjacent structures, with a peripheral layer of palisading stratified squamous epithelium. The papillary type is usually a discrete encapsulated mass, with solid sheets of well-differentiated squamous epithelium.[126]

Clinical presentation Clinical presentation includes visual disturbances, headaches, and growth hormone deficiency in 75%. Hypothalamic obesity is a common symptom of Crn.[127]

Imaging Crn presents as a partially calcified, mixed solid, and cystic extra-axial suprasellar mass. CT is the examination of choice for the evaluation of calcifications, which are seen in 87% of cases. The signal intensity of the cystic component varies from hypointense to hyperintense on T1WI and variably hyperintense on T2WI. The solid component enhances after contrast administration (**Fig. 34**). On MRS, prominent lipid peaks centered at 1 to 1.5 ppm have been reported, correlating with high amounts of cholesterol within the cystic component.[128]

Differential diagnosis Differential diagnosis includes Rathke cleft cyst, hypothalamic astrocytoma, and pituitary adenoma, dermoid, and epidermoid cyst.

Therapy and prognosis Therapy of choice in patients with favorable tumor localization is complete resection, with a specific focus on maintaining functions of the optic nerve and hypothalamic-pituitary axis. In cases of limited resection, local irradiation is recommended. The overall survival rates are high (92%), but relapses and reduced quality of life in survivors are also frequent.[129]

Brain Metastasis

Terminology
Brain metastasis (BM) is a complication of cancer, with formidable consequences.

Epidemiology BMs are the most common type of intracranial neoplasms. They outnumber primary brain tumors by a ratio of 10:1 and occur in about 25% of all patients with cancer.[130] Sixty percent of patients with BM are aged between 50 and 70 years. Metastases accounts for 6% of all CNS tumors in children.

Location Brain metastases are located in the cerebral hemispheres in about 80%, in the cerebellum in 15%, and in the brainstem in 5% of patients. Unlike primary brain tumors, metastatic lesions rarely involve the corpus callosum or cross the midline.[131] Metastases in the meninges or in the epidural intracranial space can also occur.

Pathology BMs are rounded, firm, and well demarcated. BMs show histologic features similar to those in their primary sites. Regardless of the cell type, neovascularity is evident within the tumor parenchyma characterized by immature vessels. Most brain metastases originate from lung (40%–50%), breast (15%–25%), melanoma (5%–20%), and kidney (5%–10%).[132]

Clinical presentation Clinical presentation is similar to any intracranial mass lesion and include headache (70%), seizures (30%–60%), cognitive impairment (30%), papilledema (8%), and miscellaneous focal neurologic deficits.[132]

Imaging On CT, metastases may be hypodense, isodense, or hyperdense compared with the brain. Acutely hemorrhagic metastases appear hyperdense to brain tissue. Hemorrhagic metastases are usually derived from melanoma, choriocarcinoma, renal

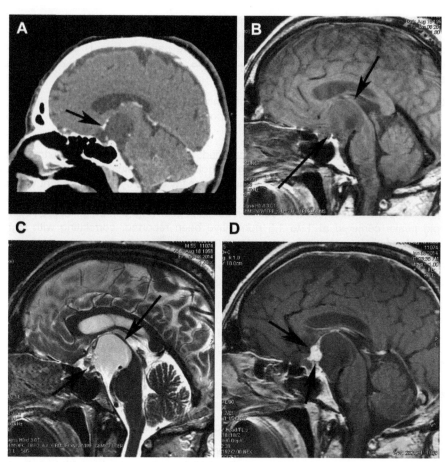

Fig. 34. Crn in a 55-year-old man. CT scan, sagittal reconstruction (*A*) shows a cystic supra-sellar mass with calcified rim (*arrow*). On T1WI (*B*), the lesion is hypointense (*arrows*) and on T2WI (*C*) hyperintense (*arrows*). Postcontrast T1WI (*D*) shows nodular and ringlike enhancement, whereas the cystic component is nonenhanced (*arrows*).

cell carcinoma, and lung and thyroid cancer.[5] On postcontrast CT, brain metastases show ring, nodular, or solid enhancement. Contrast-enhanced CT is less sensitive than contrast-enhanced brain MRI. On MRI, metastases are usually isointense or hypointense on T1IWI and hyperintense on T2WI and show avid enhancement (**Fig. 35**). Some metastases, such as melanoma, are T1WI hyperintense as a result of the paramagnetic effects of melanin. Hemorrhagic metastases may also show T1 signal hyperintensity, depending on the age of hemorrhage (**Fig. 36**). Vasogenic edema can be substantial and is unrelated to lesion size. Some reports[133] have found a significantly increased ratio of vasogenic edema to contrast-enhancing lesion size in metastases compared with high-grade primary brain tumors, although metastases may display little or no vasogenic edema (**Fig. 37**). Gadolinium contrast enhancement is vital to detect small metastases. On MRS, the enhancing components of brain metastases show increased Cho/Cr peak ratios compared with normal brain, depressed NAA, and increased lipid and lactate peaks. Perfusion characteristics of brain metastases depend on the primary tumor as well as relative differentiation of the tumor cells.

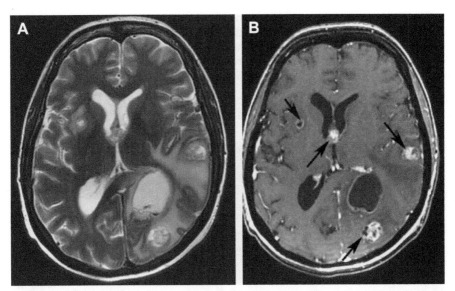

Fig. 35. Brain metastases in a woman with history of breast cancer. Axial T2WI (*A*) shows multiple heterogeneous lesions with perilesional edema. On postcontrast T1WI (*B*), nodular and rimlike enhancement is seen (*arrows*).

Thus, hypervascular metastases such as renal cell carcinoma and melanoma may show markedly increased rCBV compared with less vascular metastases.[134]

Differential diagnosis Differential diagnosis includes septic emboli, multiple embolic infarcts, multiple sclerosis, and multiple cavernous angiomas. GBM is included in case of solitary metastasis. In GBM, the metabolite profile of the T2-hyperintense,

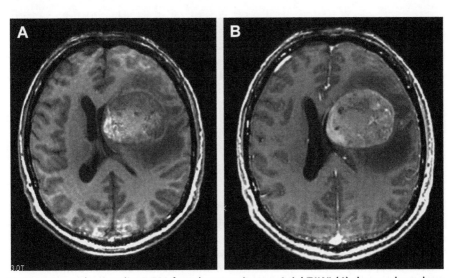

Fig. 36. Hemorrhagic solitary BM from lung carcinoma. Axial T1WI (*A*) shows a large hemorrhagic hyperintense mass in left basal ganglia. Postcontrast T1WI (*B*) shows heterogeneous enhancement. Note peritumoral edema and compressed lateral ventricle.

nonenhancing area surrounding the enhancing mass shows significantly increased Cho/Cr ratios compared with metastases. On MRS, the T2-hyperintense area around enhancing metastases shows spectra more similar to normal white matter (**Fig. 38**). GBMs show higher rCBV in the peritumoral T2-hyperintense area compared with metastases.

Treatment and prognosis Treatment of brain metastases is multidisciplinary, with radiation and chemotherapy forming the cornerstones of treatment. Patients with

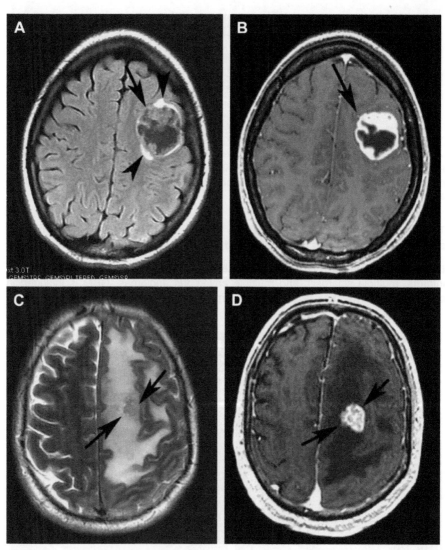

Fig. 37. Vasogenic edema is unrelated to lesion size. Axial FLAIR (*A*) and axial postcontrast T1WI (*B*) of solitary metastasis in a 20-year-old woman with osteosarcoma show an inhomogeneous peripherally enhancing lesion (*arrow*) with minimal edema (*arrowhead*). Axial T2WI (*C*) and axial postcontrast T1WI (*D*) in a 70-year-old with lung cancer show a smaller, compared with the previous patient, homogeneous enhancing metastasis (*arrows*) with extensive high signal edema.

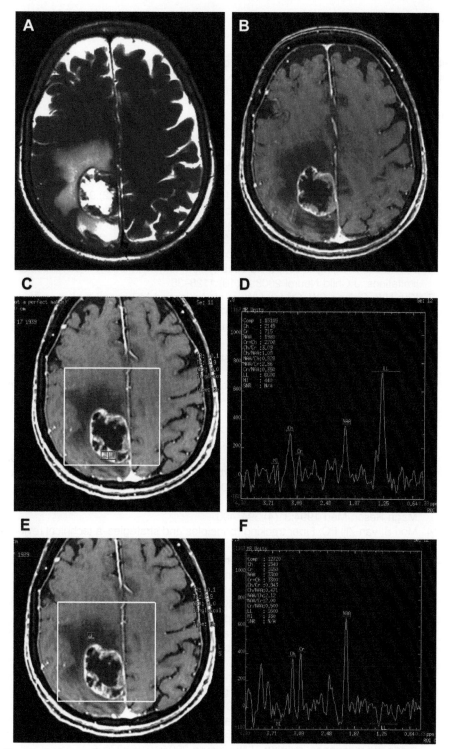

Fig. 38. Solitary metastasis in a 76-year-old woman with colon cancer. Axial T2WI (*A*) shows a right parietal parasagittal mass with peritumoral white matter edema. On axial postcontrast T1WI (*B*), the mass shows an irregular enhancing rim with central necrosis. MRS (*C, D*) shows increased Cho/Cr peak ratios, depressed NAA levels and increased lipid and lactate peaks. On peritumoral edema, MRS (*E, F*) shows normal metabolite ratios.

solitary metastasis experience improved quality of life and prolonged survival from surgical resection.

REFERENCES

1. Al-Okaili RN, Krejza J, Wang S, et al. Advanced MR imaging techniques in the diagnosis of intraaxial brain tumors in adults. Radiographics 2006;26:173–89.
2. Cha S. Neuroimaging in neuro-oncology. Neurotherapeutics 2009;63:465–77.
3. Louis DN, Ohgaki H, Wiestler OD, et al. The 2007 WHO classification of tumours of the central nervous system. Acta Neuropathol 2007;114(2):97–109.
4. Lee EJ, Lee SK, Agid R, et al. Preoperative grading of presumptive low-grade astrocytomas on MR imaging: diagnostic value of minimum apparent diffusion coefficient. AJNR Am J Neuroradiol 2008;29:1872–7.
5. Mechtler L. Neuroimaging in neuro-oncology. Neurol Clin 2009;27(1):171–201.
6. Vézina LG. Imaging of central nervous system tumors in children: advances and limitations. J Child Neurol 2008;23(10):1128–35.
7. Kao HW, Chiang SW, Chung HW, et al. Advanced MR imaging of gliomas: an update. Biomed Res Int 2013;2013:970586.
8. Wen PY, Kesari S. Malignant gliomas in adults. N Engl J Med 2008;359(5): 492–507.
9. Le Bihan D. Molecular diffusion nuclear magnetic resonance imaging. Magn Reson Q 1991;7(1):1–30.
10. Ebisu T, Tanaka C, Umeda M, et al. Discrimination of brain abscess from necrotic or cystic tumors by diffusion-weighted echo planar imaging. Magn Reson Imaging 1996;14:1113–6.
11. Bai X, Zhang Y, Liu Y. Grading of supratentorial astrocytic tumors by using the difference of ADC value. Neuroradiology 2011;53(7):533–9.
12. Stadnik TW, Chaskis C, Michotte A, et al. Diffusion-weighted MR imaging of intracerebral masses: comparison with conventional MR imaging and histologic findings. AJNR Am J Neuroradiol 2001;22:969–76.
13. Beaulieu C, Allen PS. Determinants of anisotropic water diffusion in nerves. Magn Reson Med 1994;31(4):394–400.
14. Mori S, van Zijl PC. Fiber tracking: principles and strategies–a technical review. NMR Biomed 2002;15(7–8):468–80.
15. Fernandez-Miranda JC, Pathak S, Engh J, et al. High-definition fiber tractography of the human brain: neuroanatomical validation and neurosurgical applications. Neurosurgery 2012;71(2):430–53.
16. Calamante F. Perfusion MRI using dynamic-susceptibility contrast MRI: quantification issues in patient studies. Top Magn Reson Imaging 2010;21(2):75–85.
17. Harrer JU, Parker GJ, Haroon HA, et al. Comparative study of methods for determining vascular permeability and blood volume in human gliomas. J Magn Reson Imaging 2004;20(5):748–57.
18. Direksunthorn T, Chawalparit O, Sangruchi T, et al. Diagnostic performance of perfusion MRI in differentiating low-grade and high-grade gliomas: advanced MRI in glioma. J Med Assoc Thai 2013;96(9):1183–90.
19. Maia AC Jr, Malheiros SM, da Rocha AJ, et al. Stereotactic biopsy guidance in adults with supratentorial nonenhancing gliomas: role of perfusion-weighted magnetic resonance imaging. J Neurosurg 2004;101(6):970–6.
20. Bulakbasi N, Kocaoglu M, Farzaliyev A, et al. Assessment of diagnostic accuracy of perfusion MR imaging in primary and metastatic solitary malignant brain tumors. AJNR Am J Neuroradiol 2005;26:2187–99.

21. Kim YH, Oh SW, Lim YJ, et al. Differentiating radiation necrosis from tumor recurrence in high-grade gliomas: assessing the efficacy of 18F-FDG PET, 11C-methionine PET and perfusion MRI. Clin Neurol Neurosurg 2010;112(9):758–65.
22. Marshall I, Wardlaw J, Cannon J, et al. Reproducibility of metabolite peak areas in 1H MRS of brain. Magn Reson Imaging 1996;14:281–92.
23. Calvar JA. Accurate (1)H tumor spectra quantification from acquisitions without water suppression. Magn Reson Imaging 2006;24:1271–9.
24. Moffett JR, Ross B, Arun P, et al. N-acetyl aspartate in the CNS: from neurodiagnostics to neurobiology. Prog Neurobiol 2007;81:89–131.
25. Wyss M, Kaddurah-Daouk R. Creatine and creatinine metabolism. Physiol Rev 2000;80:1107–213.
26. Devos A, Lukas L, Suykens JA, et al. Classification of brain tumours using short echo time 1H MR spectra. J Magn Reson 2004;170:164–75.
27. Li X, Vigneron DB, Cha S, et al. Relationship of MR-derived lactate, mobile lipids, and relative blood volume for gliomas in vivo. AJNR Am J Neuroradiol 2005;26:760–9.
28. Catalaa I, Henry R, Dillon WP, et al. Perfusion, diffusion and spectroscopy values in newly diagnosed cerebral gliomas. NMR Biomed 2006;19:463–75.
29. Hall WA, Martin A, Liu H, et al. Improving diagnostic yield in brain biopsy: coupling spectroscopic targeting with real-time needle placement. J Magn Reson Imaging 2001;13:12–5.
30. Lang S, Duncan N, Northoff G. Resting state fMRI: review of neurosurgical applications. Neurosurgery 2014;74(5):453–64.
31. Krieg SM, Sollmann N, Hauck T, et al. Functional language shift to the right hemisphere in patients with language-eloquent brain tumors. PLoS One 2013;8(9): e75403.
32. Dimou S, Battisti RA, Hermens DF, et al. A systematic review of functional magnetic resonance imaging and diffusion tensor imaging modalities used in presurgical planning of brain tumour resection. Neurosurg Rev 2013;36(2):205–14.
33. Koeller KK, Rushing EJ. Pilocytic astrocytoma: radiologic-pathologic correlation. Radiographics 2004;24:1693–708.
34. Cristoforidis G, Drevelengas A, Bourekas E, et al. Low grade gliomas. In: Drevelegas A, editor. Imaging of brain tumors with histological correlations. Heidelberg: Springer; 2011. p. 43–7.
35. Segal L, Darvish-Zargar M, Dilenge ME, et al. Optic pathway gliomas in patients with neurofibromatosis type 1: follow-up of 44 patients. J AAPOS 2010;14(2):155–8.
36. Hwang JH, Egnaczyk GF, Ballard E, et al. Proton MR spectroscopic characteristics of pediatric pilocytic astrocytomas. AJNR Am J Neuroradiol 1998;19:535–40.
37. Palma L, Guidetti B. Cystic pilocytic astrocytomas of the cerebral hemispheres. Surgical experience with 51 cases and long-term results. J Neurosurg 1985; 62(6):811–5.
38. Kestle J, Townsend JJ, Brockmeyer DL, et al. Juvenile pilocytic astrocytoma of the brainstem in children. J Neurosurg 2004;101:1–6.
39. Rumboldt Z, Camacho DL, Lake D, et al. Apparent diffusion coefficients for differentiation of cerebellar tumors in children. AJNR Am J Neuroradiol 2006;27(6):1362–9.
40. Yamashita Y, Kumabe T, Higano S, et al. Minimum apparent diffusion coefficient is significantly correlated with cellularity in medulloblastomas. Neurol Res 2009; 31(9):940–6.
41. Bing F, Kremer S, Lamalle L, et al. Value of perfusion MRI in the study of pilocytic astrocytoma and hemangioblastoma: preliminary findings. J Neuroradiol 2009; 36(2):82–7.

42. Liu ZL, Zhou Q, Zeng QS, et al. Noninvasive evaluation of cerebral glioma grade by using diffusion-weighted imaging-guided single-voxel proton magnetic resonance spectroscopy. J Int Med Res 2012;40(1):76–84.
43. Johannesen TB, Langmark F, Lote K. Progress in long-term survival in adult patients with supratentorial low-grade gliomas: a population-based study of 993 patients in whom tumors were diagnosed between 1970 and 1993. J Neurosurg 2003;99:854–62.
44. Osborn A, editor. Astrocytomas. In: Osborn's brain imaging pathology, and anatomy. Philadelphia: Lippincott Williams &Wilkins; 2013. p. 472–5.
45. Server A, Kulle B, Gadmar ØB, et al. Measurements of diagnostic examination performance using quantitative apparent diffusion coefficient and proton MR spectroscopic imaging in the preoperative evaluation of tumor grade in cerebral gliomas. Eur J Radiol 2011;80(2):462–70.
46. Law M, Yang S, Wang H, et al. Glioma grading: sensitivity, specificity, and predictive values of perfusion MR imaging and proton MR spectroscopic imaging compared with conventional MR imaging. AJNR Am J Neuroradiol 2003; 24(10):1989–98.
47. Hilario A, Ramos A, Perez-Nuñez A, et al. The added value of apparent diffusion coefficient to cerebral blood volume in the preoperative grading of diffuse gliomas. AJNR Am J Neuroradiol 2012;33(4):701–7.
48. Bulik M, Jancalek R, Vanicek J, et al. Potential of MR spectroscopy for assessment of glioma grading. Clin Neurol Neurosurg 2013;115(2):146–53.
49. Koukourakis GV, Kouloulias V, Zacharias G, et al. Temozolomide with radiation therapy in high grade brain gliomas: pharmaceuticals considerations and efficacy; a review article. Molecules 2009;14(4):1561–77.
50. Rees JH, Smirniotopoulos JG, Jones RV, et al. Glioblastoma multiforme: radiologic-pathologic correlation. Radiographics 1996;16:1413–38.
51. Higano S, Yun X, Kumabe T, et al. Malignant astrocytic tumors: clinical importance of apparent diffusion coefficient in prediction of grade and prognosis. Radiology 2006;241(3):839–46.
52. Lee EJ, terBrugge K, Mikulis D, et al. Diagnostic value of peritumoral minimum apparent diffusion coefficient for differentiation of glioblastoma multiforme from solitary metastatic lesions. Am J Roentgenol 2011;196(1):71–6.
53. Halshtok Neiman O, Sadetzki S, Chetrit A, et al. Perfusion-weighted imaging of peritumoral edema can aid in the differential diagnosis of glioblastoma multiforme versus brain metastasis. Isr Med Assoc J 2013;15(2):103–5.
54. Mouthuy N, Cosnard G, Abarca-Quinones J, et al. Multiparametric magnetic resonance imaging to differentiate high-grade gliomas and brain metastases. J Neuroradiol 2012;39(5):301–7.
55. Tsolaki E, Svolos P, Kousi E, et al. Automated differentiation of glioblastomas from intracranial metastases using 3T MR spectroscopic and perfusion data. Int J Comput Assist Radiol Surg 2013;8(5):751–61.
56. Tsougos I, Svolos P, Kousi E, et al. Differentiation of glioblastoma multiforme from metastatic brain tumor using proton magnetic resonance spectroscopy, diffusion and perfusion metrics at 3 T. Cancer Imaging 2012;26(12):423–36.
57. Park CK, Lee SH, Kim TM, et al. The value of temozolomide in combination with radiotherapy during standard treatment for newly diagnosed glioblastoma. J Neurooncol 2013;112(2):277–83.
58. Kelly K, Koeller KK, Rushing EJ. Oligodendroglioma and its variants: radiologic-pathologic correlation. Radiographics 2005;25:1669–88.

59. Zulfiqar M, Dumrongpisutikul N, Intrapiromkul J, et al. Detection of intratumoral calcification in oligodendrogliomas by susceptibility-weighted MR imaging. AJNR Am J Neuroradiol 2012;33:858–64.
60. White ML, Zhang Y, Kirby P, et al. Can tumor contrast enhancement be used as a criterion for differentiating tumor grades of oligodendrogliomas? AJNR Am J Neuroradiol 2005;26:784–90.
61. Lev MH, Ozsunar Y, Henson JW, et al. Glial tumor grading and outcome prediction using dynamic spin-echo MR susceptibility mapping compared with conventional contrast-enhanced MR: confounding effect of elevated rCBV of oligodendrogliomas. AJNR Am J Neuroradiol 2004;25:214–21.
62. Xu M, See SJ, Ng WH, et al. Comparison of magnetic resonance spectroscopy and perfusion-weighted imaging in presurgical grading of oligodendroglial tumors. Neurosurgery 2005;56(5):919–26.
63. Jenkinson MD, Smith TS, Brodbelt AR, et al. Apparent diffusion coefficients in oligodendroglial tumors characterized by genotype. J Magn Reson Imaging 2007;26(6):1405–12.
64. Lebrun C, Fontaine D, Ramaioli A, et al. Long-term outcome of oligodendrogliomas. Neurology 2004;62(10):1783–7.
65. Metellus P, Barrie M, Figarella-Branger D, et al. Multicentric French study on adult intracranial ependymomas: prognostic factors analysis and therapeutic considerations from a cohort of 152 patients. Brain 2007;130:1338–49.
66. Koeller KK, Sandberg GD. From the archives of the AFIP: cerebral intraventricular neoplasms: radiologic-pathologic correlation. RadioGraphics 2002;22:1473–505.
67. Mermuys K, Jeuris W, Vanhoenacker PK, et al. Best cases from the AFIP: supratentorial ependymoma. RadioGraphics 2005;25:486–90.
68. Yuh EL, Barkovich AG, Gupta N. Imaging of ependymomas: MRI and CT. Childs Nerv Syst 2009;25:1203–13.
69. Majos C, Aguilera C, Cos M, et al. In vivo proton magnetic spectroscopy of intraventricular tumors of the brain. Eur Radiol 2009;19(8):2049–59.
70. Guyotat J, Metellus P, Giorgi R, et al. Infratentorial ependymomas: prognostic factors and outcome in a multi-center retrospective series of 106 adult patients. Acta Neurochir (Wien) 2009;151(8):947–60.
71. Jaiswal S, Vij M, Mehrotra A, et al. Choroid plexus tumors: a clinico-pathological and neuro-radiological study of 23 cases. Asian J Neurosurg 2013;8(1):29–35.
72. Anderson DR, Falcone S, Bruce JH, et al. Radiologic-pathologic correlation: congenital choroid plexus papillomas. AJNR Am J Neuroradiol 1995;16:2072–6.
73. Steven DA, McGinn GJ, McClarty BM. A choroid plexus papilloma arising from an incidental pineal cyst. AJNR Am J Neuroradiol 1996;17:939–42.
74. Lafay-Cousin L, Keene D, Carret AS, et al. Choroid plexus tumors in children less than 36 months: the Canadian Pediatric Brain Tumor Consortium (CPBTC) experience. Childs Nerv Syst 2011;27(2):259–64.
75. Krieger MD, Panigrahy A, McComb JG, et al. Differentiation of choroid plexus tumors by advanced magnetic resonance spectroscopy. Neurosurg Focus 2005;18(6A):E4.
76. Zimny A, Sasiadek M. Contribution of perfusion-weighted magnetic resonance imaging in the differentiation of meningiomas and other extra-axial tumors: case reports and literature review. J Neurooncol 2011;103:777–83.
77. Meyers SP, Khademian ZP, Chuang SH, et al. Choroid plexus carcinomas in children: MRI features and patient outcomes. Neuroradiology 2004;46(9):770–80.

78. Koeller KK, Rushing EJ. From the archives of the AFIP: medulloblastoma: a comprehensive review with radiologic-pathologic correlation. RadioGraphics 2003;23:1613–37.
79. Wilms G, Drevelegas A, Demaerel P, et al. Embryonal tumors. In: Drevelegas A, editor. Imaging of brain tumors with histological correlations. 2nd edition. Heidelberg: Springer; 2011. p. 215–21.
80. Bartlett F, Kortmann R, Saran F. Medulloblastoma. Clin Oncol (R Coll Radiol) 2013;25(1):36–45.
81. da Fonte MV, Amara RP, Costa MO, et al. Medulloblastoma: correlation among findings of conventional magnetic resonance imaging, diffusion-weighted imaging and proton magnetic resonance spectroscopy. Radiol Bras 2008;41(6): 373–8.
82. Levy RA, Blaivas M, Muraszko K, et al. Desmoplastic medulloblastoma: MR findings. AJNR Am J Neuroradiol 1997;18:1364–6.
83. Neto AC, Gasparetto EL, Ono SE, et al. Adult cerebellar medulloblastoma. CT and MRI findings in eight cases. Arq Neuropsiquiatr 2003;61(2A):199–203.
84. Moreno-Torres A, Martínez-Pérez I, Baquero M, et al. Taurine detection by proton magnetic resonance spectroscopy in medulloblastoma: contribution to noninvasive differential diagnosis with cerebellar astrocytoma. Neurosurgery 2004;55(4):824–9.
85. Huang X, Xu J, Xu M, et al. Clinical features of intracranial vestibular schwannomas. Oncol Lett 2013;5(1):57–62.
86. Hamilton JD, DeMonte F, Ginsberg LE. Imaging of carotid canal sympathetic plexus schwannoma. AJNR Am J Neuroradiol 2011;32:1212–5.
87. Salzman KL, Childs AM, Davidson HC, et al. Intralabyrinthine schwannomas: imaging diagnosis and classification. AJNR Am J Neuroradiol 2012;33:104–9.
88. Stone JA, Cooper H, Castillo M, et al. Malignant schwannoma of the trigeminal nerve. AJNR Am J Neuroradiol 2001;22:505–7.
89. Muzzafar S, Ketonen L, Weinberg JS, et al. Imaging and clinical features of an intra-axial brain stem schwannoma. AJNR Am J Neuroradiol 2010;31:567–9.
90. Zagardo MT, Castellani RJ, Rees JH, et al. Radiologic and pathologic findings of intracerebral schwannoma. AJNR Am J Neuroradiol 1998;19:1290–3.
91. Tanghe H, Parizel P, Drevelegas A. Tumours of the cranial nerves. In: Drevelegas A, editor. Imaging of brain tumors with histological correlations. 2nd edition. Heidelberg: Springer; 2011. p. 229–32.
92. Wiggins RH III, Harnsberger HR, Salzman KL, et al. The many faces of facial nerve schwannoma. AJNR Am J Neuroradiol 2006;27:694–9.
93. Eldevik OP, Gabrielsen TO, Jacobsen EA. Imaging findings in schwannomas of the jugular foramen. AJNR Am J Neuroradiol 2000;21:1139–44.
94. Thamburaj K, Radhakrishnan VV, Thomas B, et al. Intratumoral microhemorrhages on T2*-weighted gradient-echo imaging helps differentiate vestibular schwannoma from meningioma. AJNR Am J Neuroradiol 2008;29(3): 552–7.
95. Babu R, Sharma R, Bagley JH, et al. Vestibular schwannomas in the modern era: epidemiology, treatment trends, and disparities in management. J Neurosurg 2013;119(1):121–30.
96. Ferri GG, Pirodda A, Ceroni AR, et al. Management of growing vestibular schwannomas. Eur Arch Otorhinolaryngol 2013;270(7):2013–9.
97. Massager N, Delbrouck C, Masudi J, et al. Hearing preservation and tumour control after radiosurgery for NF2-related vestibular schwannomas. B-ENT 2013;9(1):29–36.

98. Drevelegas A, Karkavelas G, Chourmouzi D, et al. Petridis meningeal tumors. In: Drevelegas A, editor. Imaging of brain tumors with histological correlation. 2nd edition. Heidelberg: Springer; 2011. p. 255–88.

99. Watts J, Box G, Galvin A, et al. Magnetic resonance imaging of meningiomas: a pictorial review. Insights Imaging 2014;5(1):113–22.

100. Buetow MP, Buetow PC, Smirniotopoulos JG. Typical, atypical, and misleading features in meningioma. Radiographics 1991;11(6):1087–106.

101. Sanverdi SE, Ozgen B, Oguz KK, et al. Is diffusion-weighted imaging useful in grading and differentiating histopathological subtypes of meningiomas? Eur J Radiol 2012;81(9):2389–95.

102. Todua F, Chedia S. Differentiation between benign and malignant meningiomas using diffusion and perfusion MR imaging. Georgian Med News 2012;206: 16–22.

103. Zhang H, Rödiger LA, Shen T, et al. Perfusion MR imaging for differentiation of benign and malignant meningiomas. Neuroradiology 2008;50(6):525–30.

104. Osborn A, editor. Tumors of the meninges. In: Osborn's brain imaging pathology, and anatomy. Philadelphia: Lippincott Williams &Wilkins; 2013. p. 583–95.

105. Chourmouzi D, Potsi S, Moumtzouoglou A, et al. Dural lesions mimicking meningiomas: a pictorial essay. World J Radiol 2012;4(3):75–82.

106. Singla A, Deshaies EM, Melnyk V, et al. Controversies in the role of preoperative embolization in meningioma management. Neurosurg Focus 2013;35(6):E17.

107. Maclean J, Fersht N, Short S. Controversies in radiotherapy for meningioma. Clin Oncol (R Coll Radiol) 2014;26(1):51–64.

108. Moazzam AA, Wagle N, Zada G. Recent developments in chemotherapy for meningiomas: a review. Neurosurg Focus 2013;35(6):E18.

109. Osborn A, editor. Lymphomas, hematopoietic and histiocytic tumors. In: Osborn's brain imaging pathology, and anatomy. Philadelphia: Lippincott Williams &Wilkins; 2013. p. 645–54.

110. Gerstner ER, Batchelor TT. Primary central nervous system lymphoma. Arch Neurol 2010;67:291–7.

111. Bühring U, Herrlinger U, Krings T, et al. MRI features of primary central nervous system lymphomas at presentation. Neurology 2001;57:393–6.

112. Zhang D, Hu LB, Henning TD, et al. MRI findings of primary CNS lymphoma in 26 immunocompetent patients. Korean J Radiol 2010;11:269–77.

113. Hochberg FH, Baehring JM, Hochberg EP. Primary CNS lymphoma: diagnosis. Nat Clin Pract Neurol 2007;3:24–35.

114. Adachi K, Yamaguchi F, Node Y, et al. Neuroimaging of primary central nervous system lymphoma in immunocompetent patients: comparison of recent and previous findings. J Nippon Med Sch 2013;80(3):174–83.

115. Schlegel U, Schmidt-Wolf IG, Deckert M. Primary CNS lymphoma: clinical presentation, pathological classification, molecular pathogenesis and treatment. J Neurol Sci 2000;181:1–12.

116. Zacharia TT, Law M, Naidich TP, et al. Central nervous system lymphoma characterization by diffusion-weighted imaging and MR spectroscopy. J Neuroimaging 2008;18:411–7.

117. Toh CH, Castillo M, Wong AM, et al. Primary cerebral lymphoma and glioblastoma multiforme: differences in diffusion characteristics evaluated with diffusion tensor imaging. AJNR Am J Neuroradiol 2008;29:471–5.

118. Hartmann M, Heiland S, Harting I, et al. Distinguishing of primary cerebral lymphoma from high-grade glioma with perfusion-weighted magnetic imaging. Neurosci Lett 2003;338:119–22.

119. Hakyemez B, Erdogan C, Bolca N, et al. Evaluation of different cerebral mass lesions by perfusion-weighted MR imaging. J Magn Reson Imaging 2006;24:817–24.
120. Osborn A, editor. Pineal and germ cell tumors. In: Osborn's brain imaging pathology, and anatomy. Philadelphia: Lippincott Williams &Wilkins; 2013. p. 550–8.
121. Drevelegas A, Strigaris A, Samara C. Pineal tumors. In: Drevelegas A, editor. Imaging of brain tumors with histological correlations. 2nd edition. Heidelberg: Springer; 2011. p. 203–7.
122. Tong T, Zhenwei Y, Xiaoyuan F. MRI and 1H-MRS on diagnosis of pineal region tumors. Clin Imaging 2012;36(6):702–9.
123. Dumrongpisutikul N, Intrapiromkul J, Yousem DM. Distinguishing between germinomas and pineal cell tumors on MR imaging. AJNR Am J Neuroradiol 2012;33(3):550–5.
124. Kortmann RD. Current concepts and future strategies in the management of intracranial germinoma. Expert Rev Anticancer Ther 2014;14(1):105–19.
125. Bourekas E, Slone W, Chaudhury A. Masses of the sellar and juxtasellar region. In: Drevelegas A, editor. Imaging of brain tumors with histological correlations. 2nd edition. Heidelberg: Springer; 2011. p. 335–42.
126. Osborn A, editor. Sellar neoplasms and tumorlike lesions. In: Osborn's brain imaging pathology, and anatomy. Philadelphia: Lippincott Williams &Wilkins; 2013. p. 706–12.
127. Rosenfeld A, Arrington D, Miller J, et al. A review of childhood and adolescent craniopharyngiomas with particular attention to hypothalamic obesity. Pediatr Neurol 2014;50(1):4–10.
128. Sener RN. Proton MR spectroscopy of craniopharyngiomas. Comput Med Imaging Graph 2001;25(5):417–22.
129. Müller HL. Childhood craniopharyngioma: treatment strategies and outcomes. Expert Rev Neurother 2014;14(2):187–97.
130. Saha A, Ghosh SK, Roy C, et al. Demographic and clinical profile of patients with brain metastases: a retrospective study. Asian J Neurosurg 2013;8(3):157–61.
131. Patchell RA. Metastatic brain tumors. Neurol Clin 1995;13(4):915–25.
132. Posner JB. Brain metastases: 1995. A brief review. J Neurooncol 1996;27(3):287–93.
133. Patronas N. Brain metastasis. In: Drevelegas A, editor. Imaging of brain tumors with histological correlations. 2nd edition. Heidelberg: Springer; 2011. p. 373–91.
134. Fink KR, Fink JR. Imaging of brain metastases. Surg Neurol Int 2013;2(4):209–19.

Value of Imaging in Head and Neck Tumors

Alexander J. Antoniou, MD, MA[a], Charles Marcus, MD[a],
Rathan M. Subramaniam, MD, PhD, MPH[a,b,c,d],*

KEYWORDS

- Imaging • Head and neck • Oncology

KEY POINTS

- Imaging is an integral part of management of patients with head and neck cancers. Imaging provides information for accurate staging, therapy selection, therapy assessment, detection of recurrence, and predicting survival outcomes.
- Computed tomography (CT) or magnetic resonance imaging (MRI) is useful for primary tumor staging. Ultrasonography and positron emission tomography (PET)/CT are more useful for identifying neck nodal metastasis, and PET/CT is useful for detecting distant metastasis. MRI is useful for detecting perineural spread, marrow, skull base, and intracranial involvement.
- Posttherapy assessment is performed using CT/MRI or PET/CT. PET/CT is increasingly used for posttherapy assessment because of superior sensitivity and specificity, especially in patients treated with chemoradiation therapy. Fluorodeoxyglucose PET/CT is usually performed 12 weeks after completion of therapy.
- The best value of imaging in follow-up is when it is used with clinical assessment and suspicion for disease recurrence.

INTRODUCTION: NATURE OF THE PROBLEM

Head and neck cancers constitute approximately 3% of all cancers in the United States,[1] with approximately 52,000 new cases diagnosed every year.[2] Head and

R.M. Subramaniam is supported by a Radiological Society of North America Education Scholar Grant (RSNA: ESCH1319).

[a] Russell H Morgan Department of Radiology and Radiological Sciences, Johns Hopkins School of Medicine, 601 North Caroline Street, Baltimore, MD 21287, USA; [b] Department of Oncology, Johns Hopkins School of Medicine, 401 North Broadway, Baltimore, MD 21287, USA; [c] Department of Otolaryngology-Head and Neck Surgery, Johns Hopkins School of Medicine, 601 North Caroline Street, Baltimore, MD 21287, USA; [d] Department of Health Policy and Management, Johns Hopkins Bloomberg School of Public Health, 615 North Wolfe Street, Baltimore, MD 21205, USA

* Corresponding author. Russell H Morgan Department of Radiology and Radiologic Science, Johns Hopkins Medical Institutions, JHOC 3235, 601 North Caroline Street, Baltimore, MD 21287.

E-mail address: rsubram4@jhmi.edu

neck cancer include cancers that have developed in the nasal cavity, sinuses, lips, mouth, salivary glands, paranasal sinuses, pharynx, throat, or larynx. Most head and neck cancers (90%–95%) are squamous cell carcinomas arising from mucosal linings of the upper aerodigestive tract. Other rare cancers that may involve the head and neck include salivary tumors, thyroid cancers, lymphoma, and melanoma.

Tobacco and alcohol use are the most important risk factors for most head and neck cancers. Approximately 75% of head and neck cancers are caused by tobacco and alcohol use. Infection with certain types of human papillomavirus causes more than half of all cases of oropharyngeal cancer.

Early diagnosis and accurate staging are essential for treatment planning and can strongly influence prognosis. In addition, early identification of tumor recurrence can often be treated with additional surgery or reirradiation. A combination of history, physical examination, endoscopy, and tissue sampling has historically been the mainstay of diagnosis and staging. The use of advanced imaging with computed tomography (CT), magnetic resonance imaging (MRI), and positron emission tomography (PET)/CT has greatly improved staging, therapy assessment, and monitoring for disease recurrence.

PREIMAGING PLANNING
Relevant Anatomy

The anatomy of the head and neck is a broad and complex subject, which is best appreciated when taken into context with the primary malignancy of interest. This review is by no means exhaustive but rather highlights the important structures from an imaging perspective as pertain to tumor spread and stage.

Sinonasal

- Malignant neoplasms include squamous cell carcinoma, adenoid cystic carcinoma, adenocarcinoma, olfactory neuroblastoma (esthesioneuroblastoma), melanoma, and lymphoma.
- The sinonasal cavity begins at the nostrils and ends at the posterior nasal septum, which separates it from the nasopharynx. The nasal cavity contains 3 medial bony projections, known as the turbinates, which originate in the lateral walls.[3]
- The paranasal sinuses consist of the maxillary, ethmoid, frontal, and sphenoid sinuses. The maxillary sinuses form the inferior margin of the nasal cavity, whereas the superior maxillary sinus forms the orbital floor and contains the infraorbital groove, through which the infraorbital nerve runs. The frontal sinuses anteriorly contribute to the orbital roof. The sphenoid sinus posteriorly forms the nasopharynx roof. The ethmoid sinus forms the superior lateral and medial walls of the nasal cavity.[3]
- The most common malignancy is squamous cell carcinoma. It may originate in the maxillary sinuses (60%–70%), followed by the nasal cavity (20%–30%), then the ethmoid sinuses (10%–15%), and rarely, in the frontal or sphenoid sinuses (1%).[4–7]
- The second most common malignancy, adenocarcinoma, most commonly originates in the ethmoid sinus.
- Tumor can invade in several different directions[5]:
  - From the maxillary antrum posterolaterally to the pterygoid plates, pterygopalatine fossa, and infratemporal fossa
  - From the pterygopalatine fossa to the orbit via the inferior orbital fissure or to the middle cranial fossa via the foramen rotundum

- From the maxillary antrum superiorly to the anterior cranial fossa and posterior wall of the frontal sinus via the orbital floor or the cribriform plate of the ethmoid
- Inferiorly to the maxillary ridge and hard palate
- Inferolaterally to the buccal space
- Medially to the nasal cavity

Salivary gland

- The major salivary glands consist of the parotid, submandibular, and sublingual glands, and the minor salivary glands are distributed within the mucosa of the oral cavity, palate, paranasal sinuses, pharynx, larynx, trachea, and bronchi.[8]
- Most parotid gland tumors are benign (80%), and only 20% to 25% are malignant. The probability for malignancy in the submandibular gland is about 40% to 50%. The risk of malignancy in sublingual and minor salivary glands is the highest, ranging from 50% to 81%.[8] Unlike the major salivary glands, 80% or more of minor salivary gland tumors are malignant and tend to have a great variation in presentation and histology.[9]
- The largest salivary gland, the parotid, is located in the parotid space; it is wedge shaped and is divided into superficial and deep lobes by the facial nerve and its branches for surgical planning. The facial nerve is best visualized radiographically by a line drawn from the lateral border of the posterior belly of the digastric muscle and the retromandibular vein to the lateral edge of the mandible.[8]
- The auriculotemporal nerve connects the mandibular branch of the trigeminal nerve with the facial nerve and is embedded in the gland capsule as it curves around the mandibular neck and serves as a potential route of perineural tumor spread. Between 3 and 24 lymph nodes are found within the parotid gland within the superficial portion and drain into the level 2A and 2B cervical nodes.
- The submandibular gland is located in the submandibular triangle, which is formed by the inferior border of the mandibular body and anterior and posterior bellies of the digastric muscle. The stylohyoid muscle contributes to the posterior border as well. The submandibular gland does not contain any lymph nodes or large nerves, unlike the parotid. Lymphatic drainage of the submandibular gland is mainly through 1B or submandibular and deep cervical nodes, especially 2A nodes.
- The sublingual gland is the smallest major salivary gland; it is located above the mylohyoid muscle, is covered by mucosa of the floor of the mouth, and has no capsule. Primary lymphatic drainage is into level I cervical nodes.[10]
- There are about 450 to 750 minor salivary glands in the head and neck region, which distribute into the sinonasal cavities, oropharynx, larynx, and trachea with most being found in the oral cavity. Heterotopic minor salivary glands can occur in the lymph nodes, the capsule of the thyroid gland, facial bones, and the hypophysis.[9] Benign and malignant salivary tumors can occur at any of these sites, including heterotopic locations.[9]

Nasopharynx

- The nasopharynx is located in the upper aerodigestive tract. It encompasses the superior aspect of the pharynx, which includes the lateral pharyngeal recess, the torus tubarius, and the pharyngeal tonsil[11]
- Nasopharyngeal carcinomas are classified into (1) squamous cell carcinomas, which account for 70% to 98% of nasopharyngeal malignancy, (2) differentiated

(subtype 2a) and undifferentiated (subtype 2b) nonkeratinized carcinomas, and (3) undifferentiated carcinomas.[11,12]

- The nasopharynx is bordered by the posterior nasal cavity anteriorly, the clivus posteriorly, the carotid spaces laterally, the hard palate, and the palatopharyngeal muscle inferiorly.[11]
- It is made up of 3 layers:
  - Inner mucous lining made up of ciliated pseudostratified epithelium and chorium. There is abundant lymphoid tissue in the chorium; it is a frequent site of malignancy, such as non-Hodgkin lymphoma.
  - Middle fibrous membrane or the pharyngobasilar fascia. This fascia is a tough aponeurosis, which connects the superior constrictor muscles to the skull base. The buccopharyngeal fascia is the middle layer of the deep cervical fascia, and it represents the fascial limit of the lateral and posterior portions of the nasopharynx.[11,13]
  - Outer muscular layer made up of upper, middle, and lower pharyngeal constrictor muscles, pharyngeal levator muscles (palatopharyngeal, stylopharyngeal, and salpingopharyngeal), palatoglossus, tensor palati and levator palati, and the palatopharyngeal muscle.[11]
- The nasopharynx is 2 cm in anteroposterior diameter and 4 cm long.[11]
- The sinus of Morgagni is a posterolateral defect in the pharyngobasilar fascia, which contains the paired eustachian tubes and the medial fibers of the levator veli palatini muscle.[13]
- The lateral pharyngeal recess (fossa of Rosenmüller) is posterior and superior to the torus tubarius (the distal cartilaginous end of the eustachian tube, which can be seen projecting into the lumen of the nasopharynx).[13]
- The parapharyngeal space separates the nasopharynx from the masticator space laterally and is a fibrofatty space; invasion of this space is used in staging.[13]
- The lateral retropharyngeal nodes (nodes of Rouvière) and the cervical level II nodes are the most common sites of metastasis.[13]
- Tumor invasion: 60% to 90% of the time, the tumor pushes through the pharyngobasilar fascia and invades the parapharyngeal space.[11,13] The most common direction of invasion is superiorly (48%) into the skull base, with bone destruction seen on CT in or around the clivus, foramen lacerum, middle cranial fossa, sphenoid sinus, or foramen jugularis. The second most extension is posteriorly (40%) into the prevertebral muscles toward the retropharyngeal space. Invasion into the retropharyngeal space has a higher risk of distant metastasis because of the presence of a venous plexus and lymphatics. The remaining sites of direct invasion are in the anterolateral extensions toward the masticator space and infratemporal fossa (14%) or inferiorly through the lateral walls of the pharynx or posterior tonsillar pillars into the oropharynx.[11]
- Perineural spread to the skull base can occur from the retropharyngeal space via multiple foramina, commonly with involvement of the fifth cranial nerves.[14] Also commonly involved is the nerve of the pterygoid canal, which enters the pterygopalatine fossa and joins the pterygopalatine ganglion, from which postganglionic parasympathetic fibers distribute to various structures, including the nose and palate.[11]
- The most common sites of metastasis include bone (20%), lung (13%), and liver (9%).[12]
- The nasopharynx and oropharynx overlap and an acceptable line between the 2 is the C1/C2 junction.[13]

Oral cavity and oropharynx

- The oral cavity is bordered by the maxilla and mandible and contains the lips, tongue (anterior two-thirds reside in the oral cavity), floor of the mouth, retromolar trigone, gingiva, alveolar ridges, and the hard palate.
- The nasopharynx is the most superior portion of the pharynx and extends from the skull base to the level of the hard/soft palate junction. The oropharynx consequently includes the posterior third of the tongue, the soft palate, palatine tonsils, and tonsillar pillars and extends to the level of the hyoid bone at the pharyngoepiglottic folds. The hypopharynx then extends inferiorly to the postcricoid segment, and the piriform sinuses.
- The most common sites of oral cavity cancer are the lips followed by the floor of the mouth. The common regions of involvement in the tongue include the lateral borders and the undersurface.
- Oral cavity cancers invade the pterygomandibular raphe (between the medial pterygoid plate and the mandible, separating the anterior tonsillar pillar and retromolar trigone) and extend to the temporalis muscle superiorly, the pterygopalatine fossa anteriorly, the pterygomandibular space medially, or the floor of the mouth inferiorly.
- The primary drainage site of the oral cavity is the level I submental and submandibular lymph nodes, and the level II jugular chain.

Larynx and hypopharynx

- The larynx can be divided anatomically into 3 parts: supraglottic, glottic, and subglottic.
- The hypopharynx can be divided into pyriform sinus, postcricoid area, and posterior pharyngeal wall.[15]
- Important pathways of tumor spread in the larynx occur along the paraglottic and pre-epiglottic spaces.
- Invasion of the laryngeal cartilages is generally associated with poor prognosis. It affects staging as well as surgery planning.
- Pyriform sinus carcinomas invade the paraglottic space and the laryngeal cartilages and tend to spread superiorly and inferiorly.[16,17] Tumors arising from the lateral wall of the pyriform sinus have a tendency to infiltrate the soft tissues of the neck early in the disease course.
- Postcricoid carcinomas spread submucosally, often toward the cervical esophagus.
- Posterior pharyngeal wall tumors commonly involve both the oropharynx and hypopharynx, and invasion of surrounding structures is unusual at initial presentation.[16]

Thyroid

- The thyroid gland lies at the level of the C5-T1 vertebra. It has 2 lobes, joined by an isthmus. About 30% to 50% of normal individuals have a pyramidal lobe, which is a superior extension of the thyroid tissue.[18,19]
- Extraglandular lymphatics generally follow the venous flow. The inferior portions of the lateral lobes drain along the tracheoesophageal groove into the central neck. The superior parts of the lobes drain toward the superior thyroid veins, and the isthmus may drain toward the prelaryngeal lymph nodes or central neck nodes.
- Even although it is uncommon, lymphatic drainage to the retropharyngeal region has been reported, accounting for metastasis to the skull base.

- The central lymphatics are considered the primary drainage pathway for thyroid cancer, and the lateral neck nodes are the secondary drainage pathway. Most thyroid cancers metastasize to the central compartment nodes (level VI).
- In large series, the lateral neck nodes are involved to varying degrees. Most commonly involved is level IV, followed by levels III, V, II, and I. Level I nodal metastases are rare from thyroid cancer.[19]

The most commonly involved contralateral compartment is the paratracheal region. When this finding is positive, the risk for metastases to the lateral neck is higher.[19]

RATIONALE/ISSUES FOR MODALITY SELECTION

The choice of modality selection can depend on multiple factors. Factors such as insurance coverage, availability of imaging equipment, availability of experienced readers, and the stage of a patient's malignancy can often dictate the choice of the primary modality used. CT is best suited to define the primary tumor and to identify bony invasion but can also be used for guiding tissue biopsy. MRI is best suited to delineate the extent of the primary tumor and involvement into adjacent structures. PET/CT is used to stage the locoregional lymph nodes and for systematic staging, and to assess posttherapy response or recurrence. In addition, patient contradictions such as contrast allergy (gadolinium or iodine), metallic implants (eg, pacemaker, cochlear implant), or pediatric population (concern for cumulative radiation dose) can affect choice of imaging modality. PET/MRI, although not widely available, holds promise in patients with head and neck malignancy, but research is limited compared with other imaging modalities.[20] **Tables 1–6** present the rationale for imaging modality selection and highlight the commonly recommended first choice.

INTERPRETATION/ASSESSMENT OF CLINICAL IMAGES

Table 7 shows the generally accepted features of benign and malignant tumors by choice of modality. Additional features of interpretation that are specific to the different types of head and neck malignancies are further discussed. A strong knowledge of

Table 1 Rationale/issues for modality selection in treatment of sinonasal malignancy			
Ultrasonography	CT	MRI	PET/CT
Limited role	CT provides bony detail when looking at bone invasion as well as anatomic landmarks at the skull base The detailed anatomy of the ostiomeatal complex as shown by CT provides a road map for the surgeons before endoscopic sinus surgery	Used for mapping the extent of tumor, because of its multiplanar capability, superior soft tissue contrast Modality of choice for assessing primary tumor and for assessing orbital and intracranial involvement	Useful for neck nodal and systemic staging, especially in advanced tumors and to assess tumor response after radiation therapy Imaging is typically performed 3 mo after radiation therapy to decrease the false-positive results from inflammatory processes

Table 2
Rationale/issues for modality selection in treatment of salivary cancer

Ultrasonography	CT	MRI	PET
Used for fine-needle aspiration for nodal staging Can assess tumor vascularity	Limited role; useful for bone invasion	Exact tumor localization and extent of tumor can be assessed (axial T1-weighted and T2-weighted images) Can detect perineural spread (T1-weighted axial and coronal images postgadolinium with fat suppression)	Useful for detecting locoregional and distant metastases in advanced stage[10]

anatomy and image interpretation is used for staging, according to the anatomic classification set forth by the American Joint Committee on Cancer.

Sinonasal

CT is the modality of choice for inflammatory sinonasal disease, and malignancy is often found incidentally. When the diagnosis of malignancy is known, CT plays an important role because of its high sensitivity for erosion of the sinus walls not seen on MRI, and more importantly, it can establish involvement of the cribriform plate, which is used in staging of the tumor. Interpreting the coronal CT perpendicular to the bony palate is best suited for evaluation of the ostiomeatal complexes.

MRI is the modality of choice when it comes to staging primary sinonasal malignancy, because of its superior ability to differentiate tumor from surrounding tissue and fluid. Common landmarks for assessment of tumor involvement include the skull base, orbit, pterygopalatine fossa, and infratemporal fossa. The pterygopalatine fossa

Table 3
Rationale/issues for modality selection in treatment of nasopharyngeal malignancy

Ultrasonography	CT	MRI	PET
Limited role	Inferior to MRI for invasion into surrounding soft tissue	Can detect tumor invasion into surrounding soft tissue, pharyngobasilar fascia, sinus of Morgagni, as well as skull base and intracranial invasion[13] Best to detect nerve involvement and perineural spread	Superior to MRI and CT for assessing lymph node metastasis, especially cervical nodal metastases, and distant metastases Modality of choice for therapy assessment and for follow-up with systemic staging Imaging for therapy assessment typically performed 3 mo after radiation therapy to decrease the false-positive results from inflammatory processes

Table 4
Rationale/issues for modality selection in treatment of oral cavity and oropharynx cancer

Ultrasonography	CT	MRI	PET/CT
Limited to staging with fine-needle aspiration of neck nodes	Useful in detection of mandibular involvement Degraded to a greater extent than MRI in the presence of metal artifacts Modality of choice for primary tumor staging	Better than CT to evaluate primary tongue tumor thickness[21] and for small tongue tumors Images degraded by patient motion artifacts of breathing and swallowing	Superior to MRI and CT for assessing cervical nodal metastases and distant metastases, especially with advanced stage[22,23] Modality of choice for posttherapy assessment, especially after chemoradiation therapy and in follow-up for systemic staging Posttherapy assessment imaging is typically performed 3 mo after radiation therapy to decrease the false-positive results from inflammatory processes

Table 5
Rationale/issues for modality selection in treatment of larynx and hypopharynx cancer

Ultrasonography	CT	MRI	PET/CT
Limited role. Used with fine-needle aspiration for nodal staging	Modality of choice to assess primary tumor size, tumor infiltration of surrounding structures, and laryngeal skeleton destruction	Higher incidence of nondiagnostic results because of motion artifacts (caused by swallowing), compared with CT[24]	Superior to MRI and CT for assessing cervical nodal metastases and distant metastases, especially with advanced stage Modality of choice for posttherapy assessment, especially after chemoradiation therapy and in follow-up for systemic staging. Posttherapy assessment imaging is typically performed 3 mo after radiation therapy to decrease the false-positive results from inflammatory processes

Table 6
Rationale/issues for modality selection in treatment of thyroid cancer

Ultrasonography	CT	MRI	PET/CT
Recommended modality of evaluation for contralateral lobe and cervical lymph node evaluation[25] Used with fine-needle aspiration for staging	Useful in assessing the primary tumor extension into adjacent structures and for nodal staging	Useful in assessing the primary tumor extension into adjacent structures and for nodal staging	Incidental focal FDG thyroid uptake is associated with 24%–36% malignancy risk, with papillary thyroid carcinoma being the most common cancer[26] Used in dedifferentiated papillary and follicular cancers in patients with increased thyroglobulin levels but negative radioiodine scintigraphy to detect recurrence and metastasis Shows high FDG uptake in Hurthle cell and anaplastic thyroid cancers not detected on conventional imaging.[27,28] Useful for staging, therapy response assessment, and follow-up in these cancers

is an important landmark, because invasion of the fossa is a negative prognostic factor.[6] It is by breaching the pterygopalatine fossa that intracranial extension can occur, and it is also the location where the trigeminal nerve branches pass through, making it possible for perineural spread of the primary tumor.[3] When assessing orbital exenteration, bony erosion along with breach of the periosteum is a significant finding.[5] When assessing orbital invasion, tumor adjacent to the periorbita (CT/MRI), extraocular muscle involvement (MRI), and orbital fat obliteration (CT or MRI) are sensitive predictors. On the other hand, extraocular muscle displacement and enhancement are less accurate (**Fig. 1**).[29]

Although pathology is the gold standard to confirm diagnosis, squamous cell carcinomas tend to be hypointense on T2-weighted (T2W) images, whereas adenocarcinoma is only slightly hypointense.[3] Esthesioneuroblastoma (olfactory neuroblastoma) can present with peritumoral cysts that are hypointense on T1-weighted (T1W) images and hyperintense on T2W images.[30–33]

PET/CT has superior sensitivity and specificity for nodal staging than anatomic modalities. It is the modality of choice for systemic staging, especially with advanced

Table 7				
General features of malignancy by imaging modality				
Imaging Features	Ultrasonography	CT	MRI	PET/CT
Benign	Hypoechoic or hyperechoic, well-defined, lobulated with posterior acoustic enhancement, homogeneous structure, peripheral eggshell calcifications	Hypodense, cystic soft tissue mass; preserved muscle border and bone cortex	Homogeneous signal intensity with low T1W and high T2W internal signals	Low FDG uptake compared with blood pool, generally
Malignant	Irregular shape, irregular borders, blurred margins, hypoechoic, and inhomogeneous structure; may have punctate calcifications and high vascularity	Soft tissue thickening, presence of a bulky mass and infiltration of adjacent tissue with or without bone destruction	Ill-defined, infiltrative border, heterogeneous internal signal with cystic change and necrosis; often with postcontrast heterogeneous enhancement	High FDG uptake compared with blood pool or liver uptake in FDG-avid tumors

sinonasal malignancies, and also for posttherapy assessment, when chemoradiation therapy is used.[34] In modern PET/CT scanners with 16, 64, or 128 detectors, the CT component of the PET/CT can be used for skeletal invasion; if contrast-enhanced PET/CT is performed, primary tumor assessment could also be established, similar to stand-alone CT (**Figs. 2 and 3**).[35,36]

Salivary Gland Tumors

Radiologic features of salivary gland tumors show considerable overlap between benign and malignant lesions, and it can be difficult to differentiate between the 2. Certain features of the tumor are better appreciated by a particular modality of imaging than the others. MRI seems to be the most useful in the diagnosis of the disease.

On ultrasonography, features of a malignant lesion include an irregular shape, irregular borders, blurred margins, and hypoechoic inhomogeneous structure. However, the features may not be always be present and can be seen both in benign and malignant lesions. Vascularization of the lesion is not pathognomonic, and assessment of vascularity using Doppler does not allow reliable differentiation between benign and malignant salivary gland tumors[37]

On MRI, hemorrhage, fibrosis, and proteinaceous fluid within the tumor may give intermediate T1 signal, which can be mistaken for a high-grade malignant lesion. High-grade tumors show early enhancement and slow washout. In addition, malignancy is suggested if deep infiltration into the parapharyngeal space, muscles, or bone as well as perineural spread is present. Diagnostic accuracy for perineural spread is high with MRI and is indicated by replacement of fat in neural foramina and appearance of a

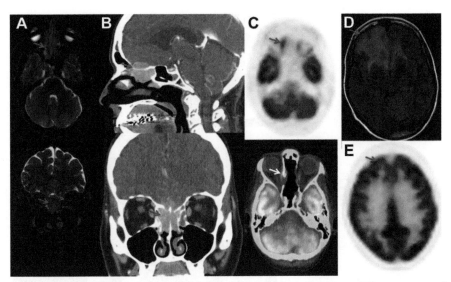

Fig. 1. Role of CT/MRI in diagnosis and FDG PET/CT in assessing treatment response and identification of postradiation necrosis in sinonasal carcinoma. Baseline axial, coronal T2-weighted MRI (*A*) and axial, coronal CT (*B*) images of a 58-year-old woman with esthesio-neuroblastoma of the ethmoid sinus, shows hyperintense mass on MRI (*arrow*), centered within the ethmoid air cells bilaterally and extending posteriorly into the sphenoid sinus. The CT images show enhancing soft tissue mass (*arrow*) in the ethmoid sinus, with associated destruction of nasal septum and cribriform plate, with intracranial extension. She underwent surgical resection of the mass, followed by radiotherapy. Axial PET and fused PET/CT images (*C*) of the restaging FDG PET/CT study performed a year after diagnosis show good treatment response (*arrow*). Axial T1-weighted (*D*) image of a follow-up MRI study performed 2 years after diagnosis showed hyperintensity (*arrow*) in the frontal lobes (left more than right). Axial PET (*E*) image of an FDG PET/CT study performed for evaluation shows corresponding hypometabolism (*arrow*), indicating probable postradiation changes.

diffuse or nodular thickened nerve with enhancement. Skip lesions on MRI my result from discontinuous neural invasion.[8]

CT has been considered an alternative modality to MRI, because certain histologic types like adenoid cystic carcinoma can lack contrast enhancement and lead to underestimation of lesions. Bone infiltration is appreciated well on CT. Malignant lymphadenopathy can be suspected with an internal heterogeneous appearance, necrosis, and extracapsular spread.[38,39]

Fluorodeoxyglucose (FDG) PET/CT has good diagnostic accuracy for determining tumor extent, nodal involvement, and distant metastases, especially in high-grade tumors showing high FDG uptake. However, differentiating between benign and malignant tumors can be difficult.[38,40] The main usefulness of FDG PET/CT in salivary gland tumors is to identify locoregional nodal metastasis and distant metastasis (**Fig. 4**).

Nasopharynx

The most common site of nasopharyngeal carcinoma is in the lateral pharyngeal recess (82%). An important point on interpretation of nasopharyngeal malignancy is taking into account the effects of aging on anatomy. With aging, there is an increase in fat tissue and inversely, a decrease in the volume of lymphoid tissues and muscle. Imaging shows an increase in size of the lateral pharyngeal recess, with a more

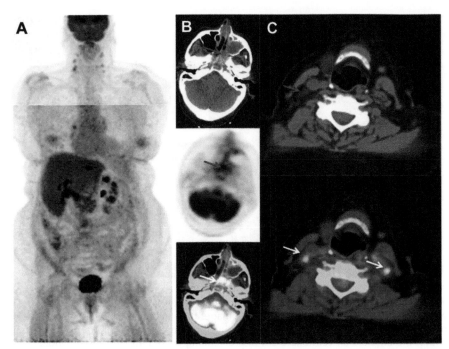

Fig. 2. Role of FDG PET/CT in restaging of sinonasal carcinoma. Anterior maximum intensity projection (MIP) (*A*), axial CT, PET, and fused PET/CT (*B*) and axial CT and fused PET/CT (*C*) images of a 78-year-old woman with squamous cell carcinoma of the nasal cavity, after concurrent chemoradiation, who underwent a staging FDG PET/CT. PET/CT showed FDG-avid (maximum SUV, 4.39), destructive soft tissue mass (*arrow*) involving the nasal cavity, sphenoid sinus, ethmoid sinus, and left maxillary sinus, consistent with residual tumor. Several enlarged/subcentimeter, metastatic cervical nodes (*arrows*) with FDG uptake (maximum SUV, 4.23) were also noted bilaterally, suggestive of active disease.

prominent torus tubarius and auditory tube ostium. This finding is physiologic and should be appreciated on imaging.[11]

MRI and CT play an important role in initial diagnosis and staging of primary tumors, whereas PET/CT is more appropriate to diagnose recurrent tumors and lymph node and distant metastasis (**Fig. 5**).[11,13] MRI sequences used include a noncontrast T1W image to detect skull base or fat plane involvement, T2W fast spin echo to detect parapharyngeal extension, paranasal sinus invasion, or cervical lymph node involvement, and T1W contrast-enhanced images with or without fat suppression to detect tumor spread, perineural spread, and intracranial extension.[12] Alternative MRI protocols used are diffusion-weighted MRI to better characterize cervical lymphadenopathy, and MRI spectroscopy, when the choline/creatine ratio is higher in metastatic nodes than musculature.

Because of the small and infiltrative nature of these tumors, fat plane obliteration and loss of muscular margins, MRI is a useful diagnostic tool to evaluate soft tissue infiltration and to differentiate lymphoid tissue from muscle.[11] The pharyngobasilar fascia is a fibrous structure; it can occasionally be seen as a thin dark line on T2W axial MRI and can outline the middle layer of the nasopharynx.[13] Parapharyngeal (between the tensor and levator veli palatini muscles) or retropharyngeal (between the nasopharyngeal mucosa anteriorly and the longus capitus colli complex posteriorly) fat infiltration presents as obliteration of the normally hyperintense fat stripe on T1W images.[14]

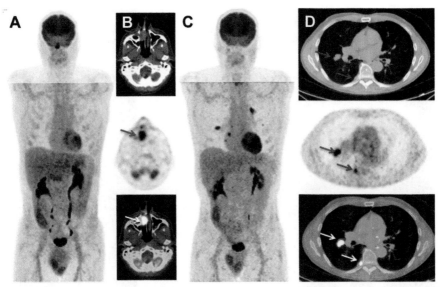

Fig. 3. Role of FDG PET/CT in the follow-up and prognostication of patients with sinonasal carcinoma. Anterior maximum intensity projection (A), axial CT, PET, and fused PET/CT images (B) of a 56-year-old man who underwent a staging FDG PET/CT for evaluation of recently diagnosed squamous cell carcinoma of the right nasal cavity. PET/CT showed hypermetabolic (maximum SUV, 9.45), large right nasal cavity mass (arrow) extending inferiorly to the soft palate, laterally into right maxillary sinus and anteriorly to the inferior nares. He underwent surgical resection of the tumor. Anterior maximum intensity projection (C), axial CT, PET, and fused PET/CT images (D) of the follow-up FDG PET/CT study performed 3 years after the initial study showed FDG-avid, bilateral lung parenchymal metastases (arrows). Despite aggressive systemic therapy, his disease progressed, resulting in death 19 months after the last study.

Perineural spread, a common theme of the suprahyoid malignancies, is an important prognostic factor. CT can reliably detect perineural spread by the secondary finding of foramina enlargement, atrophy of the muscles innervated by the trigeminal nerve, or fat infiltration of the pterygopalatine fossa. MRI, on the other hand, shows abnormal enlargement and enhancement of the involved nerve. Perineural spread is more common in adenoid cystic carcinoma than in squamous cell carcinoma.[14]

The lymph nodes of the retropharyngeal space are commonly the first nodes to be involved and can be identified between the skull base and C3.[12] Nodal spread begins at the lateral retropharyngeal lymph nodes, which are medial to the carotid artery, and then involves nodal groups along the internal jugular chain (level II–IV), spinal accessory chain (Va and Vb), and the supraclavicular nodes.[13] Nonretropharyngeal nodal involvement occurs most commonly in levels IIa and IIb, just posterior to the jugular vein.[11,13] If identified, nodal necrosis is considered 100% specific for metastatic involvement. The larger the tumor focus (usually >3 mm), the more likely necrosis can be reliably identified; it is seen as hypointense on T1W images and hyperintense on T2W images or as hypoattenuation on CT[13] or as hypometabolic areas in FDG PET/CT.[41]

Oral Cavity and Oropharynx

The primary oral cavity and oropharyngeal tumor can be best imaged with contrast-enhanced CT most of the time, and MRI is helpful for detection of small tongue tumors and to delineate extension. However, unlike other suprahyoid malignancies, multiple

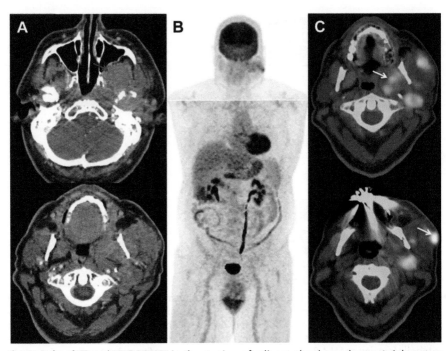

Fig. 4. Role of CT and FDG PET/CT in the staging of salivary gland neoplasms. Axial contrastenhanced CT (*A*), anterior maximum intensity projection (*B*), and axial fused FDG PET/CT (*C*) images of a 60-year-old man with left parotid adenoid cystic carcinoma. The CT images show a large left parotid mass (*arrow*) extending into the left pterygopalatine fossa, left retromolar space, and left temporomandibular joint. The PET/CT images show multifocal increased FDG uptake within the large mass, involving the left parotid gland (*top arrow*), with an adjacent intensely FDG-avid lymph node (*bottom arrow*). No FDG-avid distant metastasis was identified.

modalities are required for accurate staging and assessment of tumor extent. CT and MRI are used for evaluation of tumor invasion, especially in the tongue and mandible, whereas PET/CT and ultrasonography are better suited for evaluation of lymph node metastasis for more accurate staging (**Fig. 6**).[41] In advanced stages, PET/CT provide accurate systemic staging. In a large prospective study, PET showed the highest specificity for staging of oral cavity malignancy, whereas ultrasound-guided fine-needle aspiration had the highest sensitivity and accuracy compared with CT or MRI. However, maximum accuracy still remains low (76%), which maintains elective neck treatment as an option for many patients.[42,43]

Imaging findings play a large role in surgical planning. Two such examples are involvement of the tongue or mandible. When tumor involves the tongue, careful delineation of tumor extent is important, because the posterior base of the tongue is critical for swallowing, whereas the anterior portion is critical for phonation.[14] Mandibular invasion often leads to marginal resection or segmental mandibulectomy. Squamous cell carcinoma commonly invades the mandible via the alveolar crest.[44]

When there is suspicion of bone invasions of the mandible or maxilla, multiplanar images are required to adequately assess the extent of invasion. It is most commonly assessed with CT, and fusion with PET can increase sensitivity.[45] On MRI, the signal intensity of tumor replaces the hypointense cortical bone and the hyperintense medullar bone.[46] Involvement of the bone marrow is hypointense on T1W images and

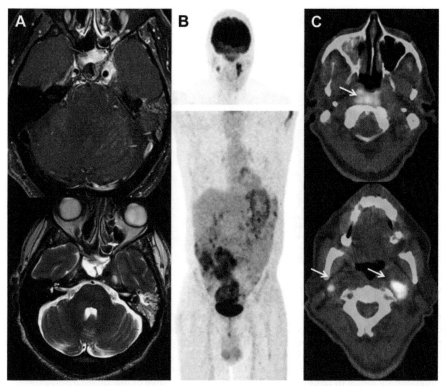

Fig. 5. Role of MRI and FDG PET/CT in the staging of nasopharyngeal carcinoma. Axial T1W and T2W MRI (*A*), anterior maximum intensity projection (*B*), and axial fused FDG PET/CT (*C*) images of a 62-year-old man with a recent diagnosis of nasopharyngeal carcinoma, who underwent baseline imaging. The T1W and T2W axial MRI images show an enhancing soft tissue mass (*arrow*) along the lateral wall of the nasopharynx, with extension of tumor via perineural spread into the left cavernous sinus as well as the pterygopalatine fossa. The PET/CT study shows an intensely FDG-avid nasopharyngeal mass (*top arrow*), with bilateral hypermetabolic, metastatic cervical lymphadenopathy (*bottom arrows*). No FDG-avid distant metastasis was identified.

hyperintense on T2W images with fat suppression. Although invasion of the mandible has been shown to be more sensitive when assessed with MRI, there is no difference in accuracy, and most centers still opt for CT.[47]

On the other hand, an image finding of tumor fixation to the prevertebral fascia seen as T2W hyperintensity and enhancement denotes irresectability. On T1W images, the preservation of the retropharyngeal fat plane reliably predicts absence of prevertebral fixation.[21]

Evidence of sublingual extension, especially in large (>2 cm) tumors, is associated with involvement of the neurovascular bundle in oral cavity malignancy.[48] Additional image findings of submucosal spread and mucosal lesions are typically correlated and confirmed with findings from endoscopy. Moreover, in cases of unknown primary, a negative PET study does not preclude panendoscopy with biopsy.[49,50]

Larynx and Hypopharynx

In cancers of the larynx and hypopharynx, cross-sectional imaging with CT provides valuable information regarding primary tumor staging and treatment

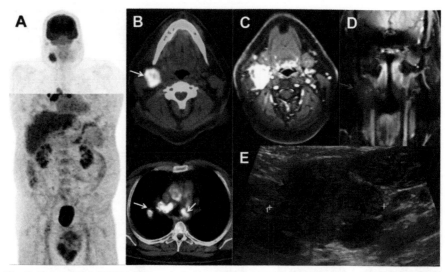

Fig. 6. Role of FDG PET/CT, MRI and ultrasonography in the staging of oropharyngeal cancer. Anterior maximum intensity projection (A), axial fused PET/CT (B), axial and coronal T1W MRI (C, D), and ultrasonographic (E) images of a 40-year-old man, recently diagnosed with squamous cell carcinoma of the left tonsil, after tonsillectomy, who underwent baseline imaging evaluation. The FDG PET/CT images show metastatic disease involving the bilateral lungs and mediastinum (arrows), and cervical lymph nodes. The MRI images show a heterogeneously enhancing mass (arrow) in the right cervical region abutting the right sternocleidomastoid muscle and cervical internal and external carotid arteries. Ultrasonography showed a right cervical conglomerate group of nodes (arrow), with features suggestive of malignant involvement.

planning. PET/CT has been shown to have an increasing impact in the management of these patients, especially in the staging of advanced disease, detection of distant metastases, and providing prognostic information (**Fig. 7**).

MRI predicts cervical esophagus invasion by identifying esophageal wall thickening, effacement of adjacent fat plane, and T2 signal abnormality.[51,52] Deep soft tissue extension is seen in the periglottic space, the laryngeal cartilages, and the base of tongue on CT and MRI. Gross cartilage invasion can be detected on CT; however, early cartilage abnormalities are detected better on MRI. Areas of cartilage involvement result in high signal intensity on T2W images and contrast-enhanced T1W images.

In hypopharyngeal cancers, prevertebral space invasion should be suspected when there is obliteration of the retropharyngeal fat plane on cross-sectional imaging.[16] Because hypopharyngeal cancer presents in advanced stages with nodal metastasis, FDG PET/CT is performed for accurate locoregional nodal and distant metastasis staging. PET/CT seems to be useful in nodal staging, identifying distant metastases. A pretreatment standardized uptake value (SUV) of less than 9.0 in the primary tumor has been shown to be associated with less frequency of disease recurrence and improved disease-free survival.[53] Pretreatment metabolic tumor volume has also been found to be an independent prognostic factor in patients with locoregionally advanced squamous cell carcinoma of the larynx and hypopharynx.[53,54]

Thyroid

In cancers of the thyroid glands, ultrasonography, CT, MRI, radioiodine whole body scintigraphy, and FDG PET/CT have all proved useful in different aspects in the management of the disease, as described later (**Fig. 8**).

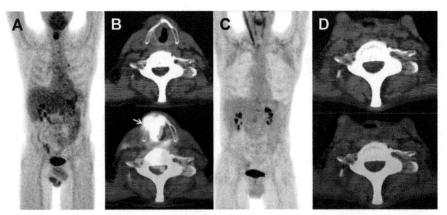

Fig. 7. Role of FDG PET/CT in the staging and therapy assessment of laryngeal malignancy. Anterior maximum intensity projection (*A*), axial CT, and fused FDG PET/CT (*B*) images of a 53-year-old man with laryngeal squamous cell carcinoma who underwent a baseline staging PET/CT study. The images show a large hypermetabolic laryngeal mass (*bottom arrow*). The patient underwent total laryngectomy, neck dissection, and radiation therapy. The anterior maximum intensity projection (*C*), axial CT, and fused PET/CT (*D*) images of the restaging FDG PET/CT study performed 8 months after the previous study showed a negative study for recurrent or metastatic disease, consistent with complete response to treatment.

Ultrasonographic features of malignant cervical nodes include width of the node being more than half that of the length of the node, heterogeneity, and necrosis.[55] Factors to be examined in evaluation of lesions include calcification, cyst formation, necrosis, hemorrhage, tumor margins, extraglandular extension, and metastatic

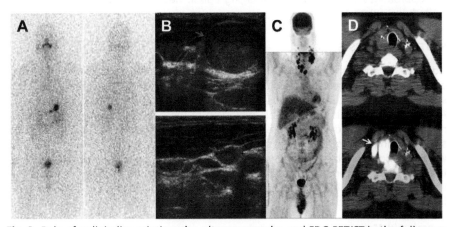

Fig. 8. Role of radioiodine scintigraphy, ultrasonography, and FDG PET/CT in the follow-up of differentiated thyroid cancer. Anterior and posterior planar images of the radioiodine scintigraphy (*A*), ultrasonography (*B*), anterior maximum intensity projection (*C*), axial CT, and fused PET/CT (*D*) images of a 37-year-old man with papillary thyroid cancer, after thyroidectomy and radioiodine ablation. At follow-up, his radioiodine scintigraphy was negative; however, his serum thyroglobulin was 24 ng/mL, and he had palpable cervical nodes on clinical examination. Ultrasonography and FDG PET/CT performed for evaluation showed bilateral cervical lymphadenopathy (*arrows*) and metabolically active recurrent disease (*arrows*) in the thyroid bed with nodal metastases.

lymph nodes. Calcifications can be punctate, linear, eggshell, amorphous, and nodular. Although these calcifications are observed both in benign and malignant lesions, fine, punctate calcifications are more often encountered in malignant lesions.

Cross-sectional imaging with CT or MRI provides valuable information regarding tumor extent and lymph node metastases, which has an impact on surgical planning. CT has good diagnostic accuracies in diagnosing cervical lymph node metastases, especially for deep nodal stations. In MRI, lesions with a high thyroglobulin concentration show high signal intensities in T1W and T2W images, whereas cystic lesions show low signal intensity. Hemorrhagic necrosis, often accompanied with a high signal intensity pattern on T1W images, is commonly associated with malignant lesions.

Most commonly, thyroid carcinomas metastasize to lymph nodes in the paratracheal and supraclavicular area (levels IV and V) and inferior and midjugular vein lymph nodes (levels III and II). Less commonly, thyroid carcinoma may metastasize to the upper neck lymph nodes (level II), parapharyngeal, and retropharyngeal spaces and should be actively evaluated in patients with suspected thyroid cancer by cross-sectional imaging. Metastatic nodes may show enhancement secondary to hypervascularity, show increased signal intensity on T1W images, and have punctate calcifications.[19]

Incidental focal thyroid uptake on PET has a high risk of malignancy and should be evaluated appropriately[26] with ultrasonography. However, the role of FDG PET/CT in the pretherapy staging is limited in differentiated thyroid cancers, because whole body iodine study is more sensitive.[56] FDG PET/CT can identify local or distant metastases not identified by radioiodine imaging. In anaplastic thyroid carcinoma, FDG PET can identify primary and metastatic disease at staging.

Radioactive isotopes of iodide are used to identify remnant thyroid tissue, either at the primary site or locoregional/distant metastases, and help guide the selection of therapeutic I^{131} dose, because functioning thyroid tissue concentrates radioiodine. I^{123} approaches the ideal thyroid imaging agent, because of its short half-life and limited particulate emissions.[57]

POSTTHERAPY ASSESSMENT

Additional imaging after completion of treatment (surgery, radiation, or chemotherapy or combination) is used to assess the efficacy of therapy chosen, whereas follow-up/surveillance imaging is primarily used to evaluate for tumor recurrence or metastasis. After surgery, there is considerable distortion of the normal anatomic architecture, more evident in head and neck malignancy, because of the complex anatomy and small imaging field of view. This observation is true with radiation therapy as well, which has considerable subsequent inflammation, which can last from several weeks to several years. In regards to imaging, anatomic distortion and posttherapy inflammation obscure the traditional prestaging image findings and can often lead to unwanted false-positive results.

Suprahyoid Malignancy

PET/CT is emerging as the modality of choice in posttherapy assessment, especially when chemoradiation therapy is used. However, the diagnostic potential of PET/CT is particularly evident in disease recurrence with higher specificity and overall diagnostic accuracy compared with CT.[58,59] PET is thus commonly used for restaging, because it has been shown to change management in up to 35% of patients.[60–62] PET is better than CT or MRI for detection of cervical nodal metastasis.[22,23] MRI is accurate in delineating marrow involvement, skull base extension, and perineural spread. However, both PET/CT and MRI can be false-positive, and thus, a biopsy is mandatory, in most cases, when PET/CT or MRI results are positive. After radiation, there is increased FDG uptake for several weeks, with most centers recommending 12 weeks imaging-free interval after treatment. Similarly, after chemotherapy, which can show increased uptake in the bone marrow, some investigators recommend a minimum of 2 weeks for posttherapy imaging.[63] At our institution, we recommend an imaging-free interval of 1 week after needle biopsy, 3 weeks after chemotherapy, 6 weeks after surgery, and 3 months after radiation therapy. In addition, a negative PET/CT result has excellent negative predictive value (>90%) and predicts survival advantage compared with patients with a positive PET/CT.[64]

Infrahyoid Malignancy

In the assessment of treatment response and detection of recurrence of infrahyoid malignancies, CT and MRI play a superior role, especially in evaluating the deep spaces of the head and neck, not possible to evaluate using ultrasonography. In thyroid cancer, administration of iodinated contrast for CT imaging may interfere with the treatment planning using radioiodine. MRI has a better application in this context and can detect locoregional metastases seen as hyperintense lesions on T1W imaging.[65] The role of FDG PET/CT in posttherapy assessment depends on histology. In treated patients who have differentiated thyroid cancer with an increased thyroglobulin level but negative radioiodine whole body scan, the diagnostic accuracy of FDG PET/CT increases with the level of serum thyroglobulin. The level of FDG uptake and the number of FDG-avid lesions can provide prognostic information. In patients with Hurthle cell carcinoma and anaplastic thyroid carcinoma, FDG PET is used more frequently, because of the reduced frequency of iodine-avid disease in these tumors. Similarly, FDG PET/CT is used in patients with medullary thyroid carcinoma, especially in those patients with an increased serum calcitonin and carcinoembryonic antigen level.[35,66]

In evaluation of malignancies of the larynx and hypopharynx, FDG PET/CT has an established role in assessment of therapy response, identifying disease recurrence (3–6 months after radiation therapy), and predicting prognosis. A decrease in pretreatment FDG activity after chemoradiation is associated with greater tumor response, survival, and local control.[53] CT imaging has not been warranted in asymptomatic patients, after treatment, but can be used in special situations like endoscopically detected recurrent disease. Focal masses on CT or MRI can help identify recurrent disease in the background of postinflammatory changes. Characteristics such as tumor volume, vocal cord mobility, sclerosis of laryngeal cartilage on CT, and abnormal signal intensity of laryngeal cartilage on MRI have been found to have prognostic value.[16]

SUMMARY

The role of imaging in head and neck malignancy is an integral part of patient management, because stage is often altered and treatment options change based on the image findings. Malignancies of the oropharynx, larynx, and hypopharynx are primarily imaged with CT, because of lower image degradation from breathing and swallowing during examination. Malignancies of the sinonasal, nasopharynx, and salivary gland are primarily imaged with MRI, because of superior delineation of tumor extension. Malignancies of the thyroid are first approached using ultrasonography as an inexpensive first diagnostic modality and potential for sonographic biopsy. PET/CT is used in advanced stage disease ($\geq$T2) for detection of locoregional nodal metastasis and distant metastasis. Posttherapy assessment depends on whether chemoradiation therapy is used and the level of suspicion for risk of recurrence. Generally, PET/CT is the modality of choice for therapy assessment and is performed 12 weeks after completion of chemoradiation. If marrow or skull base involvement or perineural spread is suspected, MRI is particularly useful. There is no clear consensus or guideline for the frequency of imaging in a posttherapy setting. Imaging has the best value when performed in the context of clinical assessment and suspicion rather than routinely.

REFERENCES

1. Jemal A, Siegel R, Xu J, et al. Cancer statistics, 2010. CA Cancer J Clin 2010; 60(5):277–300.
2. American Cancer Society. Cancer facts and figures 2012. Atlanta (GA): American Cancer Society; 2012. Available at: http://www.cancer.org/acs/groups/content/@epidemiologysurveilance/documents/document/acspc-031941.pdf. Accessed December 26, 2012.
3. Das S, Kirsch CF. Imaging of lumps and bumps in the nose: a review of sinonasal tumours. Cancer Imaging 2005;5:167–77.
4. Howlader N, Noone AM, Krapcho M, et al, editors. SEER cancer statistics review, 1975-2009. Bethesda (MD): National Cancer Institute; 2012. Available at: http://www.seer.cancer.gov/csr/1975_2009/.
5. Madani G, Beale TJ, Lund VJ. Imaging of sinonasal tumors. Semin Ultrasound CT MR 2009;30(1):25–38.
6. Maghami E, Kraus DH. Cancer of the nasal cavity and paranasal sinuses. Expert Rev Anticancer Ther 2004;4(3):411–24.
7. Weymuller EA, Gal TJ. Neoplasms of the nasal cavity. In: Cummings CW, Flint PW, Harker LA, editors. Otolaryngology–head and neck surgery. 4th edition. Philadelphia: Elsevier Mosby; 2005. p. 3199–206.
8. Thoeny HC. Imaging of salivary gland tumours. Cancer Imaging 2007;7:52–62.
9. Strick MJ, Kelly C, Soames JV, et al. Malignant tumours of the minor salivary glands–a 20 year review. Br J Plast Surg 2004;57(7):624–31.
10. Friedman ER, Saindane AM. Pitfalls in the staging of cancer of the major salivary gland neoplasms. Neuroimaging Clin N Am 2013;23(1):107–22.
11. Yamashiro I, Souza RP. Imaging diagnosis of nasopharyngeal tumors. Radiol Bras 2007;40(1):45–52.
12. Razek A, King A. MRI and CT of nasopharyngeal carcinoma. AJR Am J Roentgenol 2012;198(1):11–8.
13. Chan JY, Wei WI. Current management strategy of hypopharyngeal carcinoma. Auris Nasus Larynx 2013;40(1):2–6.
14. Yousem DM, Chalian AA. Oral cavity and pharynx. Radiol Clin North Am 1998; 36(5):967–81.
15. Rubin P. Cancer of the head and neck. Hypopharynx and larynx. 1. JAMA 1972; 221(1):68–72.
16. Becker M, Burkhardt K, Dulquerov P, et al. Imaging of the larynx and hypopharynx. Eur J Radiol 2008;66(3):460–79.
17. Bertagna F, Biasiotto G, Orlando E, et al. Role of 18F-fluorodeoxyglucose positron emission tomography/computed tomography in patients affected by differentiated thyroid carcinoma, high thyroglobulin level, and negative 131I scan: review of the literature. Jpn J Radiol 2010;28(9):629–36.
18. Hansen JT. Netter's clinical anatomy. Philadelphia: Saunders Elsevier; 2010.
19. Newman JG, Chalian AA, Shaha AR. Surgical approaches in thyroid cancer: what the radiologist needs to know. Neuroimaging Clin N Am 2008;18(3): 491–504, viii.

20. Buchbender C, Heusner TA, Lauenstein TC, et al. Oncologic PET/MRI, part 1: tumors of the brain, head and neck, chest, abdomen, and pelvis. J Nucl Med 2012;53(6):928–38.

21. Hsu WC, Loevner LA, Karpati R, et al. Accuracy of magnetic resonance imaging in predicting absence of fixation of head and neck cancer to the prevertebral space. Head Neck 2005;27(2):95–100.

22. Kim SY, Roh JL, Kim JS, et al. Utility of FDG PET in patients with squamous cell carcinomas of the oral cavity. Eur J Surg Oncol 2008;34(2):208–15.

23. Ng SH, Yen TC, Chang JT, et al. Prospective study of [18F] fluorodeoxyglucose positron emission tomography and computed tomography and magnetic resonance imaging in oral cavity squamous cell carcinoma with palpably negative neck. J Clin Oncol 2006;24(27):4371–6.

24. Keberle M, Kenn W, Hahn D. Current concepts in imaging of laryngeal and hypopharyngeal cancer. Eur Radiol 2002;12(7):1672–83.

25. Niu LJ, Hao YZ, Zhou CW. Diagnostic value of ultrasonography in thyroid lesions. Zhonghua Er Bi Yan Hou Tou Jing Wai Ke Za Zhi 2006;41(6):415–8 [in Chinese].

26. Treglia G, Bertagna F, Sadeghi R, et al. Focal thyroid incidental uptake detected by 18F-fluorodeoxyglucose positron emission tomography. Meta-analysis on prevalence and malignancy risk. Nuklearmedizin 2013;52(4):130–6.

27. Pryma DA, Schoder H, Gonen M, et al. Diagnostic accuracy and prognostic value of 18F-FDG PET in Hurthle cell thyroid cancer patients. J Nucl Med 2006;47(8):1260–6.

28. Treglia G, Muoio B, Giovanella L, et al. The role of positron emission tomography and positron emission tomography/computed tomography in thyroid tumours: an overview. Eur Arch Otorhinolaryngol 2013;270(6):1783–7.

29. Eisen MD, Yousem DM, Loevner LA, et al. Preoperative imaging to predict orbital invasion by tumor. Head Neck 2000;22:456–62.

30. Broski SM, Hunt CH, Johnson GB, et al. The added value of 18F-FDG PET/CT for evaluation of patients with esthesioneuroblastoma. J Nucl Med 2012;53(8): 1200–6. http://dx.doi.org/10.2967/jnumed.112.102897.

31. Loevner LA, Sonners AI. Imaging of neoplasms of the paranasal sinuses. Magn Reson Imaging Clin N Am 2002;10:467–93.

32. Loevner LA, Sonners AI. Imaging of neoplasms of the paranasal sinuses. Neuroimaging Clin N Am 2004;14(4):625–46.

33. Loevner LA, Sonners AI, Schulman BJ, et al. Reinterpretation of cross-sectional images in patients with head and neck cancer in the setting of a multidisciplinary cancer center. AJNR Am J Neuroradiol 2002;23(10):1622–6.

34. Paidpally V, Chirindel A, Chung CH, et al. FDG Volumetric Parameters and Survival Outcomes After Definitive Chemoradiotherapy in Patients With Recurrent Head and Neck Squamous Cell Carcinoma. AJR Am J Roentgenol 2014; 203(2):W139–45.

35. Subramaniam RM, Agarwal A, Colucci A, et al. Impact of concurrent diagnostic level CT with PET/CT on the utilization of stand-alone CT and MRI in the management of head and neck cancer patients. Clin Nucl Med 2013;38(10):790–4.

36. Subramaniam RM, Truong M, Peller P, et al. Fluorodeoxyglucose-positron-emission tomography imaging of head and neck squamous cell cancer. AJNR Am J Neuroradiol 2010;31(4):598–604.

37. Bialek EJ, Jakubowski W, Zajkowski P, et al. US of the major salivary glands: anatomy and spatial relationships, pathologic conditions, and pitfalls. Radiographics 2006;26(3):745–63.

38. Ettl T, Schwarz-Furlan S, Gosau M, et al. Salivary gland carcinomas. Oral Maxillofac Surg 2012;16(3):267–83.

39. Lee YY, Wong KT, King AD, et al. Imaging of salivary gland tumours. Eur J Radiol 2008;66(3):419–36.

40. Hadiprodjo D, Ryan T, Truong MT, et al. Parotid gland tumors: preliminary data for the value of FDG PET/CT diagnostic parameters. AJR Am J Roentgenol 2012;198(2):W185–90.

41. Tahari AK, Alluri KC, Quon H, et al. FDG PET/CT imaging of oropharyngeal squamous cell carcinoma: characteristics of human papillomavirus-positive and -negative tumors. Clin Nucl Med 2014;39(3):225–31.

42. Stuckensen T, Kovacs AF, Adams S, et al. Staging of the neck in patients with oral cavity squamous cell carcinomas: a prospective comparison of PET, ultrasound, CT and MRI. J Craniomaxillofac Surg 2000;28(6):319–24.

43. Van den Brekel MW, Castelijns JA, Stel HV, et al. Modern imaging techniques and ultrasound-guided aspiration cytology for the assessment of neck node metastases: a prospective comparative study. Eur Arch Otorhinolaryngol 1993; 250(1):11–7.

44. Huntley TA, Busmanis I, Desmond P, et al. Mandibular invasion by squamous cell carcinoma: a computed tomographic and histological study. Br J Oral Maxillofac Surg 1996;34(1):69–74.

45. Babin E, Desmonts C, Hamon M, et al. PET/CT for assessing mandibular invasion by intraoral squamous cell carcinomas. Clin Otolaryngol 2008;33(1): 47–51.

46. Bolzoni A, Cappiello J, Piazza C, et al. Diagnostic accuracy of magnetic resonance imaging in the assessment of mandibular involvement in oral-oropharyngeal squamous cell carcinoma: a prospective study. Arch Otolaryngol Head Neck Surg 2004;130(7):837–43.

47. Vidiri A, Guerrisi A, Pellini R, et al. Multi-detector row computed tomography (MDCT) and magnetic resonance imaging (MRI) in the evaluation of the mandibular invasion by squamous cell carcinomas (SCC) of the oral cavity. Correlation with pathological data. J Exp Clin Cancer Res 2010;29:73.

48. Lam P, Au-Yeung KM, Cheng PW, et al. Correlating MRI and histologic tumor thickness in the assessment of oral tongue cancer. AJR Am J Roentgenol 2004;182(3):803–8.

49. Miller FR, Karnad AB, Eng T, et al. Management of the unknown primary carcinoma: long-term follow-up on a negative PET scan and negative panendoscopy. Head Neck 2008;30(1):28–34.

50. Minn H, Paul R, Ahonen A. Evaluation of treatment response to radiotherapy in head and neck cancer with fluorine-18 fluorodeoxyglucose. J Nucl Med 1988; 29(9):1521–5.

51. Hermans R. Staging of laryngeal and hypopharyngeal cancer: value of imaging studies. Eur Radiol 2006;16(11):2386–400.

52. Rumboldt Z, Gordon L, Gordon L, et al. Imaging in head and neck cancer. Curr Treat Options Oncol 2006;7(1):23–34.

53. Joshi VM, Wadhwa V, Mukherji SK, et al. Imaging in laryngeal cancers. Indian J Radiol Imaging 2012;22(3):209–26.

54. Park GC, Kim JS, Roh JL, et al. Prognostic value of metabolic tumor volume measured by 18F-FDG PET/CT in advanced-stage squamous cell carcinoma of the larynx and hypopharynx. Ann Oncol 2013;24(1):208–14.

55. Hopkins CR, Reading CC. Thyroid and parathyroid imaging. Semin Ultrasound CT MR 1995;16(4):279–95.

56. Marcus C, Whitworth PW, Surasi DS, et al. PET/CT in the management of thyroid cancers. AJR Am J Roentgenol 2014;202(6):1316–29.
57. Intenzo CM, Dam HQ, Manzone TA, et al. Imaging of the thyroid in benign and malignant disease. Semin Nucl Med 2012;42(1):49–61.
58. Abgral R, Querellou S, Potard G, et al. Does 18F-FDG PET/CT improve the detection of posttreatment recurrence of head and neck squamous cell carcinoma in patients negative for disease on clinical follow-up? J Nucl Med 2009; 50(1):24–9.
59. Giorgetti A, Volterrani D, Mariani G. Clinical oncological applications of positron emission tomography (PET) using fluorine-18-fluoro-2-deoxy-D-glucose. Radiol Med 2002;103(4):293–318.
60. Fleming AJ Jr, Smith SP Jr, Paul CM, et al. Impact of [18F]-2-fluorodeoxyglucose-positron emission tomography/computed tomography on previously untreated head and neck cancer patients. Laryngoscope 2007;117(7):1173–9.
61. Lamarre ED, Scharpf J, Batra PS, et al. Role of 18F-FDG PET in management of sinonasal neoplasms. Otolaryngol Head Neck Surg 2008;139(Suppl 2):P44.
62. Otsuka H, Graham MM, Kogame M, et al. The impact of FDG-PET in the management of patients with salivary gland malignancy. Ann Nucl Med 2005; 19(8):691–4.
63. Goerres GW, von Schulthess GK, Hany TF. Positron emission tomography and PET CT of the head and neck: FDG uptake in normal anatomy, in benign lesions, and in changes resulting from treatment. AJR Am J Roentgenol 2002;179: 1337–43.
64. Paidpally V, Tahari AK, Lam S, et al. Addition of 18F-FDG PET/CT to clinical assessment predicts overall survival in HNSCC: a retrospective analysis with follow-up for 12 years. J Nucl Med 2013;54(12):2039–45.
65. Loevner LA, Kaplan SL, Cunnane ME, et al. Cross-sectional imaging of the thyroid gland. Neuroimaging Clin N Am 2008;18(3):445–61, vii.
66. Palaniswamy SS, Subramanyam P. Diagnostic utility of PETCT in thyroid malignancies: an update. Ann Nucl Med 2013;27(8):681–93.

Imaging of Thoracic Cavity Tumors

Sara A. Hayes, MD, Andrew J. Plodkowski, MD, Michelle S. Ginsberg, MD*

KEYWORDS

- Computed tomography (CT)
- Fluorine-18–fluorodeoxyglucose positron emission tomography (^{18}F-FDG PET/CT)
- Magnetic resonance imaging (MRI) • Lung cancer • Mediastinal mass
- Pleural tumor

KEY POINTS

- Computed tomography (CT) is the primary imaging modality used in the diagnosis, staging, and follow-up of most thoracic cavity tumors.
- Fluorine-18–fluorodeoxyglucose positron emission tomography (^{18}F-FDG PET)/CT has established itself as a supplementary tool to CT in lung cancer staging and in the assessment for distant metastases of many thoracic tumors.
- Magnetic resonance imaging is an important adjunctive imaging modality in thoracic oncologic imaging and is used as a problem-solving tool to assess for chest wall invasion, intraspinal extension, and cardiac/vascular invasion.

INTRODUCTION

Thoracic tumors, of which lung cancer is the most common, are an important global health issue. Lung cancer is the most common cancer worldwide, with an estimated 1.8 million cases diagnosed in 2012, of which more than half (58%) were in the developing world.[1] Globally, lung cancer is the most common cause of death from cancer, accounting for almost 1 in 5 cancer deaths (1.59 million deaths, 19.4% of total). Although the 1-year relative survival for this malignancy has increased from 37% in 1975 to 1979 to 44% in 2005 to 2008, the overall 5-year survival rate for all stages of lung cancer remains low at 16%.[1] Worldwide, lung cancer rates have peaked for men; but rates for women continue to increase and are closely linked to smoking rates.[2]

Funding: None.
Disclosures: None.
Department of Radiology, Memorial Sloan Kettering Cancer Center, 1275 York Avenue, New York, NY 10065, USA
* Corresponding author.
E-mail address: ginsberm@mskcc.org

Primary mediastinal neoplasms, with the exception of lymphoma, are rare tumors that can arise from any cell precursor. Because of their low incidence and heterogeneity, diagnosis can be difficult. Staging and treatment pathways are often not well defined.[3] This point is particularly true for thymic epithelial tumors, the most common tumor of the anterior mediastinum.[4–6]

Tumors involving the pleura are largely caused by metastatic disease, whereas only 10% are considered true primary pleural tumors.[7] The most common primary neoplasms include fibrous tumor of the pleura and malignant pleural mesothelioma. These disease processes can manifest as pleural effusion, pleural thickening, or mass, which can be detected on computed tomography (CT) or magnetic resonance imaging (MRI). In particular, the incidence of malignant pleural mesothelioma (MPM) is increasing worldwide and is expected to peak in industrialized countries in 2010 to 2020.[8]

LUNG CANCER
Diagnosis

Many advances have been made in recent decades in the imaging of lung cancer and molecular diagnostics; however, most new patients with lung cancer still have advanced stage disease at the time of presentation. The 5-year survival rate for localized disease is 53%; but only 15% of lung cancers are diagnosed at this early, potentially resectable stage. New targeted treatments of lung cancer have failed to achieve a significant reduction in mortality; therefore, early diagnosis will remain a crucial aim in the battle against this disease.

Histologic subtypes

Non–small cell lung cancer (NSCLC) represents 85% of cases, and small cell lung cancer (SCLC) accounts for approximately 15%. Adenocarcinoma is the most prevalent subtype of lung cancer in the United States, having replaced squamous cell carcinoma as the most common cell type in recent years.[2,9] The typical appearance of adenocarcinoma of the lung is that of a solitary pulmonary nodule or mass, often peripheral (**Fig. 1**). Peripheral adenocarcinomas can invade the pleura and grow in a

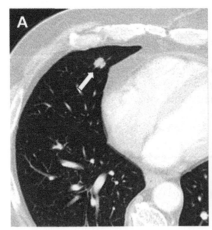
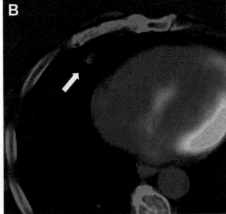

Fig. 1. A 74-year-old male former smoker. Incidental finding of 1.3-cm right middle lobe nodule on CT (A, axial CT [arrow]). Fluorine-18–fluorodeoxyglucose positron emission tomography (^{18}F-FDG PET)/CT showed mild FDG uptake with the nodule (B, axial fused PET/CT [arrow]). Pathology demonstrated adenocarcinoma with lymphovascular invasion.

circumferential manner around the lung, sometimes mimicking a malignant mesothelioma.[10]

In 2011, The International Association for the Study of Lung Cancer (IASLC), the American Thoracic Society, and the European Respiratory Society published new guidelines for the classification of lung adenocarcinoma, which placed an increased emphasis on imaging characteristics.[11] The terms *bronchioloalveolar cell carcinoma* and *mixed subtype adenocarcinoma* were eliminated. They introduced the pathologic subtypes of adenocarcinoma in situ (AIS) and minimally invasive adenocarcinoma (MIA) to define a subset of patients who would have close to 100% disease-specific survival rates following a complete resection. AIS refers to small adenocarcinomas with purely lepidic growth. If an invasive component of 5 mm or less is present, the term *MIA* is applied. Both typically appear as ground-glass nodules on CT (**Fig. 2**) with the presence of a solid component raising suspicion for invasion. In 2013, the Fleischner Society published recommendations for the follow-up of subsolid pulmonary nodules, taking into account the often-indolent growth of subsolid adenocarcinomas and the risk of an invasive component.[12]

Squamous cell carcinoma is now the second most common histologic subtype and accounts for 24% of cases. Squamous cell carcinoma is strongly associated with smoking. Approximately two-thirds of these tumors are centrally located,[10] and they often have associated postobstructive atelectasis or pneumonia. The remaining third are peripheral and can rarely be distinguished from adenocarcinoma based on imaging alone, although squamous cell carcinomas are more likely to be cavitary lesions (**Fig. 3**). Large cell carcinoma is an uncommon histologic subtype of NSCLC, accounting for less than 3% of all cases,[9] and commonly presents as a large peripheral mass.

The incidence of SCLC has been decreasing for many years, currently representing approximately 15% of all lung cancer cases in the United States.[9] Like squamous cell carcinoma, SCLC usually arises centrally, often a large lobulated mass at time of diagnosis, with frequent mediastinal and hilar invasion (**Fig. 4**). Distant metastases are common at presentation.

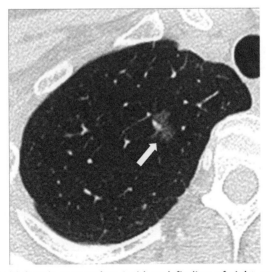

Fig. 2. A 67-year-old female nonsmoker. Incidental finding of right apical ground-glass nodule on CT chest (axial CT, *arrow*). Pathology demonstrated a 1.2-cm minimally invasive adenocarcinoma with lepidic and acinar pattern.

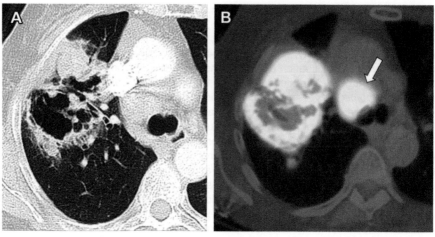

Fig. 3. A 75-year-old female smoker with nonproductive cough. Large, irregular, cavitating mass in the right upper lobe on CT chest (*A*, axial CT). Fluorine-18–fluorodeoxyglucosepositron emission tomography (^{18}F-FDG PET)/CT (*B*, axial fused PET/CT) demonstrated FDG avidity within the lesion and in mediastinal nodal metastases (*arrow*). Pathology confirmed squamous cell carcinoma.

Screening

An effective screening test for the detection of early lung cancer has been a goal of cancer researchers for several decades. Early randomized screening trials using chest radiography raised concerns about the rate of false-positive results and were inconclusive in demonstrating a mortality benefit from screening.[13,14] On November 5, 2010, the results of the National Lung Screening Trial (NLST) were published, which was the first trial to show that screening could decrease lung cancer mortality.[15] Their

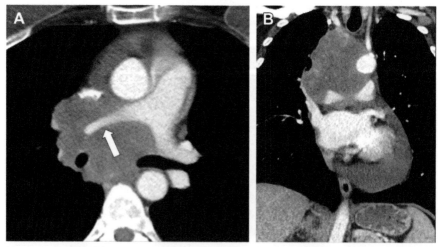

Fig. 4. A 54-year-old woman with shortness of breath and chest discomfort. Contrast-enhanced CT chest (*A*, axial CT) (*B*, coronal CT) demonstrated a mediastinal mass and confluent mediastinal adenopathy, narrowing the right pulmonary artery (*arrow*). Pathology demonstrated small cell carcinoma.

results demonstrated a significant reduction in the mortality rate from lung cancer (20%) in patients who were screened annually with low-dose CT (LDCT). They also found a 6.7% reduction in mortality from any cause.

In July 2013, the US Preventative Services Task Force published new guidelines for lung cancer screening, concluding that there was now strong evidence that LDCT screening can reduce lung cancer and all-cause mortality.[16,17] Their new guidelines recommend annual screening with LDCT in adults aged 55 to 80 years who have a 30 pack-year smoking history and currently smoke or have quit within the previous 15 years.

LDCT chest for lung cancer screening is performed without intravenous contrast. The low-dose technique results in increased image noise[17]; but newer reconstruction algorithms are now available for CT, which can improve the image quality of low-dose studies, including adaptive statistical image reconstruction, iterative reconstruction in image space, and the newer model-based iterative reconstruction (MBIR) techniques.[18–20] The use of MBIR in particular could potentially allow diagnostic quality scans to be performed at even lower doses than are currently being used for screening,[20] but this will require validation with larger studies in the future.

Evaluation of pulmonary nodules

Despite the high spatial and contrast resolution offered by CT, pulmonary nodules are still often missed, for reasons including small size, subsolid composition, location adjacent to vessels, and adjacent parenchymal disease.[21–24] Computer-aided detection (CAD) is increasingly recognized as a method for increasing the detection of small pulmonary nodules on CT and has been shown to have good sensitivity in the detection of small lung tumors, including those missed on the initial read by a radiologist.[25–27] However, most lung CAD systems are optimized for the detection of solid, spherical nodules; the sensitivity of these systems for the detection of subsolid nodules remains poor.[26,28,29]

Although lung CAD can improve the detection of pulmonary nodules on CT, there remains a need to develop more robust strategies to help differentiate benign and malignant pulmonary nodules, as most small pulmonary nodules are benign. The current follow-up guidelines for solid nodules, as recommended by the Fleischner Society, are based solely on size criteria (**Table 1**).[30] The high false-positive rate of screening CT

Table 1		
Fleischner guidelines for follow-up and management of incidentally detected pulmonary nodules less than 8 mm		
Nodule Size (mm)	**Low-Risk Patients**	**High-Risk Patients**
≤4	No follow-up needed	CT at 12 mo; if unchanged, no further follow-up
>4–6	CT at 12 mo; if unchanged, no further follow-up	Initial follow-up CT at 6–12 mo, then at 18–24 mo if no change
>6–8	Initial follow-up CT at 6–12 mo, then at 18–24 mo if no change	Initial follow-up CT at 3–6 mo, then at 9–12 and 24 mo if no change
>8	Follow-up CT at around 3, 9, and 24 mo; dynamic contrast-enhanced CT, PET, +/− biopsy	Same as for low-risk patients

Abbreviation: PET, positron emission tomography.

Adapted from MacMahon H, Austin JH, Gamsu G, et al. Guidelines for management of small pulmonary nodules detected on CT scans: a statement from the Fleischner Society. Radiology 2005;237(2):398.

chests remains a concern, as it often leads to unnecessary further imaging studies, biopsies, or surgery. In the NLST trial, only 3.6% of the positive CT studies for pulmonary nodules were subsequently proven to represent lung cancer.[15]

Fluorine-18–fluorodeoxyglucose positron emission tomography (^{18}F-FDG PET)/CT is an important tool in the assessment of pulmonary nodules but should not be relied on when the nodule size is less than 8 mm. Overall, the lack of FDG uptake in a pulmonary nodule on ^{18}F-FDG PET/CT predicts a less than 5% chance of malignancy.[31–33] The degree of FDG uptake within a malignant nodule may also have implications for prognosis.[34]

MRI in lung cancer diagnosis

MRI, because of its lower inherent spatial resolution, is not usually used in the evaluation of pulmonary nodules. Studies have suggested that, although the sensitivity of MRI in nodule detection is lower than that of CT, it is more sensitive in detecting malignant than benign nodules[35]; MRI diffusion-weighted imaging may be of use in differentiating benign from malignant lesions.[36]

Tissue diagnosis

Percutaneous CT-guided biopsy is the most commonly used method for obtaining a sample for tissue diagnosis of a lung mass. The diagnosis yield for a percutaneous needle biopsy is 36% to 84%, depending on factors such as the size of the lesion, technique used, and lesion location. The sensitivity of a CT-guided biopsy is 94%, with a specificity of 99%.[37] Flexible bronchoscopy with transbronchial needle aspiration is an alternative method for obtaining a biopsy specimen but is best suited for lesions in a central location or those with endobronchial extension. Navigational bronchoscopy uses standard CT images to create a virtual 3-dimensional (3D) bronchoscopy, which can assist in locating lesions in the lung periphery during flexible bronchoscopy.

Staging

Accurate staging in lung cancer is vital for determining appropriate clinical management. Imaging studies play a key role. The seventh edition of the TNM staging handbook, published in 2009, made substantial changes to the staging of NSCLC.[38] The IASLC proposed a new lymph node map in 2009 (Fig. 5), which grouped lymph node stations into zones.[39] The now ubiquitous use of multidetector CT for the staging of lung cancer has been supplemented in the past 2 decades by ^{18}F-FDG PET/CT, and it is well recognized that the use of newer imaging modalities can supplement CT findings (Table 2) and has resulted in clinically relevant stage migration for patients.

The current guidelines of the National Comprehensive Cancer Network for staging of both NSCLC and SCLC recommend a CT scan (preferably contrast enhanced) of the chest and upper abdomen for initial staging.[40,41] An integrated ^{18}F-FDG PET/CT scan is recommended for all patients with NSCLC and for suspected limited stage patients with SCLC to assess for nodal and distant metastases. Integrated ^{18}F-FDG PET/CT has been found to be more accurate for staging NSCLC than ^{18}F-FDG PET alone, CT alone, or in comparison with separate PET and CT studies.[42] The positive predictive value of ^{18}F-FDG PET/CT for nodal metastases is better than that of CT (80%–90% compared with approximately 50%).

When the ^{18}F-FDG PET/CT findings suggest nodal metastases in NSCLC, pathologic confirmation is recommended by mediastinoscopy, mediastinotomy, endobronchial ultrasound (US), or CT-guided biopsy. In patients with NSCLC who are clinically T1N0, the absence of nodal uptake on ^{18}F-FDG PET obviates histologic correlation with invasive mediastinal node sampling.[40]

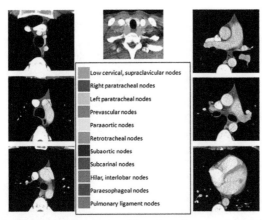

Low cervical, supraclavicular nodes
Right paratracheal nodes
Left paratracheal nodes
Prevascular nodes
Paraaortic nodes
Retrotracheal nodes
Subaortic nodes
Subcarinal nodes
Hilar, interlobar nodes
Paraesophageal nodes
Pulmonary ligament nodes

Fig. 5. Summary of IASLC's new international lymph node maps. (*Data from* Rusch VW, Asamura H, Watanabe H, et al. The IASLC lung cancer staging project: a proposal for a new international lymph node map in the forthcoming seventh edition of the TNM classification for lung cancer. J Thorac Oncol 2009;4(5):568–77.)

CT has some limitations in the staging of lung cancer, particularly in assessing for chest wall or mediastinal invasion. The role of MRI in staging of lung cancer is small, but it can be used to assess for vascular or cardiac invasion or invasion of vertebral bodies in suspected T4 tumors. MRI of the brachial plexus is occasionally useful when staging Pancoast tumors (**Fig. 6**). Potential future uses for MRI in lung cancer staging include the use of diffusion-weighted imaging to assess for nodal metastases, which several studies have suggested is superior to ^{18}F-FDG PET/CT in nodal staging.[43–47] MRI is the preferred imaging modality to assess for brain metastases.

Treatment

Despite many recent advances in treatment of primary lung cancer, surgery remains the current standard of treatment of early stage disease. Recently, nonsurgical treatments, including stereotactic body radiation (SBRT) for stage I NSCLC have become more commonly used, particularly in patients who are poor candidates for surgery. In SBRT, several fractions of very-high-dose radiation therapy are administered to small lung tumors, which must be remote from the central mediastinal vessels, esophagus, and main bronchi. The use of SBRT requires careful pretreatment planning with respiratory-correlated CT scans and image guidance of radiation delivery. Accelerated or hyperfractionated radiotherapy regimes have also been proven to confer a

Table 2		
The use of different imaging modalities in lung cancer staging		
Modality	**Uses**	
CT	Preferred modality for assessing tumor size, location of tumor, proximity to other structures, and presence of pulmonary metastasis	
^{18}F-FDG PET/CT	Mediastinal nodal staging Evaluation for distant metastases	
MRI	Assessment of superior sulcus tumors for brachial plexus and subclavian vessel invasion Assessment of vertebral body invasion Evaluation for brain metastases	

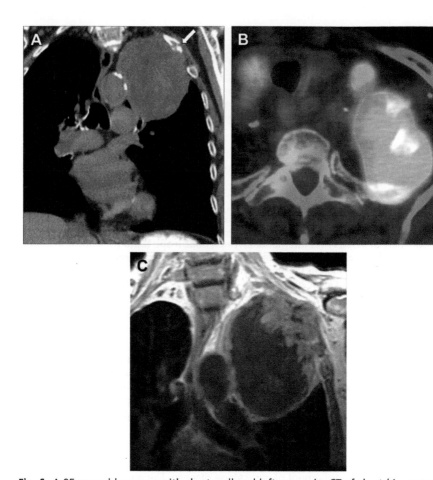

Fig. 6. A 95-year-old woman with chest wall and left arm pain. CT of chest (*A*, coronal CT) revealed a large left upper lobe Pancoast tumor, with pathologic fracture of an adjacent rib (*arrow*). ^{18}F-FDG PET/CT (*B*, axial fused PET/CT) demonstrated FDG avidity within the lesion. MRI of brachial plexus (*C*; coronal T1-weighted, postgadolinium) demonstrated the extent of chest wall invasion with involvement of the inferior left brachial plexus. Pathology was consistent with poorly differentiated non–small cell carcinoma.

survival advantage over conventional radiotherapy regimes in patients with locally advanced lung cancers.[48,49] ^{18}F-FDG PET/CT is an important modality in the pretreatment evaluation of radiotherapy; its use can result in smaller subsequent radiation fields, potentially allowing for radiation dose escalation with fewer side effects.[50,51] ^{18}F-FDG PET/CT integration has also been proven to reduce the variability among radiation oncologists in delineation of the primary tumor[52–54] and can facilitate automatic tumor delineation.[55]

Radiofrequency (RF) ablation is an alternative treatment option for early stage tumors in patients who are not suitable candidates for surgery and can also be used in the treatment of lung metastases as well as in the palliative treatment of chest wall masses.[56–58] Pretreatment imaging in RF ablation helps to guide access trajectory and can also influence probe choice and the use of adjunctive imaging modalities, such as US and CT fluoroscopy.

Follow-up

The evaluation of tumor response to nonsurgical therapy has become an important topic in recent years, particularly since the advent of targeted therapies to specific molecular targets in lung cancer. CT has traditionally been the most widely used diagnostic tool in assessing tumor response, but the utility of molecular imaging is becoming increasingly recognized because of its potential to characterize tumor tissue by its biochemical and biological characteristics. Alterations in cellular metabolism usually precede change in tumor size, and the metabolic response on PET has been shown to correlate better with outcome than size response on CT.[59] In addition to monitoring for the response to standard chemotherapy, PET can also be used to assess the response to biological therapies, such as the epidermal growth factor receptor (EGFR) kinase inhibitor erlotinib. Recent studies have shown that ^{18}F-FDG PET/CT can separate metabolic responders from nonresponders as early as 2 weeks following initiation of targeted therapy.[60–62]

Evolving techniques with potential for clinical use include the development of new molecular tracers targeting different aspects of tumor biology, such as ^{18}F-fluorothymidine,[63] and the assessment of EGFR and EGFR tyrosine kinase overexpression in tumors by PET imaging. In vivo a priori determination of the efficacy of EGFR-targeted drug therapy is a promising imaging tool for the future and may ultimately help in the development of individualized treatment plans for patients.[64,65] Posttreatment tumor response has also been investigated using various MRI techniques, such as diffusion-weighted and perfusion imaging and magnetization transfer.

Newer nonsurgical treatment modalities, such as RF ablation and SBRT, have made it essential for the radiologist to be familiar with the expected, treatment-attributable changes in the lung parenchyma on follow-up imaging. Immediately following RF ablation, a region of focal ground-glass change surrounds the lesion on CT. This ground-glass change usually resolves within a month. Occasionally, these lesions cavitate but with a gradual decrease in size of the cavity on subsequent follow-up.[66] On postablation ^{18}F-FDG PET/CT, a rim of FDG-avid inflamed tissue is often seen surrounding the treated lesion. This uptake may persist for several months.[67] However, increasing FDG uptake within the ablated lesion over time is suspicious for local recurrence of tumor rather than posttreatment inflammation.[68]

Radiation-induced lung changes after SBRT differ from those seen following conventional radiotherapy. Changes in CT lung density, particularly masslike consolidation, are common post-SBRT[69,70] and can cause overestimation of tumor recurrence.[71] Distinguishing between radiation-induced changes and local recurrence is of paramount importance. The current practices mainly rely on CT for follow-up, but the adjunct use of ^{18}F-FDG PET/CT is increasingly recognized where local recurrence is suspected, although its use remains controversial.[70,72]

Careful imaging follow-up is required in all patients with lung cancer to detect local recurrences at an earlier stage in the initial years following treatment and to evaluate for the development of a second primary lung tumor in later years. The risk of developing a second primary lung cancer is substantial: approximately 1% to 2% per year following resection of an NSCLC and 6% in patients who have survived SCLC. The risk increases to greater than 10% per patient per year 10 years following the initial treatment of SCLC. Death from a second primary tumor is, thus, common in lung cancer survivors.[40] The current recommendations for follow-up after the treatment of NSCLC recommend a contrast-enhanced CT scan every 4 to 6 months for the first 2 years to optimally evaluate for mediastinal recurrence, followed by a yearly non–contrast-enhanced CT scan to assess for new lesions in the lung parenchyma.[40]

Other Primary Lung Tumors

Bronchopulmonary carcinoid tumors are relatively rare malignant tumors, most indolent in behavior, but with variability depending on tumor grade. All have the potential for invasion and metastases. Approximately 25% present as a central mass, often involving a lobar or segmental bronchus (**Fig. 7**). Peripheral carcinoids are generally well-circumscribed, homogeneous, slow-growing masses. A contrast-enhanced CT scan is essential for the evaluation of a central carcinoid tumor, to assess the relationship with hilar structures, and to identify lymphadenopathy suggesting nodal metastases. The role of ^{18}F-FDG PET/CT is not well established in the imaging of carcinoid tumors and has a wide range of quoted sensitivity (14%–100%). One-third of carcinoid tumors are somatostatin-receptor negative; the remainder exhibits only weak uptake on octreotide scans, so routine use of octreotide scanning is not recommended.

MEDIASTINAL TUMORS
Relevant Anatomy

The mediastinum is demarcated superiorly by the thoracic inlet, inferiorly by the diaphragm, and laterally by the pleural cavities. The mediastinum is classically divided into 3 compartments based on anatomic landmarks: the anterior, middle, and posterior mediastinum. These divisions are not separated by fascial planes and communicate freely with one another.

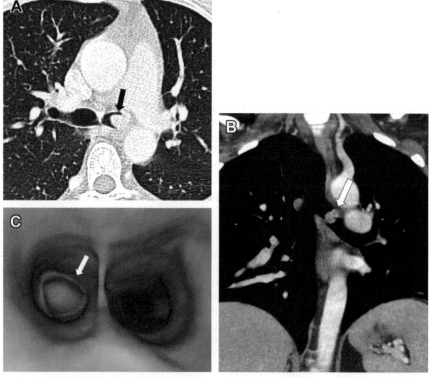

Fig. 7. A 36-year-old woman with wheezing and intermittent stridor. CT revealed an endobronchial mass within the left main bronchus (*arrows*) (*A*, axial CT; *B*, coronal CT; *C*, reconstructed 3D virtual bronchoscopy). Pathology was consistent with an atypical carcinoid tumor.

The anterior mediastinum contains the thymus, lymph nodes, and fat. The middle mediastinum contains the heart, pericardium, great vessels, tracheobronchial tree, and lymph nodes; the posterior mediastinum contains the esophagus, descending thoracic aorta, azygous vein, autonomic ganglia and nerves, lymph nodes, and fat. The location of a mass within the mediastinum is one of the key factors influencing the differential diagnosis. Although at least two-thirds of mediastinal tumors are benign, masses in the anterior compartment are much more likely to be malignant.[73]

Diagnosis

Many mediastinal tumors are detected as incidental findings on chest radiography or CT scan. A posteroanterior and lateral chest radiograph can provide information about the size and location of the mass, but contrast-enhanced CT of the chest offers far superior information about the composition of the lesion and its relationship to surrounding structures. MRI is a valuable imaging tool in the initial assessment of mediastinal masses. It is of particular help when assessing a cystic lesion[74] but can also be used in the evaluation of posterior mediastinal neurogenic tumors[75] and assessing for vertebral body invasion. Where cardiac or vascular involvement is a concern, cardiac MRI can help to assess the degree of invasion.[76,77] Sestamibi is indicated when ectopic parathyroid tissue is suspected.[78] ^{18}F-FDG PET/CT scans are increasingly used as part of the initial evaluation and staging of mediastinal tumors.

Tissue diagnosis will almost always be required as part of the work-up of a mediastinal mass. If the mass is likely to be benign, surgical resection can proceed without biopsy. If the cause is unclear, a diagnostic biopsy specimen can be obtained by CT-guided percutaneous biopsy or by transbronchial biopsy, which has the added advantage of allowing endobronchial US evaluation of the mass. Fine-needle aspirate biopsy has been shown to be 78% accurate in the diagnosis of mediastinal masses[79] but has limitations, particularly in differentiating thymoma and lymphoma. Core biopsy specimens have greater diagnostic sensitivity and specificity compared with fine-needle aspirate specimens. In some cases, biopsy specimens can also be obtained through open surgical biopsy; with varying techniques depending on location of the mass.

Pretreatment Evaluation

CT is the most frequently used imaging modality in the staging of mediastinal tumors. The heterogeneity of these tumors, and the rarity of most, means that staging systems are usually not well defined. Two-thirds of mediastinal tumors are benign; for many lesions, such as bronchogenic and enteric duplication cysts, regional imaging of the chest with contrast-enhanced CT and/or MRI and ^{18}F-FDG PET/CT is sufficient. Malignant lesions generally require further work-up to evaluate the local extent of disease and to assess for distant disease/metastases.

Thymic Tumors

Thymomas are one of the most common mediastinal tumors, accounting for 20% of masses in the anterior mediastinum.[4,6] The typical CT appearance of thymoma is that of a smooth round or ovoid mass in the anterior mediastinum (**Fig. 8**), although they can appear lobulated and locally invasive, with vascular encasement. The system most commonly used in the staging of thymomas is the Masaoka system, which is based on intraoperative and histologic findings.[80] CT is the modality of choice in preoperative imaging of thymoma; the size and shape of the tumor on CT, as well as its relationship to adjacent structures, have been shown to correlate with invasiveness and a higher Masaoka stage.[81] Thymic carcinomas are more aggressive than thymomas and are often heterogeneous on CT, with areas of necrosis and calcification.

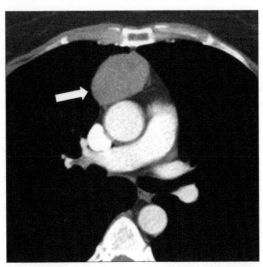

Fig. 8. A 52-year-old woman with dizziness and fatigue. CT demonstrated an anterior mediastinal mass (axial CT, *arrow*). Pathology confirmed a World Health Organization type AB thymoma, Masaoka stage 1.

In selected cases, MRI has a role in the evaluation of anterior mediastinal masses and thymic lesions, mainly in the differentiation of a thymic cyst or thymic hyperplasia from a thymic epithelial tumor. The improved contrast resolution of MRI as compared with CT can aid in distinguishing between a congenital cyst in the anterior mediastinum or a cystic thymic epithelial tumor, by delineating internal solid components. It has also been suggested that chemical shift imaging in MRI can be used to distinguish between thymic hyperplasia and true thymic tumors because of the presence of intralesional fat in hyperplasia.[82] MRI findings in thymic epithelial tumors are nonspecific,[82] and MRI as a modality in these patients is mostly reserved to evaluate the mediastinal vessels or for use in cases when a contrast-enhanced CT cannot be obtained because of a contrast allergy.

FDG uptake in thymic epithelial tumors is variable on PET imaging, and nuclear medicine in general does not currently play an important role in the evaluation of thymoma and other anterior mediastinal masses. FDG uptake has not yet proven helpful in differentiating early (stage I or II) from late-stage thymoma (stage III or IV).[83–85]

Lymphoma

Primary mediastinal lymphoma is a rare entity, accounting for only 10% of lymphoma involving mediastinum. It tends to occur in the anterior mediastinum; Hodgkin lymphoma is most common, representing 50% to 70% of mediastinal cases (**Fig. 9**). As most patients with mediastinal lymphoma have systemic disease, further imaging is needed to assess for involvement in other sites. The work-up generally involves PET for staging and follow-up, which has been shown to be superior to conventional staging with CT, bone scan, and clinical findings.[86]

Germ Cell Tumors

Primary mediastinal germ cell tumors (GCT) compose 15% of anterior mediastinal masses in adults. Testicular GCT is far more common than primary mediastinal

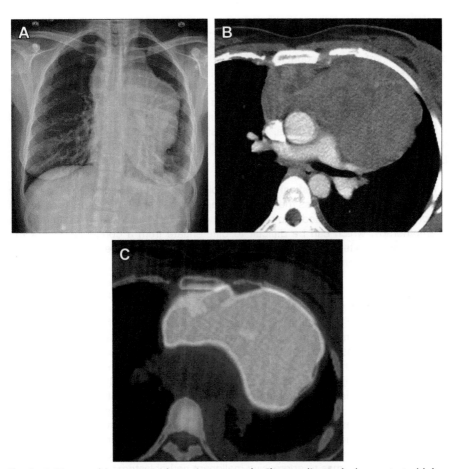

Fig. 9. A 30-year-old woman with persistent cough. Chest radiograph demonstrated lobulated mediastinal widening (A, posteroanterior chest radiograph), and CT chest confirmed a large anterior mediastinal mass (B, axial CT), which was FDG avid on ^{18}F-FDG PET/CT (C, axial fused PET/CT). Pathology was consistent with classic Hodgkin lymphoma, nodular sclerosing type.

GCT. Both gonadal and retroperitoneal GCT can metastasize to the mediastinum; therefore, a biopsy result suggesting mediastinal GCT should prompt a search for an extrathoracic primary. Scrotal US and abdominopelvic CT is recommended in all of these patients. Mediastinal GCTs are divided by cell type into mature teratomas, seminomas, and nonseminomatous GCT. Malignant teratomas are more frequent in men, whereas mature teratomas are equally common in both sexes.[4]

The CT findings of a mature mediastinal teratoma are often characteristic, containing varying amounts of soft tissue, fat, fluid, or calcium; no further work-up is generally needed before surgical resection. Seminomas are usually large, lobulated, homogeneous masses; metastatic disease is common at the time of presentation.[87] Nonseminomatous GCTs are a histologically heterogeneous group of tumors that occur predominantly in men and are usually associated with elevated alpha fetoprotein levels.

Mediastinal Cysts

Mediastinal cysts are true congenital cysts and are most commonly found in the middle mediastinum. They account for 12% to 25% of all mediastinal masses.[88] Bronchogenic cysts are most common (40%–50%), followed by esophageal duplication cysts. The cysts are usually incidental findings on CT or occasionally on chest radiograph and are generally distinguishable from a solid mass from CT findings alone, typically appearing as a round, well-circumscribed, fluid-filled lesion.[74] Occasionally, the wall may contain mural calcifications. Bronchogenic cysts occasionally develop an air-fluid level as a result of infection or communication with the tracheobronchial tree. Endoscopic US is accurate in the diagnosis of mediastinal cysts and can facilitate diagnostic/therapeutic aspiration.[89]

If the fluid within a mediastinal cyst is complex, it may appear solid on CT, in which case MRI is helpful to assess the internal composition. Malignant primary mediastinal tumors can occasionally undergo cystic degeneration, particularly after treatment with chemotherapy, which can be difficult to differentiate from a congenital cyst if the degeneration is extensive.[74] Pericardial cysts are usually diagnosed from CT findings alone and are generally observed if asymptomatic.

Neurogenic Tumors

Neurogenic tumors and esophageal tumors are the most common masses in the posterior mediastinum.[88] Most (70%–80%) are benign, and nearly half are asymptomatic. Nerve sheath tumors are most common and account for 40% to 65% of neurogenic tumors of the mediastinum. Radiographically and on CT, nerve sheath tumors are usually well-defined spherical masses adjacent to the spine. There may be erosion and deformity of the adjacent vertebrae and ribs. Approximately 10% of nerve sheath tumors involve the intervertebral foramina, giving the characteristic dumbbell-shape appearance.[90] MRI is indicated in these cases to rule out intraspinal extension of tumor. Malignant nerve sheath tumors of the posterior mediastinum include malignant neurofibromas, malignant schwannomas, and neurogenic fibrosarcomas.

Masses arising from the autonomic nervous system form a spectrum, ranging from benign ganglioneuromas to aggressive malignant neuroblastomas. CT is the primary imaging modality used to evaluate these mediastinal lesions, again with MRI in certain cases to assess for local invasion or intraspinal extension (**Fig. 10**). Neuroblastoma is a highly aggressive, metastasizing tumor that affects young children. Ninety-five percent of cases occur in patients younger than 5 years. Half of neuroblastomas arise in the adrenal glands; but 30% arise in the mediastinum, typically as an elongated paraspinal mass, which is frequently calcified.[91] In addition to MRI to evaluate for intraspinal involvement, radionuclide imaging with iodine-123 metaiodobenzylguanidine is recommended to detect primary and metastatic disease (**Fig. 11**).

PLEURAL TUMORS
Relevant Anatomy

The pleural space is composed of 2 pleural layers, the parietal and visceral pleura. The parietal pleural covers the ribs, diaphragm, and mediastinum, whereas the visceral pleural invests each lung and interlobar fissures. The 2 layers join at the hila and extend caudad as the inferior pulmonary ligament.

Diagnosis

Although CT is commonly used to evaluate pleural tumors, definitive diagnosis is accomplished by obtaining a tissue sample. There is large overlap in the imaging

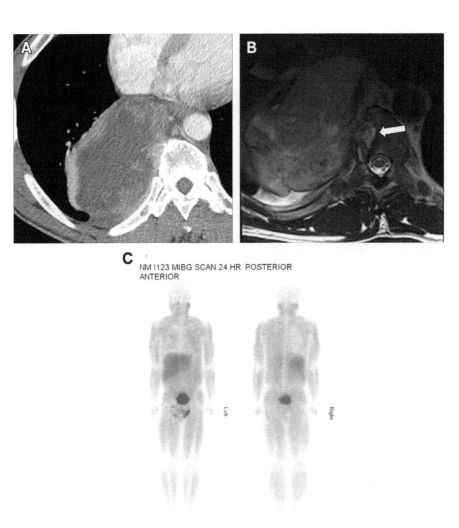

Fig. 10. A 49-year-old man with weight loss. CT chest demonstrated a heterogeneous paraspinal mass adjacent to the right lower lobe (*A*, axial CT). MRI confirmed local invasion into the adjacent T8 vertebral body (*B*, axial T2-weighted MRI [*arrow*]). The mass was non–metaiodobenzylguanidine (MIBG) avid on iodine-123 MIBG scintigraphy (*C*). Pathology demonstrated a composite paraganglioma and ganglioneuroma.

findings of malignant and benign pleural masses. Although some findings, such as circumferential pleural thickening or diffuse pleural nodularity, can suggest malignancy, many malignant tumors present with nonspecific findings, such as a pleural effusion.

CT-guided percutaneous biopsy can aid in the diagnosis of pleural lesions and can be performed with relative safety, with lower complication rates than for CT-guided lung biopsy. However, performing a single core biopsy or fine-needle aspirate can give the physician a false sense of assurance, given the heterogeneity of some tumors. For example, MPM can present as a biphasic tumor, containing both epithelioid and sarcomatoid subtypes. If only one sample is take in the area of the tumor with

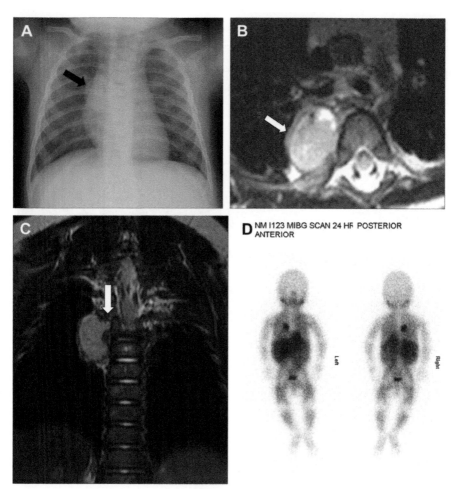

Fig. 11. A 6-month-old boy with incidental finding of right paraspinal mass on chest radiograph (*A*, anteroposterior chest radiograph [*arrow*]). MRI of chest confirmed a right paraspinal mass (*B*, axial T2-weighted MRI [*arrow*]) and demonstrated extension into the adjacent intervertebral foramen (*C*; coronal T1-weighted MRI, postgadolinium [*arrow*]). The mass was metaiodobenzylguanidine (MIBG) avid on iodine-123 MIBG scintigraphy (*D*).

epithelioid cells, the physician can be tricked into a false sense that the tumor is resectable.[92] Adequate sampling with either percutaneous or surgical biopsy is required, especially if MPM is suspected.

Pretreatment Evaluation

Given that the most common cause of a pleural-based mass is metastatic disease, it is imperative to exclude a primary tumor. If the tumor is thought to be primary and possibly a malignant pleural mesothelioma, the patient needs to be properly staged to evaluate for surgical resection. This evaluation includes CT of the chest and abdomen plus ^{18}F-FDG PET/CT scan for detection of distant metastatic disease; however, understaging is common with [18]FDG-PET/CT.[93] MRI with diffusion-weighted imaging has shown the potential to categorize some histologic subtypes of MPM[94] and could be used in the future to guide needle biopsies to more aggressive areas of the tumor.

Malignant Pleural Mesothelioma

MPM is a rare neoplasm but has been increasing in incidence in recent decades, related to an increase in asbestos exposure in industrialized countries.[95] The survival rate remains poor with 4% to 7% at 5 years.[96] The initial evaluation for MPM is primarily by contrast-enhanced CT, which can demonstrate unilateral pleural effusion and nodular pleural thickening in early stage disease. As the disease progresses, nodular pleural thickening can advance to a rindlike appearance (**Fig. 12**). However, the absence of pleural thickening does not exclude a neoplastic diagnosis.[97] Radiologically occult tumor can exist and proper staging requires surgery.

Pretreatment evaluation is needed to determine the resectability of MPM. On a contrast-enhanced CT, tumor characteristics that determine unresectability include multifocal tumor or extension into the chest wall, diaphragm, contralateral pleura, mediastinal organs, spine, myocardium, or internal surface of the pericardium,[98] as evidenced by soft tissue infiltration or obliteration of the surrounding pleural fat planes. CT and MRI both have high sensitivity in determining resectability,[99] but MRI has been demonstrated to be superior to CT with regard to identifying invasion of the diaphragm and endothoracic fascia.[100]

Fibrous Pleural Tumor

Solitary fibrous tumor of the pleura is a rare tumor[101] that includes both benign and malignant variants. CT is the primary imaging method, which often demonstrates a large pleural-based pedunculated mass (**Fig. 13**). CT findings suggestive of malignancy include a diameter larger than 10 cm, central necrosis, and ipsilateral pleural effusion (**Fig. 14**).[102] Recently, Cardillo and colleagues[103] demonstrated that the tumor size does not correlate with prognosis. In addition to CT, ^{18}F-FDG PET/CT can be useful, as increased FDG uptake is associated with an increased likelihood for

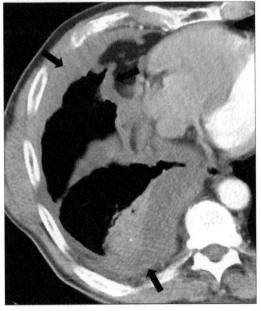

Fig. 12. A 71-year-old man with persistent cough. Contrast-enhanced CT demonstrates right circumferential pleural mass (axial CT, *arrows*). Pathology demonstrated malignant mesothelioma, epithelioid type.

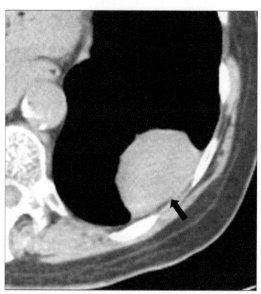

Fig. 13. A 77-year-old woman with incidental mass on routine chest radiograph. Unenhanced CT demonstrates a homogenous pleural-based mass (axial CT, *arrow*). Pathology demonstrated benign solitary fibrous tumor.

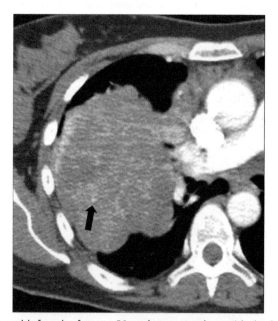

Fig. 14. A 51-year-old female former 30-pack-year smoker with back pain. Contrast-enhanced CT demonstrates a large multi-lobulated heterogeneous pleural-based tumor with internal vascularity (axial CT, *arrow*). Pathology demonstrated malignant solitary fibrous tumor.

malignancy.[104] After resection, 15% of these tumors recur; therefore, imaging follow-up is suggested.[105]

SUMMARY

Thoracic cavity tumors are a disparate group of diseases dominated by the high prevalence and mortality rates of lung cancer. Imaging is central to the diagnosis and staging of thoracic tumors, and CT remains the modality of choice for most diseases. Recent advances in techniques and the increasing tide of lung cancer screening will improve early diagnosis; but more research is needed in many areas, particularly in the imaging characterization of pulmonary nodules. ^{18}F-FDG PET/CT has established itself as an important adjunctive tool in the imaging arsenal for many thoracic tumors. The role of MRI in the evaluation of thoracic tumors remains limited to certain specific situations, but research suggests its scope will continue to expand.

REFERENCES

1. Ferlay J, Soerjomataram I, Ervik M, et al. GLOBOCAN 2012 v1.0, Cancer incidence and mortality worldwide: IARC cancer base No. 11 [Internet]. 2012. Available at: http://globocan.iarc.fr. Accessed January 24, 2014.
2. Devesa SS, Bray F, Vizcaino AP, et al. International lung cancer trends by histologic type: male:female differences diminishing and adenocarcinoma rates rising. Int J Cancer 2005;117(2):294–9.
3. Weissferdt A, Moran CA. Staging of primary mediastinal tumors. Adv Anat Pathol 2013;20(1):1–9.
4. Duwe BV, Sterman DH, Musani AI. Tumors of the mediastinum. Chest 2005; 128(4):2893–909.
5. Gerein AN, Srivastava SP, Burgess J. Thymoma: a ten year review. Am J Surg 1978;136(1):49–53.
6. Mullen B, Richardson JD. Primary anterior mediastinal tumors in children and adults. Ann Thorac Surg 1986;42(3):338–45.
7. Weyant MJ, Flores RM. Imaging of pleural and chest wall tumors. Thorac Surg Clin 2004;14(1):15–23.
8. Pinto C, Ardizzoni A, Betta PG, et al. Expert opinions of the first Italian consensus conference on the management of malignant pleural mesothelioma. Am J Clin Oncol 2011;34(1):99–109.
9. Howlader N, Noone AM, Krapcho M, et al. SEER cancer statistics review, 1975–2010. Based on November 2012 SEER data submission, posted to the SEER Web site. 2013. Available at: http://seer.cancer.gov/csr/1975_2010/. Accessed January 18, 2014.
10. Rosado-de-Christenson ML, Templeton PA, Moran CA. Bronchogenic carcinoma: radiologic-pathologic correlation. Radiographics 1994;14(2):429–46 [quiz: 447–8].
11. Travis WD, Brambilla E, Noguchi M, et al. International Association for the Study of Lung Cancer/American Thoracic Society/European Respiratory Society International multidisciplinary classification of lung adenocarcinoma. J Thorac Oncol 2011;6(2):244–85.
12. Naidich DP, Bankier AA, MacMahon H, et al. Recommendations for the management of subsolid pulmonary nodules detected at CT: a statement from the Fleischner Society. Radiology 2013;266(1):304–17.
13. Marcus PM, Bergstralh EJ, Fagerstrom RM, et al. Lung cancer mortality in the Mayo Lung Project: impact of extended follow-up. J Natl Cancer Inst 2000; 92(16):1308–16.

14. Melamed MR. Lung cancer screening results in the National Cancer Institute New York study. Cancer 2000;89(Suppl 11):2356–62.
15. Aberle DR, Adams AM, Berg CD, et al. Reduced lung-cancer mortality with low-dose computed tomographic screening. N Engl J Med 2011;365(5):395–409.
16. Humphrey LL, Deffebach M, Pappas M, et al. Screening for lung cancer with low-dose computed tomography: a systematic review to update the US Preventive Services Task Force recommendation. Ann Intern Med 2013;159(6):411–20.
17. Donnelly EF. Technical parameters and interpretive issues in screening computed tomography scans for lung cancer. J Thorac Imaging 2012;27(4):224–9.
18. Hu XH, Ding XF, Wu RZ, et al. Radiation dose of non-enhanced chest CT can be reduced 40% by using iterative reconstruction in image space. Clin Radiol 2011;66(11):1023–9.
19. Leipsic J, Nguyen G, Brown J, et al. A prospective evaluation of dose reduction and image quality in chest CT using adaptive statistical iterative reconstruction. AJR Am J Roentgenol 2010;195(5):1095–9.
20. Neroladaki A, Botsikas D, Boudabbous S, et al. Computed tomography of the chest with model-based iterative reconstruction using a radiation exposure similar to chest X-ray examination: preliminary observations. Eur Radiol 2013;23(2):360–6.
21. Gurney JW. Missed lung cancer at CT: imaging findings in nine patients. Radiology 1996;199(1):117–22.
22. Kakinuma R, Ohmatsu H, Kaneko M, et al. Detection failures in spiral CT screening for lung cancer: analysis of CT findings. Radiology 1999;212(1):61–6.
23. Ko JP, Rusinek H, Naidich DP, et al. Wavelet compression of low-dose chest CT data: effect on lung nodule detection. Radiology 2003;228(1):70–5.
24. White CS, Romney BM, Mason AC, et al. Primary carcinoma of the lung overlooked at CT: analysis of findings in 14 patients. Radiology 1996;199(1):109–15.
25. Armato SG 3rd, Li F, Giger ML, et al. Lung cancer: performance of automated lung nodule detection applied to cancers missed in a CT screening program. Radiology 2002;225(3):685–92.
26. Godoy MC, Cooperberg PL, Maizlin ZV, et al. Detection sensitivity of a commercial lung nodule CAD system in a series of pathologically proven lung cancers. J Thorac Imaging 2008;23(1):1–6.
27. Li F, Arimura H, Suzuki K, et al. Computer-aided detection of peripheral lung cancers missed at CT: ROC analyses without and with localization. Radiology 2005;237(2):684–90.
28. Yanagawa M, Honda O, Yoshida S, et al. Commercially available computer-aided detection system for pulmonary nodules on thin-section images using 64 detectors-row CT: preliminary study of 48 cases. Acad Radiol 2009;16(8):924–33.
29. Yuan R, Vos PM, Cooperberg PL. Computer-aided detection in screening CT for pulmonary nodules. AJR Am J Roentgenol 2006;186(5):1280–7.
30. MacMahon H, Austin JH, Gamsu G, et al. Guidelines for management of small pulmonary nodules detected on CT scans: a statement from the Fleischner Society. Radiology 2005;237(2):395–400.
31. Christensen JA, Nathan MA, Mullan BP, et al. Characterization of the solitary pulmonary nodule: 18F-FDG PET versus nodule-enhancement CT. AJR Am J Roentgenol 2006;187(5):1361–7.
32. Gupta NC, Maloof J, Gunel E. Probability of malignancy in solitary pulmonary nodules using fluorine-18-FDG and PET. J Nucl Med 1996;37(6):943–8.

33. Lowe VJ, Fletcher JW, Gobar L, et al. Prospective investigation of positron emission tomography in lung nodules. J Clin Oncol 1998;16(3):1075–84.
34. Erasmus JJ, McAdams HP, Patz EF Jr. Non-small cell lung cancer: FDG-PET imaging. J Thorac Imaging 1999;14(4):247–56.
35. Sommer G, Tremper J, Koenigkam-Santos M, et al. Lung nodule detection in a high-risk population: comparison of magnetic resonance imaging and low-dose computed tomography. Eur J Radiol 2013;83(3):600–5.
36. Li B, Li Q, Chen C, et al. A systematic review and meta-analysis of the accuracy of diffusion-weighted MRI in the detection of malignant pulmonary nodules and masses. Acad Radiol 2014;21(1):21–9.
37. Hiraki T, Mimura H, Gobara H, et al. CT fluoroscopy-guided biopsy of 1,000 pulmonary lesions performed with 20-gauge coaxial cutting needles: diagnostic yield and risk factors for diagnostic failure. Chest 2009;136(6):1612–7.
38. Sobin LH, Gospodarowicz MK, Wittekind C, editors. UICC International Union Against Cancer. Lung and pleural tumours. TNM classification of malignant tumours. 7th edition. Oxford (England): Wiley-Blackwell; 2009.
39. Rusch VW, Asamura H, Watanabe H, et al. The IASLC lung cancer staging project: a proposal for a new international lymph node map in the forthcoming seventh edition of the TNM classification for lung cancer. J Thorac Oncol 2009;4(5):568–77.
40. National Comprehensive Cancer Network. Non-small cell lung cancer. 2014. 2.2014. Available at: http://www.nccn.org/professionals/physician_gls/pdf/nscl.pdf. Accessed January 22, 2014.
41. National Comprehensive Cancer Network. Small cell lung cancer. 2014. 2.2014. Available at: http://www.nccn.org/professionals/physician_gls/pdf/sclc.pdf. Accessed January 22, 2014.
42. Lardinois D, Weder W, Hany TF, et al. Staging of non-small-cell lung cancer with integrated positron-emission tomography and computed tomography. N Engl J Med 2003;348(25):2500–7.
43. Hasegawa I, Boiselle PM, Kuwabara K, et al. Mediastinal lymph nodes in patients with non-small cell lung cancer: preliminary experience with diffusion-weighted MR imaging. J Thorac Imaging 2008;23(3):157–61.
44. Nomori H, Mori T, Ikeda K, et al. Diffusion-weighted magnetic resonance imaging can be used in place of positron emission tomography for N staging of non-small cell lung cancer with fewer false-positive results. J Thorac Cardiovasc Surg 2008;135(4):816–22.
45. Ohno Y, Koyama H, Yoshikawa T, et al. N stage disease in patients with non-small cell lung cancer: efficacy of quantitative and qualitative assessment with STIR turbo spin-echo imaging, diffusion-weighted MR imaging, and fluorodeoxyglucose PET/CT. Radiology 2011;261(2):605–15.
46. Usuda K, Sagawa M, Motono N, et al. Advantages of diffusion-weighted imaging over positron emission tomography-computed tomography in assessment of hilar and mediastinal lymph node in lung cancer. Ann Surg Oncol 2013;20(5):1676–83.
47. Usuda K, Zhao XT, Sagawa M, et al. Diffusion-weighted imaging is superior to positron emission tomography in the detection and nodal assessment of lung cancers. Ann Thorac Surg 2011;91(6):1689–95.
48. Hatton MQ, Martin JE. Continuous hyperfractionated accelerated radiotherapy (CHART) and non-conventionally fractionated radiotherapy in the treatment of non-small cell lung cancer: a review and consideration of future directions. Clin Oncol (R Coll Radiol) 2010;22(5):356–64.

49. Mauguen A, Le Pechoux C, Saunders MI, et al. Hyperfractionated or accelerated radiotherapy in lung cancer: an individual patient data meta-analysis. J Clin Oncol 2012;30(22):2788–97.

50. Nestle U, Kremp S, Grosu AL. Practical integration of [18F]-FDG-PET and PET-CT in the planning of radiotherapy for non-small cell lung cancer (NSCLC): the technical basis, ICRU-target volumes, problems, perspectives. Radiother Oncol 2006;81(2):209–25.

51. van Der Wel A, Nijsten S, Hochstenbag M, et al. Increased therapeutic ratio by 18FDG-PET CT planning in patients with clinical CT stage N2-N3M0 non-small-cell lung cancer: a modeling study. Int J Radiat Oncol Biol Phys 2005;61(3): 649–55.

52. Caldwell CB, Mah K, Ung YC, et al. Observer variation in contouring gross tumor volume in patients with poorly defined non-small-cell lung tumors on CT: the impact of 18FDG-hybrid PET fusion. Int J Radiat Oncol Biol Phys 2001;51(4): 923–31.

53. Steenbakkers RJ, Duppen JC, Fitton I, et al. Reduction of observer variation using matched CT-PET for lung cancer delineation: a three-dimensional analysis. Int J Radiat Oncol Biol Phys 2006;64(2):435–48.

54. Werner-Wasik M, Nelson AD, Choi W, et al. What is the best way to contour lung tumors on PET scans? Multiobserver validation of a gradient-based method using a NSCLC digital PET phantom. Int J Radiat Oncol Biol Phys 2012;82(3):1164–71.

55. van Baardwijk A, Bosmans G, Boersma L, et al. PET-CT-based auto-contouring in non-small-cell lung cancer correlates with pathology and reduces interobserver variability in the delineation of the primary tumor and involved nodal volumes. Int J Radiat Oncol Biol Phys 2007;68(3):771–8.

56. Fernando HC. Radiofrequency ablation to treat non-small cell lung cancer and pulmonary metastases. Ann Thorac Surg 2008;85(2):S780–4.

57. Herrera LJ, Fernando HC, Perry Y, et al. Radiofrequency ablation of pulmonary malignant tumors in nonsurgical candidates. J Thorac Cardiovasc Surg 2003; 125(4):929–37.

58. Pennathur A, Luketich JD, Abbas G, et al. Radiofrequency ablation for the treatment of stage I non-small cell lung cancer in high-risk patients. J Thorac Cardiovasc Surg 2007;134(4):857–64.

59. Mac Manus MP, Hicks RJ, Matthews JP, et al. Positron emission tomography is superior to computed tomography scanning for response-assessment after radical radiotherapy or chemoradiotherapy in patients with non-small-cell lung cancer. J Clin Oncol 2003;21(7):1285–92.

60. Aukema TS, Kappers I, Olmos RA, et al. Is 18F-FDG PET/CT useful for the early prediction of histopathologic response to neoadjuvant erlotinib in patients with non-small cell lung cancer? J Nucl Med 2010;51(9):1344–8.

61. Benz MR, Herrmann K, Walter F, et al. (18)F-FDG PET/CT for monitoring treatment responses to the epidermal growth factor receptor inhibitor erlotinib. J Nucl Med 2011;52(11):1684–9.

62. Mileshkin L, Hicks RJ, Hughes BG, et al. Changes in 18F-fluorodeoxyglucose and 18F-fluorodeoxythymidine positron emission tomography imaging in patients with non-small cell lung cancer treated with erlotinib. Clin Cancer Res 2011;17(10):3304–15.

63. Zander T, Scheffler M, Nogova L, et al. Early prediction of nonprogression in advanced non-small-cell lung cancer treated with erlotinib by using [(18)F]fluorodeoxyglucose and [(18)F]fluorothymidine positron emission tomography. J Clin Oncol 2011;29(13):1701–8.

64. Basu S. The scope and potentials of functional radionuclide imaging towards advancing personalized medicine in oncology: emphasis on PET-CT. Discov Med 2012;13(68):65–73.
65. Mishani E, Abourbeh G, Eiblmaier M, et al. Imaging of EGFR and EGFR tyrosine kinase overexpression in tumors by nuclear medicine modalities. Curr Pharm Des 2008;14(28):2983–98.
66. Bojarski JD, Dupuy DE, Mayo-Smith WW. CT imaging findings of pulmonary neoplasms after treatment with radiofrequency ablation: results in 32 tumors. AJR Am J Roentgenol 2005;185(2):466–71.
67. Kang S, Luo R, Liao W, et al. Single group study to evaluate the feasibility and complications of radiofrequency ablation and usefulness of post treatment position emission tomography in lung tumours. World J Surg Oncol 2004;2:30.
68. Singnurkar A, Solomon SB, Gonen M, et al. 18F-FDG PET/CT for the prediction and detection of local recurrence after radiofrequency ablation of malignant lung lesions. J Nucl Med 2010;51(12):1833–40.
69. Matsuo Y, Nagata Y, Mizowaki T, et al. Evaluation of mass-like consolidation after stereotactic body radiation therapy for lung tumors. Int J Clin Oncol 2007;12(5): 356–62.
70. Takeda A, Kunieda E, Takeda T, et al. Possible misinterpretation of demarcated solid patterns of radiation fibrosis on CT scans as tumor recurrence in patients receiving hypofractionated stereotactic radiotherapy for lung cancer. Int J Radiat Oncol Biol Phys 2008;70(4):1057–65.
71. Dunlap NE, Yang W, McIntosh A, et al. Computed tomography-based anatomic assessment overestimates local tumor recurrence in patients with mass-like consolidation after stereotactic body radiotherapy for early-stage non-small cell lung cancer. Int J Radiat Oncol Biol Phys 2012;84(5):1071–7.
72. Vahdat S, Oermann EK, Collins SP, et al. CyberKnife radiosurgery for inoperable stage IA non-small cell lung cancer: 18F-fluorodeoxyglucose positron emission tomography/computed tomography serial tumor response assessment. J Hematol Oncol 2010;3:6.
73. Strollo DC, Rosado de Christenson ML, Jett JR. Primary mediastinal tumors. Part 1: tumors of the anterior mediastinum. Chest 1997;112(2):511–22.
74. Jeung MY, Gasser B, Gangi A, et al. Imaging of cystic masses of the mediastinum. Radiographics 2002;22(Spec No):S79–93.
75. Sakai F, Sone S, Kiyono K, et al. Intrathoracic neurogenic tumors: MR-pathologic correlation. AJR Am J Roentgenol 1992;159(2):279–83.
76. Goldman M, Matthews R, Meng H, et al. Evaluation of cardiac involvement with mediastinal lymphoma: the role of innovative integrated cardiovascular imaging. Echocardiography 2012;29(8):E189–92.
77. Thomas A, Shanbhag S, Haglund K, et al. Characterization and management of cardiac involvement of thymic epithelial tumors. J Thorac Oncol 2013;8(2): 246–9.
78. Kebebew E, Arici C, Duh QY, et al. Localization and reoperation results for persistent and recurrent parathyroid carcinoma. Arch Surg 2001;136(8):878–85.
79. Assaad MW, Pantanowitz L, Otis CN. Diagnostic accuracy of image-guided percutaneous fine needle aspiration biopsy of the mediastinum. Diagn Cytopathol 2007;35(11):705–9.
80. Masaoka A, Monden Y, Nakahara K, et al. Follow-up study of thymomas with special reference to their clinical stages. Cancer 1981;48(11):2485–92.
81. Marom EM, Milito MA, Moran CA, et al. Computed tomography findings predicting invasiveness of thymoma. J Thorac Oncol 2011;6(7):1274–81.

82. Inaoka T, Takahashi K, Mineta M, et al. Thymic hyperplasia and thymus gland tumors: differentiation with chemical shift MR imaging. Radiology 2007;243(3): 869–76.

83. Benveniste MF, Moran CA, Mawlawi O, et al. FDG PET-CT aids in the preoperative assessment of patients with newly diagnosed thymic epithelial malignancies. J Thorac Oncol 2013;8(4):502–10.

84. Shibata H, Nomori H, Uno K, et al. 18F-fluorodeoxyglucose and 11C-acetate positron emission tomography are useful modalities for diagnosing the histologic type of thymoma. Cancer 2009;115(11):2531–8.

85. Terzi A, Bertolaccini L, Rizzardi G, et al. Usefulness of 18-F FDG PET/CT in the pre-treatment evaluation of thymic epithelial neoplasms. Lung Cancer 2011; 74(2):239–43.

86. Schiepers C, Filmont JE, Czernin J. PET for staging of Hodgkin's disease and non-Hodgkin's lymphoma. Eur J Nucl Med Mol Imaging 2003;30(Suppl 1):S82–8.

87. Bokemeyer C, Nichols CR, Droz JP, et al. Extragonadal germ cell tumors of the mediastinum and retroperitoneum: results from an international analysis. J Clin Oncol 2002;20(7):1864–73.

88. Davis RD Jr, Oldham HN Jr, Sabiston DC Jr. Primary cysts and neoplasms of the mediastinum: recent changes in clinical presentation, methods of diagnosis, management, and results. Ann Thorac Surg 1987;44(3):229–37.

89. Chen VK, Eloubeidi MA. Endoscopic ultrasound-guided fine-needle aspiration of intramural and extraintestinal mass lesions: diagnostic accuracy, complication assessment, and impact on management. Endoscopy 2005;37(10):984–9.

90. Aughenbaugh GL. Thoracic manifestations of neurocutaneous diseases. Radiol Clin North Am 1984;22(3):741–56.

91. Stark DD, Moss AA, Brasch RC, et al. Neuroblastoma: diagnostic imaging and staging. Radiology 1983;148(1):101–5.

92. Ettinger DS, Akerley W, Borghaei H, et al. Malignant pleural mesothelioma. J Natl Compr Canc Netw 2012;10(1):26–41.

93. Pilling J, Dartnell JA, Lang-Lazdunski L. Integrated positron emission tomography-computed tomography does not accurately stage intrathoracic disease of patients undergoing trimodality therapy for malignant pleural mesothelioma. Thorac Cardiovasc Surg 2010;58(4):215–9.

94. Gill RR, Umeoka S, Mamata H, et al. Diffusion-weighted MRI of malignant pleural mesothelioma: preliminary assessment of apparent diffusion coefficient in histologic subtypes. AJR Am J Roentgenol 2010;195(2):W125–30.

95. Park EK, Takahashi K, Hoshuyama T, et al. Global magnitude of reported and unreported mesothelioma. Environ Health Perspect 2011;119(4):514–8.

96. Gatta G, Ciccolallo L, Kunkler I, et al. Survival from rare cancer in adults: a population-based study. Lancet Oncol 2006;7(2):132–40.

97. Leung AN, Muller NL, Miller RR. CT in differential diagnosis of diffuse pleural disease. AJR Am J Roentgenol 1990;154(3):487–92.

98. Rusch VW. A proposed new international TNM staging system for malignant pleural mesothelioma. From the International Mesothelioma Interest Group. Chest 1995;108(4):1122–8.

99. Patz EF Jr, Shaffer K, Piwnica-Worms DR, et al. Malignant pleural mesothelioma: value of CT and MR imaging in predicting resectability. AJR Am J Roentgenol 1992;159(5):961–6.

100. Heelan RT, Rusch VW, Begg CB, et al. Staging of malignant pleural mesothelioma: comparison of CT and MR imaging. AJR Am J Roentgenol 1999;172(4): 1039–47.

101. Al-Izzi M, Thurlow NP, Corrin B. Pleural mesothelioma of connective tissue type, localized fibrous tumour of the pleura, and reactive submesothelial hyperplasia. An immunohistochemical comparison. J Pathol 1989;158(1):41–4.
102. Ferretti GR, Chiles C, Choplin RH, et al. Localized benign fibrous tumors of the pleura. AJR Am J Roentgenol 1997;169(3):683–6.
103. Cardillo G, Carbone L, Carleo F, et al. Solitary fibrous tumors of the pleura: an analysis of 110 patients treated in a single institution. Ann Thorac Surg 2009; 88(5):1632–7.
104. Kohler M, Clarenbach CF, Kestenholz P, et al. Diagnosis, treatment and long-term outcome of solitary fibrous tumours of the pleura. Eur J Cardiothorac Surg 2007;32(3):403–8.
105. Hussein-Jelen T, Bankier AA, Eisenberg RL. Solid pleural lesions. AJR Am J Roentgenol 2012;198(6):W512–20.

Emerging Modalities in Breast Cancer Imaging

Shadi Aminololama-Shakeri, MD[a], Vijay P. Khatri, MBChB, MBA[b],*

KEYWORDS

- Breast • Cancer • Imaging • Modalities

KEY POINTS

- Although each of the emerging imaging techniques has advantages compared with standard mammography, they are not perfect, and each has inherent limitations.
- To date, no imaging techniques have been studied by large randomized clinical trials to match the proven benefits of screening mammography; namely the reduction of mortality caused by breast cancer by nearly 30%.
- More research into breast cancer imaging modalities is required.

INTRODUCTION

Breast cancer continues to be the most frequently diagnosed malignancy and the second leading cause of death caused by cancer in women in the United States.[1] Nearly 3 million women were estimated to be living with breast cancer in the United States in 2011. Approximately, 230,000 new cases and 40,000 deaths caused by breast cancer are estimated to occur in 2014. At present, a woman living in the United States has a 1 in 8 (12.3%) risk of developing breast cancer during her lifetime.[2] Today, standard-of-care breast imaging techniques include digital mammography (DM), targeted ultrasonography, and dynamic contrast-enhanced magnetic resonance imaging (MRI).

Mammography has been the mainstay of breast cancer screening programs in the United States and many European countries since the 1990s. Although mammography remains the only imaging modality shown to reduce mortality caused by breast cancer by nearly 30% in multiple large randomized clinical trials, it has several shortcomings. A well-known limitation of mammography is its decreased sensitivity in breasts with predominantly dense parenchyma.[3] Some of the deficiencies of

---

The authors have nothing to disclose.
[a] Department of Radiology, University California, Davis Health System, Sacramento, CA, USA;
[b] Division of Surgical Oncology, Department of Surgery, University of California, Davis Comprehensive Cancer Center, University California, Davis Health System, 4501 X Street, Suite 3010D, Sacramento, CA 95817, USA
* Corresponding author.
E-mail address: vijay.khatri@ucdmc.ucdavis.edu

mammography are caused by the depiction of the three-dimensional (3D) breast in a two-dimensional (2D) format. As a result, overlapping tissue may cloak a potential cancer or create a fictitious lesion with features suspicious of a malignancy that is not present. As a result, further unnecessary work-ups and interventions, including needle and excisional biopsies, are performed, incurring both monetary costs and emotional distress to the patient and society. Another important limitation of mammography is the need for breast compression to perform a high-quality study. Breast compression is perhaps the most frequent cause of patient discomfort and anxiety, particularly after recent radiation therapy.

Efforts to overcome these shortcomings of routine mammography have led to the development of newer breast imaging modalities. Apart from targeted ultrasonography, the ubiquitous adjunct to mammography for diagnostic work-up, breast MRI has evolved over the past decade and is now an established modality in breast imaging. Lack of ionizing radiation and high sensitivity when combined with mammography are some of the advantages of MRI. However, lower specificity, requirement of intravenous contrast, high cost, lower patient tolerance, and lack of access have prevented this technique from replacing routine mammograms. With continued improvements in technique, MRI has become established as the modality of choice for specific indications.[4] At present, MRI is most commonly used as a screening supplement to mammography in women at high risk of developing breast cancer.[4] Other common indications for MRI are evaluation of extent of disease and treatment monitoring such as patients receiving neoadjuvant chemotherapy for locally advanced breast cancer. Earlier in the development of this technology, there was prevalent use of MRI for surgical planning, which has now subsided, primarily because of studies with conflicting results regarding desired outcomes such as lowered reexcision and local recurrence rates as well as a paucity of data for survival outcomes. The exact criteria of use beyond screening of high-risk women remains a topic of controversy. Techniques and clinical indications for this modality with an expanding body of evidence for its utility are reviewed elsewhere.[5]

Other breast imaging modalities continue to be developed with hopes of overcoming the challenges of mammography, MRI, and ultrasonography. These modalities include automated whole-breast ultrasonography (AWBUS), digital breast tomosynthesis (DBT), dedicated breast computed tomography (bCT), contrast-enhanced DM (CEDM), and nuclear medicine studies such as positron emission mammography (PEM) and breast-specific gamma imaging (BSGI). These emerging breast imaging technologies show promise in improving the current standards of practice of breast imaging and are the subject of this article.

ULTRASONOGRAPHY REFINEMENTS

Targeted ultrasonography has been a long-standing adjunct to mammography for problem solving and biopsy planning. The advantages of ultrasonography are wide availability, lack of ionizing radiation, and lower cost compared with other techniques such as breast MRI. With increasing awareness of the limitations of mammography, ultrasonography has gained popularity as a supplemental screening tool. Many states such as Texas, New York, Connecticut, and California now have legislation mandating that women be informed of their breast density, encouraging a dialogue between the patient and her referring physician regarding the need for additional screening. Legislation in at least 1 state, Connecticut, has more specific language regarding screening ultrasonography that mandates insurance companies to pay for the examination if recommended by a physician. Whether legislation is the best way to improve clinical outcomes is debatable because there are always unintended consequences resulting from mandates and regulations.

Several studies have shown an incremental cancer detection rate of up to 4.2 cancers per 1000 women screened when ultrasonography is added to mammography screening.[6–9] The largest trial of screening ultrasonography was performed in 2637 women with increased risk for breast cancer as part of The American College of Radiology Imaging Network (ACRIN) 6666. The addition of a single screening whole-breast ultrasonography to screening mammogram increased the cancer yield from 7.6 to 11.8 per 1000 screened. This gain was balanced by a lower specificity and positive predictive value (PPV) for ultrasonography (8.9%) compared with mammography (22.6%). The call-back rate from the physician-performed examination using hand-held ultrasonography was 5.4% in the ACRIN 6666, which is lower than mammography (5%–12%). The recall rate with screening ultrasonography for additional needed imaging may increase with AWBUS, because the physician is not able to evaluate the findings in real time during scanning. Moreover, ultrasonography is costly in terms of time management, requiring adjustments in the practice workflow and additional qualified personnel. In the ACRIN 6666 trial, along with most other screening ultrasonography studies, a physician using a hand-held device performed the examination. The median time to perform screening breast ultrasonography was 19 minutes, which significantly adds time spent per patient doing a screening study. Similar outcomes have been reported by technologist-performed studies.[9,10] This labor-intensive and time-consuming protocol has been a major obstacle to widespread implementation of ultrasonography screening.

AWBUS is a recent refinement in technique compared with hand-held ultrasonography that offers some advantages. In AWBUS, the ultrasonography probe is attached to and controlled by a mechanized arm that scrolls over the breast section by section. Physician time is spent on the interpretation of images rather than on acquiring them. Given the automated nature of the examination, dependence on operator skill at the time of acquisition is eliminated. The average examination times are 15 minutes and the technique is limited in large-breasted women, in whom manual scan times are anticipated to take longer. One system approved by the US Food and Drug Administration (FDA) for screening is currently available in the United States. High false-positive rates and low PPV remain obstacles to widespread implementation of AWBUS.

In addition to having a poorer PPV than mammography, there is currently no established Current Procedural Terminology (CPT) code that specifically applies to either method of screening ultrasonography. The performance and interpretation of this lengthier and more laborious screening examination than its more focused targeted counterpart are reimbursed at the same rate using the same CPT codes at this time.

DBT

DBT (also referred to as 3D mammography) is a modified mammographic technique designed to increase lesion visibility by decreasing superimposition of adjacent parenchyma. Unlike conventional mammography, in which the x-ray tube and receptor are stationary, producing a single image, in DBT the x-ray source moves through a limited angle range (15°–60°) relative to the receptor and breast in standard projection (**Fig. 1**).[11] A series of low-dose images are produced through the compressed breast and reconstructed into a volumetric 3D dataset. Images reconstructed at selected thinness ranging from 1 to 10 mm may be viewed individually or as a cine-loop.[12] Separating the breast tissue into a stack of thinly reconstructed images minimizes the effects of tissue overlap.[13] Several manufacturers have developed their own

Digital Tomosynthesis

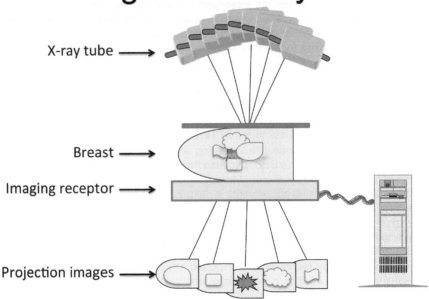

Fig. 1. In DBT, the x-ray tube moves through a limited angle, producing a series of low-dose projection images of the compressed breast that are reconstructed into multiple thin-slice images.

models with variations on the same theme. The tomosynthesis units currently in clinical use have the capability of obtaining 2D DM and tomosynthesis views of the breast during the same compression in standard craniocaudal (CC) and mediolateral oblique (MLO) projections. In 2011, the FDA approved this DM/DBT combination (Selenia Dimensions, Hologic) for clinical practice in the United States.[14]

Early experimental clinical studies have shown an increase in screening sensitivity, decrease in false-positives, and improved performance of DM in combination with DBT compared with DM alone.[14] Several small studies of lesions including masses and microcalcifications showed physician preference for tomosynthesis image quality compared with DM.[15–17] Interim results from several ongoing trials have shown the potential for DBT to decrease false-positive recall rates with equal or improved cancer detection rates to DM. The Oslo Tomosynthesis Screening Trial is one of the largest prospective single-center tomosynthesis studies performed to date. Skaane and colleagues[18] reported initial results for 12,631 women, aged 50 to 70 years, who were invited for biennial screening comparing standard 2-view DM (2v DM) alone with combined 2v DM and 2-view DBT (Selenia Dimensions, Hologic). They reported a significant 27% increase in cancer detection (8.0 vs 6.1 per 1000 examinations) for DM plus DBT compared with DM alone. False-positive rates decreased from 61.1 to 53.1 per 1000 patients screened with DM alone compared with DM plus DBT; a decrease of 15% in screening recall rates. Similar results were reported by the Screening with Tomosynthesis or standard Mammography (STORM) trial, a prospective Italian screening study of women 48 years of age or older.[19] Eight radiologists interpreted the 2v DM (Selenia Dimensions, Hologic) screening study followed by the 2v DM plus DBT in 7294 subjects. An incremental cancer detection rate of 2.7 cancers per

1000 patients (33.9%) attributable to an integrated DM and DBT screening approach relative to 2v DM alone was reported. The decrease in the false-positive recall rate of 2% based on DM alone to 1% with the addition of DBT supports the results of previous studies. The latest study in the United States retrospectively evaluated 454,850 screening examinations from 13 sites interpreted by 139 radiologists.[20] The evaluation included 281,187 (61.8%) DM performed in the year before implementation of tomosynthesis and 173,663 (38.2%) DM plus DBT in the year following. The cancer detection rate increased from 4.2 per 1000 patients screened with DM to 5.4 per 1000 patients screened with DM plus DBT. The investigators reported a model-adjusted false-positive rate per 1000 screens of 107 with DM versus 91 for mammography combined with tomosynthesis. These studies add to a growing body of evidence that DBT in combination with DM reduces false-positive examinations and improves cancer detection rates.

Several studies have suggested that there may be a role for DBT in standard diagnostic work-up of symptomatic patients and screening callback examinations (**Fig. 2**). In a reader study of 67 subjects with 30 malignant and 37 benign breast masses, Noroozian and colleagues[21] compared DBT with standard mammographic spot compression views. They reported no significant difference in accuracy but slightly better mass visibility with DBT. Tagliafico and colleagues[22] showed no statistical difference between DM spot compression views and DBT in a small prospective study of 52 screening recalls of noncalcified lesions. However, lesion conspicuity was better for DBT (4.1) than for spot compression views (2.9). A more recent retrospective analysis of 217 noncalcified lesions was designed to compare the diagnostic performance of DBT and DM for 8 readers. Receiver operating characteristic curves offer a way to measure the trade-off between sensitivity and specificity for a diagnostic test. The area under the curve (AUC) is a metric of better performance as it approaches a value

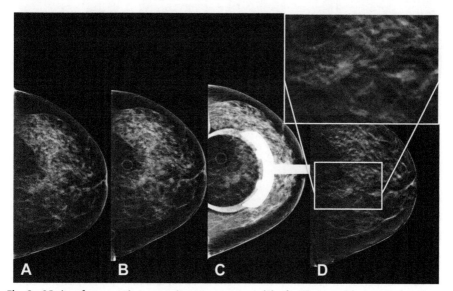

Fig. 2. CC view from routine screening mammogram (*B*) of a 73-year-old woman showing a subtle developing asymmetry in posterior breast just medial to the nipple line compared with prior year (*A*). Spot compression view (*C*) shows that the asymmetry persists. Tomosynthesis in CC view (*D*) shows a spiculated, suspicious mass shown to be an invasive ductal carcinoma on histopathology.

of 1.00. Using this analysis, tomosynthesis (AUC, 0.87) significantly outperformed conventional supplemental diagnostic views (AUC, 0.83) in its performance measuring probability of malignancy.[23] Additional studies have also suggested the potential for DBT to replace standard mammographic diagnostic views (**Fig. 3**).[24–26]

Many challenges remain to be addressed before tomosynthesis can gain wide acceptance into clinical practice. These challenges include the optimal number of DBT views, with or without conventional DM; DBT performance in detection and

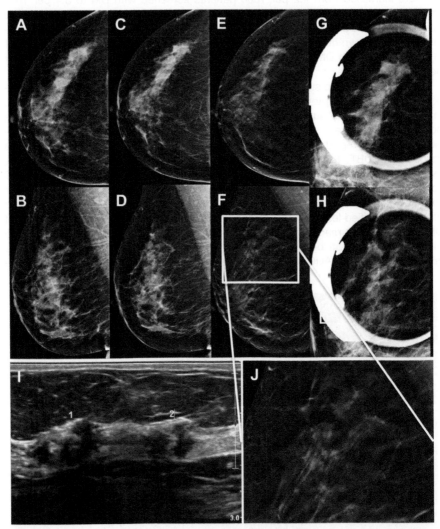

Fig. 3. CC (*C*) and MLO (*D*) views from screening mammogram of a 53-year-old woman compared with prior year CC (*A*) and MLO (*B*) shows subtle possible architectural distortion that does not persist on spot compression views in CC (*G*) and MLO (*H*) projections. CC (*E*) and MLO (*F*) tomosynthesis views clearly show a large area of architectural distortion in at least 3 lesions in close proximity. Inset from MLO DBT shows the 3 areas of architectural distortion in greater detail (*J*). Ultrasonography (*I*) shows 2 highly suspicious hypoechoic, irregular masses (third mass not shown), which were proved on biopsy to be invasive ductal carcinoma grade 2.

characterization of calcifications; concerns of increased radiation dose; and work-flow issues.

Characterization of calcifications remains a challenging area for tomosynthesis. Several trials have compared DM and DBT for calcification evaluation with mixed results.[15,27,28] So far, there is no robust evidence that tomosynthesis is advantageous compared with 2D mammography for detection and characterization of calcifications.

Although multiple preliminary studies have been performed with a variety of numbers and combinations of DM and DBT views, consensus has yet to be reached regarding an optimized protocol. As expected, the greatest improvements in accuracy are found when 2v DBT is added to 2v DM.[14,18,19,29] This combination, which is essentially a double mammogram, also has the highest radiation dose compared with other algorithms that include fewer images of one or the other imaging techniques. Toward this goal, manufacturers have been developing a synthesized 2D mammogram from the 3D DBT data. Recent results from early studies comparing the performance of DBT and synthesized 2D mammogram are promising.[30] Gur and colleagues[31] showed a similar sensitivity of DBT plus DM (0.83) compared with DBT and synthesized DM (0.77).

There are other issues to consider, such as increased examination interpretation time, cost-effectiveness, and development of interventional capabilities for lesions only seen by DBT. The reading time of a screening mammogram nearly doubles with the addition of DBT.[16,18,32] There is no approved CPT code and no standard reimbursement yet.

Although there has been mounting evidence for the utility of tomosynthesis in the practice of breast imaging care, its role is not clear. Although there seems to be a surge in the literature in support of DBT, a recent survey of breast imaging specialists in the United States found that only about a third are using this technology.[33] Development of guidelines to assist clinical practice are needed to determine the optimal role for tomosynthesis in breast imaging.

DEDICATED BCT

Compared with conventional mammography (2D), and tomosynthesis (quasi-3D) depiction of the breast, dedicated bCT is a fully 3D modality. As such, this investigational tool has the potential to improve breast cancer detection and reduce the number of false-positives and biopsies.

In one dedicated bCT prototype the patient is placed prone with the breast pendant through an opening in the tabletop. The x-ray tube and flat panel detector rotate 360° around the breast in the horizontal plane, producing approximately 500 projection images (**Fig. 4**).[34] These images are acquired in less than 20 seconds with techniques chosen to deliver the same radiation dose as a 2-view mammogram.[34] The images may be reconstructed in any plane but are routinely reviewed with specialized software in axial, sagittal, and coronal planes akin to breast MRI viewing software (**Fig. 5A**). Maximum intensity projections can be reconstructed and viewed similarly to a breast MRI display (see **Fig. 5B**). An important feature of the bCT viewing software is the ability to dynamically adjust slice thickness in all 3 directions. This ability gives the interpreting physician the ability to trade off slice thickness (along the line of sight) with x-ray quantum noise visible in the images. Precise measurements of lesion volume can be made with this visualization tool, because the variable magnification issues are factored out in the reconstruction process.

Several clinical trials comparing bCT with other breast imaging modalities have been reported. Early work in 69 women with suspicious lesions designated as Breast Imaging Reporting and Data System (BI-RADS) 4 or 5 diagnoses based on standard

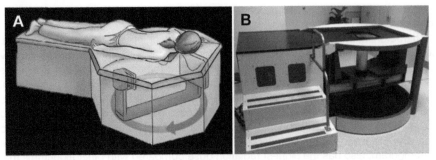

Fig. 4. The bCT system. The woman lies prone with the breast to be imaged in pendant position (*A*). In the third prototype bCT system, open access for biopsy and radiofrequency ablation are available (*B*). (*From* Lindfors KK, Boone JM, Newell MS, et al. Dedicated breast computed tomography: the optimal cross-sectional imaging solution? Radiol Clin North Am 2010;48(5):1046. http://dx.doi.org/10.1016/j.rcl.2010.06.001; with permission.)

imaging showed that unenhanced bCT was significantly better for visualization of masses (*P*<.002), but that mammography outperformed bCT for visualization of calcifications (*P*<.006).[35] Prompted by the need for improved detection of early stage breast cancers, including ductal carcinoma in situ (DCIS), compared with standard 2D mammography the investigators studied the use of intravenous contrast to increase the sensitivity of bCT. In 54 reported BI-RADS 4 or 5 breast lesions, malignancies were seen significantly better with contrast-enhanced bCT (CE-bCT) compared with unenhanced bCT (*P*<.001) or mammography (*P*<.001).[36] Malignant lesions enhanced an average of 55.9 Hounsfield units (HU), whereas benign lesions enhanced 17.6 HU (*P*<.001) (**Fig. 6**).

In a more recent study of suspicious microcalcifications recommended for biopsy by conventional work-up (BI-RADS 4 or 5), malignant microcalcifications were equally well seen on CE-bCT and mammography, both of which are significantly superior to unenhanced bCT for DCIS visualization (**Fig. 7**).[37] In the same study, benign

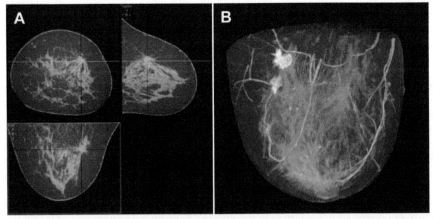

Fig. 5. Display software shows full 3D image from orthogonal views (*A*). An infiltrating ductal carcinoma at the 1 o'clock position is shown. (*B*). Maximum intensity projection shows the index cancer and a second lesion anterior to it. (*From* Lindfors KK, Boone JM, Newell MS, et al. Dedicated breast computed tomography: the optimal cross-sectional imaging solution? Radiol Clin North Am 2010;48(5):1043–54. http://dx.doi.org/10.1016/j.rcl.2010.06.001; with permission.)

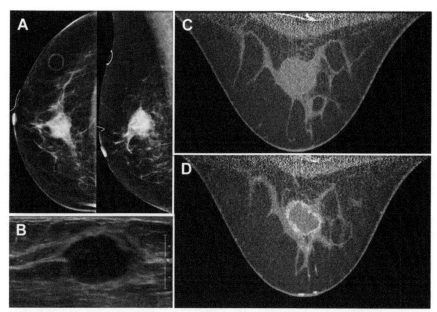

Fig. 6. CC and MLO mammographic views show a mass in the 12 o'clock position (*A*). High-resolution ultrasonography shows the mass to be predominantly anechoic with low-level internal echoes (*B*). Axial noncontrast bCT (*C*) shows the corresponding mass that shows irregular rim enhancement after contrast injection (*D*) and a hypodense center. Biopsy reveals poorly differentiated invasive ductal carcinoma with central necrosis.

calcifications were significantly better seen on mammography than on either enhanced or unenhanced bCT. Quantitative enhancement of malignant calcifications (mean of nearly 60 HU) was significantly greater than enhancement of benign calcifications. All malignant calcifications enhanced, whereas most benign lesions showed no enhancement, suggesting that enhanced bCT has the potential to reduce benign breast biopsies.

Comparisons of bCT with other modalities, including tomosynthesis and MRI, are underway. One early study showed that, in 103 BI-RADS 4 or 5 lesions, malignant masses had significantly greater conspicuity on CE-bCT than on mammography or

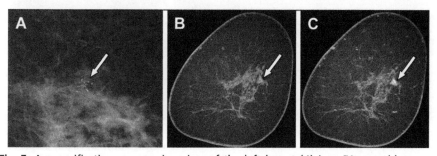

Fig. 7. A magnification compression view of the left breast (*A*) in a 51-year-old woman shows a 5-mm focus of pleomorphic microcalcifications at the 2 o'clock position (*arrow*). A coronal unenhanced bCT (*B*) shows faint microcalcifications (*arrow*). The corresponding contrast-enhanced bCT (*C*) shows a 5-mm focus of enhancement (*arrow*) at the site of the calcifications. DCIS with focus of microinvasion was shown on core biopsy.

tomosynthesis (P<.05) and benign calcifications showed significantly lower conspicuity on CE-bCT than mammography or tomosynthesis (P<.05).[38] Benign masses and malignant calcifications were seen equally well on all 3 modalities.

In a comparative study of 24 cancers and 33 benign lesions, CE-bCT was equivalent to MRI in diagnostic performance.[39] Among 5 radiologist readers, enhanced bCT correctly classified 83.6% of the benign lesions and 94.2% of the cancers. MRI correctly classified 86.1% of the benign lesions and 93.3% of the cancers (P>.63). These results suggest that CE-bCT may be an alternative to MRI in the evaluation of breast lesions (**Fig. 8**).

In addition to early clinical data, mathematical analyses of bCT breast images show that the anatomic texture produced by thin sections is more conducive to mass-lesion detection than DM or DBT.[40,41] Physiologic information can be obtained when intravenous contrast is used, increasing both the sensitivity and specificity of bCT.

The expected cost of bCT should be lower than MRI, and the compact footprint and lower siting costs should allow wide bCT system deployment in most breast imaging clinics. Although currently in development, bCT is a promising new tool that will add

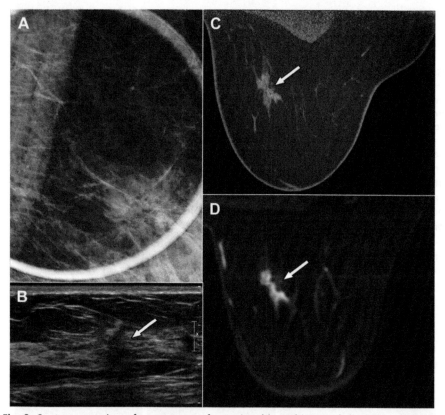

Fig. 8. Spot compression of a new area of questionable architectural distortion and mass (*arrows*). (*A*) Suspicious hypoechoic mass as seen on ultrasonography. (*B*) Highly suspicious enhancing irregular mass with distortion of the parenchyma seen almost identically on CE-bCT (*C*) and MRI (*D*) that was shown to be an invasive ductal carcinoma by core biopsy. (*From* Lindfors KK, Boone JM, Newell MS, et al. Dedicated breast computed tomography: the optimal cross-sectional imaging solution? Radiol Clin North Am 2010;48(5):1043–54. http://dx.doi.org/10.1016/j.rcl.2010.06.001; with permission.)

considerable flexibility to both screening and diagnostic breast examination. Image-guided biopsy and radiofrequency ablation are potential future applications of the bCT platform and are under development.

NUCLEAR MEDICINE AND BREAST IMAGING

Over the past decade nuclear medicine imaging of the breast has advanced from its singular role in sentinel lymph node identification using technetium 99m-labeled sulfur colloid. With the development of breast-optimized gamma cameras, BSGI, an update to scintimammography, has been studied as a complementary tool to mammography. In BSGI, images of both breasts may be obtained using a gamma camera with a small field of view device after injection of technetium 99m sestamibi.

The sensitivity and specificity of BSGI have been reported as 91% to 96% and 96% to 77% respectively in several studies.[42,43] In one multicenter patient registry, the greatest impact of BSGI was in patients with negative or indeterminate mammograms.[42] One small study compared the performance of BSGI with MRI in 23 women with indeterminate breast findings and there was no significant difference between the two modalities.[44]

Proposed applications for BSGI include evaluation of extent of disease in patients unable to undergo MRI, evaluation of lesions considered for short-interval follow-up (BI-RADS 3) in patients not thought to be reliable to return in 6 months and unwilling to have a biopsy evaluation, palpable abnormality in the setting of normal mammography and ultrasonography, any indications for MRI in which the patient is unable to tolerate the examination, or lack of access.

Another developing technique is PEM, which most commonly involves injection of 18F-fluorodeoxyglucose radionuclide in a fasting patient and imaging on a high-resolution positron emission tomography scanner. Images may be acquired in a seated position with the breast positioned similarly to mammography or in a prone position. Berg and colleagues[45] showed 90% sensitivity, 86% specificity, and PPV of 88% for breast cancer in a series of 77 women with known breast cancer or suspicious lesions. Some proposed roles for PEM include evaluation of extent of disease and aid in preoperative planning, problem solving in indeterminate mammographic lesions, and possibly as a supplemental screening tool.

The single most important barrier to the widespread adoption of these methods for routine breast imaging is radiation dose to the whole body. The lifetime attributable risk of fatal cancer caused by a single PEM or BSGI examination is 20 to 30 times greater than that of imaging with mammography.[46] There are currently no recommendations for use of molecular breast imaging. The high radiation doses compared with conventional breast imaging are prohibitive for annual examinations.

CEDM

The addition of intravenous contrast in breast imaging brings physiologic information to images that otherwise display only anatomic information. This principle is the basis of techniques such as MRI and CE-bCT, which are designed to take advantage of tumor neovascularity to display malignancy. An extension of this concept to DM is the basis for CEDM.[47,48] Hypervascular lesions are displayed when nonenhancing background is digitally removed from the final image. There are 2 main methods of performing CEDM: temporal subtraction and dual-energy imaging.

Temporal CEDM is performed by obtaining a precontrast image of the compressed breast followed by a series of images at regular intervals after contrast injection. The precontrast image is then digitally subtracted from the serial images, leaving only enhancing structures.[48,49] A major disadvantage of this technique is being limited to a single projection of the breast; for example, in the MLO view, thereby making it more suitable for problem solving rather than screening applications. This technique is also prone to errors of misregistration of the image pairs caused by motion between the precontrast and serial images.

Dual-energy CEDM is performed with modified mammography units capable of producing images obtained at 2 different energies.[50] Conventional mammographic images using lower kilovolts as well as images produced at energies higher than the attenuation coefficient of iodine (K_{iodine}; 33.2 keV) are acquired of the compressed breast after intravenous contrast injection. Digital subtraction of these two sets of images highlights areas of iodine distribution. Unlike temporal CEDM, with dual energy both breasts can be imaged with 1 contrast injection at the cost of losing kinetic data.

Early clinical feasibility studies showed a sensitivity of 80% to 85%.[48,50,51] In a retrospective cancer-enriched study of 85 lesions, 5 readers compared DM alone with DM and CEDM. Sensitivity was improved from 0.81 to 0.86 with the addition of CEDM but these results were significant for only 2 of the 5 readers. Dromain and colleagues[52] showed a significant increase in sensitivity of dual-energy CEDM (93%) compared with mammography (78%) in 120 women with 142 suspicious findings. A second clinical trial by the same group showed a significant increase in diagnostic performance of 6 readers when CEDM (AUC 0.87) was added to DM with or without ultrasonography compared with DM with or without ultrasonography (AUC 0.83).[53] Investigations of CEDM performance compared with DM and MRI are underway with promising initial results.[54] In addition to the need for compression with this modality, other limitations reported thus far include both false-negative and false-positive examinations.[55]

CEDM may be a useful adjunct to DM with a potential role in the evaluation of extension of breast cancer lesions, diagnostic evaluation of indeterminate lesions by conventional work-up, and in women unable to undergo MRI. Although early studies have been encouraging, the role of CEDM in clinical practice remains to be determined.

SUMMARY

Although each of these emerging imaging techniques has advantages compared with standard mammography, they are not perfect, and each has inherent limitations. To date, none have been studied by large randomized clinical trials to match the proven benefits of screening mammography; namely the reduction of mortality caused by breast cancer by nearly 30%.

REFERENCES

1. US Cancer Statistics Working Group. United States cancer statistics: 1999–2010 incidence and mortality web-based report. Atlanta (GA): US Department of Health and Human Services; Centers for Disease Control and Prevention and National Cancer Institute; 2013. Available at: http://www.cdc.gov/uscs.

2. Howlader N, Noone AM, Krapcho M, et al. SEER cancer statistics review, 1975-2011. Bethesda (MD): National Cancer Institute; 2014. Available at: http://seer.cancer.gov/csr/1975_2011/.

3. Mandelson MT, Oestreicher N, Porter PL, et al. Breast density as a predictor of mammographic detection: comparison of interval- and screen-detected cancers. J Natl Cancer Inst 2000;92(13):1081–7.

4. Saslow D, Boetes C, Burke W, et al. American Cancer Society guidelines for breast screening with MRI as an adjunct to mammography. CA Cancer J Clin 2007;57(2): 75–89.

5. Weinstein S, Rosen M. Breast MR imaging: current indications and advanced imaging techniques. Radiol Clin North Am 2010;48(5):1013–42.
6. Kolb TM, Lichy J, Newhouse JH. Comparison of the performance of screening mammography, physical examination, and breast US and evaluation of factors that influence them: an analysis of 27,825 patient evaluations. Radiology 2002; 225(1):165–75.
7. Berg WA, Blume JD, Cormack JB, et al. Combined screening with ultrasound and mammography vs mammography alone in women at elevated risk of breast cancer. JAMA 2008;299(18):2151–63.
8. Corsetti V, Houssami N, Ferrari A, et al. Breast screening with ultrasound in women with mammography-negative dense breasts: evidence on incremental cancer detection and false positives, and associated cost. Eur J Cancer 2008;44(4):539–44.
9. Kaplan SS. Clinical utility of bilateral whole-breast US in the evaluation of women with dense breast tissue. Radiology 2001;221(3):641–9.
10. Hooley RJ, Greenberg KL, Stackhouse RM, et al. Screening US in patients with mammographically dense breasts: initial experience with Connecticut Public Act 09-41. Radiology 2012;265(1):59–69.
11. Niklason LT, Christian BT, Niklason LE, et al. Digital tomosynthesis in breast imaging. Radiology 1997;205(2):399–406.
12. Park JM, Franken EA Jr, Garg M, et al. Breast tomosynthesis: present considerations and future applications. Radiographics 2007;27(Suppl 1):S231–40.
13. Alakhras M, Bourne R, Rickard M, et al. Digital tomosynthesis: a new future for breast imaging? Clin Radiol 2013;68(5):e225–36.
14. Available at: http://breasttomo.com/sites/default/files/010-WP-00060-Rev2_June2012-TomoWhitePaper.pdf.
15. Poplack SP, Tosteson TD, Kogel CA, et al. Digital breast tomosynthesis: initial experience in 98 women with abnormal digital screening mammography. AJR Am J Roentgenol 2007;189(3):616–23.
16. Good WF, Abrams GS, Catullo VJ, et al. Digital breast tomosynthesis: a pilot observer study. AJR Am J Roentgenol 2008;190(4):865–9.
17. Andersson I, Ikeda DM, Zackrisson S, et al. Breast tomosynthesis and digital mammography: a comparison of breast cancer visibility and BIRADS classification in a population of cancers with subtle mammographic findings. Eur Radiol 2008;18(12):2817–25.
18. Skaane P, Bandos AI, Gullien R, et al. Comparison of digital mammography alone and digital mammography plus tomosynthesis in a population-based screening program. Radiology 2013;267(1):47–56.
19. Ciatto S, Houssami N, Bernardi D, et al. Integration of 3D digital mammography with tomosynthesis for population breast-cancer screening (STORM): a prospective comparison study. Lancet Oncol 2013;14(7):583–9.
20. Friedewald SM, Rafferty EA, Rose SL, et al. Breast cancer screening using tomosynthesis in combination with digital mammography. JAMA 2014;311(24):2499–507.
21. Noroozian M, Hadjiiski L, Rahnama-Moghadam S, et al. Digital breast tomosynthesis is comparable to mammographic spot views for mass characterization. Radiology 2012;262(1):61–8.
22. Tagliafico A, Astengo D, Cavagnetto F, et al. One-to-one comparison between digital spot compression view and digital breast tomosynthesis. Eur Radiol 2012;22(3):539–44.
23. Zuley ML, Bandos AI, Ganott MA, et al. Digital breast tomosynthesis versus supplemental diagnostic mammographic views for evaluation of noncalcified breast lesions. Radiology 2013;266(1):89–95.

24. Brandt KR, Craig DA, Hoskins TL, et al. Can digital breast tomosynthesis replace conventional diagnostic mammography views for screening recalls without calcifications? A comparison study in a simulated clinical setting. AJR Am J Roentgenol 2013;200(2):291–8.

25. Waldherr C, Cerny P, Altermatt HJ, et al. Value of one-view breast tomosynthesis versus two-view mammography in diagnostic workup of women with clinical signs and symptoms and in women recalled from screening. AJR Am J Roentgenol 2013;200(1):226–31.

26. Hakim CM, Chough DM, Ganott MA, et al. Digital breast tomosynthesis in the diagnostic environment: a subjective side-by-side review. AJR Am J Roentgenol 2010;195(2):W172–6.

27. Spangler ML, Zuley ML, Sumkin JH, et al. Detection and classification of calcifications on digital breast tomosynthesis and 2D digital mammography: a comparison. AJR Am J Roentgenol 2011;196(2):320–4.

28. Kopans D, Gavenonis S, Halpern E, et al. Calcifications in the breast and digital breast tomosynthesis. Breast J 2011;17(6):638–44.

29. Gur D, Bandos AI, Rockette HE, et al. Localized detection and classification of abnormalities on FFDM and tomosynthesis examinations rated under an FROC paradigm. AJR Am J Roentgenol 2011;196(3):737–41.

30. Zuley ML, Guo B, Catullo VJ, et al. Comparison of two-dimensional synthesized mammograms versus original digital mammograms alone and in combination with tomosynthesis images. Radiology 2014;271(3):664–71.

31. Gur D, Zuley ML, Anello MI, et al. Dose reduction in digital breast tomosynthesis (DBT) screening using synthetically reconstructed projection images: an observer performance study. Acad Radiol 2012;19(2):166–71.

32. Gur D, Abrams GS, Chough DM, et al. Digital breast tomosynthesis: observer performance study. AJR Am J Roentgenol 2009;193(2):586–91.

33. Hardesty LA, Kreidler SM, Glueck DH. Digital breast tomosynthesis utilization in the United States: a survey of physician members of the society of breast imaging. J Am Coll Radiol 2014;11(6):594–9.

34. Boone JM, Nelson TR, Lindfors KK, et al. Dedicated breast CT: radiation dose and image quality evaluation. Radiology 2001;221(3):657–67.

35. Lindfors KK, Boone JM, Nelson TR, et al. Dedicated breast CT: initial clinical experience. Radiology 2008;246(3):725–33.

36. Prionas ND, Lindfors KK, Ray S, et al. Contrast-enhanced dedicated breast CT: initial clinical experience. Radiology 2010;256(3):714–23.

37. Aminololama-Shakeri S, Prionas ND, Lindfors KK, et al. Detection of DCIS with dedicated breast CT. Annual RSNA Meeting. 2011.

38. Aminololama-Shakeri S, Nosratieh A, Lindfors KK, et al. Is contrast-enhanced dedicated breast CT superior to DBT or DM in the evaluation of BIRADS 4 and 5 breast lesions? Annual RSNA Meeting. Chicago, 2013.

39. Zuley ML, Sumkin JH, Ganott MA, et al. Comparison of contrast-enhanced cone beam CT to CE-MRI in the categorization of breast lesions. Annual RSNA Meeting. Chicago, 2011.

40. Chen L, Abbey CK, Nosratieh A, et al. Anatomical complexity in breast parenchyma and its implications for optimal breast imaging strategies. Med Phys 2012;39(3):1435–41.

41. Abbey CK, Nosrateih A, Sohl-Dickstein J, et al. Non-gaussian statistical properties of breast images. Med Phys 2012;39(11):7121–30.

42. Weigert JM, Bertrand ML, Lanzkowsky L, et al. Results of a multicenter patient registry to determine the clinical impact of breast-specific gamma imaging, a

molecular breast imaging technique. AJR Am J Roentgenol 2012;198(1): W69–75.

43. Brem RF, Floerke AC, Rapelyea JA, et al. Breast-specific gamma imaging as an adjunct imaging modality for the diagnosis of breast cancer. Radiology 2008; 247(3):651–7.

44. Brem RF, Petrovitch I, Rapelyea JA, et al. Breast-specific gamma imaging with 99mTc-sestamibi and magnetic resonance imaging in the diagnosis of breast cancer–a comparative study. Breast J 2007;13(5):465–9.

45. Berg WA, Weinberg IN, Narayanan D, et al. High-resolution fluorodeoxyglucose positron emission tomography with compression ("positron emission mammography") is highly accurate in depicting primary breast cancer. Breast J 2006; 12(4):309–23.

46. Hendrick RE. Radiation doses and cancer risks from breast imaging studies. Radiology 2010;257(1):246–53.

47. Skarpathiotakis M, Yaffe MJ, Bloomquist AK, et al. Development of contrast digital mammography. Med Phys 2002;29(10):2419–26.

48. Dromain C, Balleyguier C, Muller S, et al. Evaluation of tumor angiogenesis of breast carcinoma using contrast-enhanced digital mammography. AJR Am J Roentgenol 2006;187(5):W528–37.

49. Diekmann F, Diekmann S, Jeunehomme F, et al. Digital mammography using iodine-based contrast media: initial clinical experience with dynamic contrast medium enhancement. Invest Radiol 2005;40(7):397–404.

50. Lewin JM, Isaacs PK, Vance V, et al. Dual-energy contrast-enhanced digital subtraction mammography: feasibility. Radiology 2003;229(1):261–8.

51. Jong RA, Yaffe MJ, Skarpathiotakis M, et al. Contrast-enhanced digital mammography: initial clinical experience. Radiology 2003;228(3):842–50.

52. Dromain C, Thibault F, Muller S, et al. Dual-energy contrast-enhanced digital mammography: initial clinical results. Eur Radiol 2011;21(3):565–74.

53. Dromain C, Thibault F, Diekmann F, et al. Dual-energy contrast-enhanced digital mammography: initial clinical results of a multireader, multicase study. Breast Cancer Res 2012;14(3):R94.

54. Jochelson MS, Dershaw DD, Sung JS, et al. Bilateral contrast-enhanced dual-energy digital mammography: feasibility and comparison with conventional digital mammography and MR imaging in women with known breast carcinoma. Radiology 2013;266(3):743–51.

55. Badr S, Laurent N, Regis C, et al. Dual-energy contrast-enhanced digital mammography in routine clinical practice in 2013. Diagn Interv Imaging 2014;95(3):245–58.

Imaging of Pancreatic Neoplasms

Aparna Balachandran, MD[a],*, Priya R. Bhosale, MD[a], Chuslip Charnsangavej, MD[b],†, Eric P. Tamm, MD[a]

KEYWORDS

- Pancreatic adenocarcinoma • Pancreatic neuroendocrine neoplasms • Imaging
- Cystic pancreatic neoplasms • Pancreatic neoplasms • Radiology

KEY POINTS

- Adenocarcinoma of the pancreas has a high mortality rate. Imaging plays a critical role in determining patients who are surgically resectable.
- Pancreatic neuroendocrine neoplasms encompass diverse clinical entities. These neoplasms show distinctive patterns of spread, which is important to recognize on imaging.
- Pancreatic cysts are increasingly detected because of the increased utility of imaging. Recent updates to management need to be incorporated into the management of these patients.
- Imaging plays a central role in diagnosing and characterizing pancreatic neoplasms. Preoperative high-quality imaging is essential in planning surgery.

INTRODUCTION

Imaging is critical in the assessment of all pancreatic neoplasms. Pancreatic neoplasms can be divided into solid and cystic neoplasms. The most common solid neoplasm is pancreatic ductal adenocarcinoma (PDAC) accounting for 85% to 90% of all solid pancreatic neoplasms, and it is the fourth leading cause of cancer-related deaths.[1] PDAC is a diagnostic challenge in terms of early detection, imaging of exact extent of spread, disease response assessment, and postoperative follow-up because of the nonspecific symptoms associated with ductal adenocarcinoma in the early stages of the disease and because of the ill-defined appearance and infiltrative nature of the spread of the disease.[2] The treatment of ductal adenocarcinoma requires multidisciplinary planning so as to optimize the management of patients, especially in the selection of patients to undergo surgery.

The authors have nothing to disclose.
[a] Abdominal Imaging, The University of Texas MD Anderson Cancer Center, 1515 Holcombe Boulevard, Unit 1473, Houston, TX 77030, USA; [b] Abdominal Imaging, The University of Texas MD Anderson Cancer Center, 1515 Holcombe Boulevard, Houston, TX 77030, USA
† Deceased.
* Corresponding author.
E-mail address: abalachandran@mdanderson.org

Surg Oncol Clin N Am 23 (2014) 751–788
http://dx.doi.org/10.1016/j.soc.2014.07.002
1055-3207/14/$ – see front matter © 2014 Elsevier Inc. All rights reserved.

surgonc.theclinics.com

The next most common solid neoplasm arising from the pancreas is the pancreatic neuroendocrine tumor (PanNET), which accounts for 5% to 10% of all pancreatic solid tumors. PanNETs are a diverse group of tumors and comprise both functional tumors and nonfunctional tumors. Functional tumors produce high levels of different hormones, and this leads to patients presenting with a hormone-related syndrome. On imaging, these tumors typically have a distinct appearance when compared with PDAC. These tumors tend to be well defined and hypervascular. The importance in correctly identifying these tumors is based on the different prognosis of PanNET when compared with PDAC.

Pancreatic cystic neoplasms are increasingly detected as incidental findings.[3] These neoplasms can vary from the benign serous cystadenoma to the premalignant or malignant mucinous neoplasms and intraductal papillary mucinous neoplasms (IPMN). Imaging plays an important role in the surveillance of these cystic neoplasms when they are small and in defining anatomy, additional lesions, and invasive features when they are larger.

ANATOMY

The pancreas is a J-shaped retroperitoneal organ that is closely associated with peritoneal[4] ligaments (**Fig. 1**). There is a small portion of the tail of the pancreas that

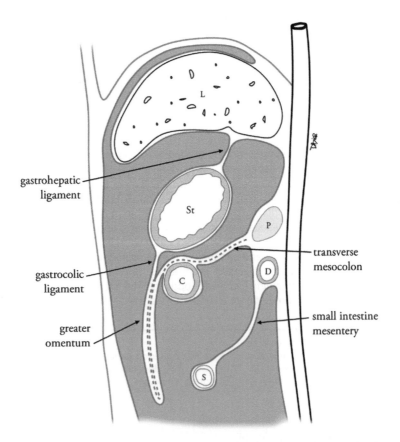

Fig. 1. The relationship of the pancreas to the peritoneum. C, colon; D, duodenum; P, pancreas; S, small bowel; St, stomach.

extends into the lienorenal ligament and is intraperitoneal. The pancreas is divided into the head, uncinate, neck, body, and tail of the pancreas. The head is the largest portion of the pancreas and is located in the curve of the duodenum and develops from both the ventral and dorsal pancreatic buds. The uncinate process is a triangular extension of the pancreas and is situated behind the superior mesenteric vessels. The neck of the pancreas is located anterior to the superior mesenteric vessels. The body and tail of the pancreas constitute the rest of the pancreas. There is no clear anatomic division between the body and tail of the pancreas.

Histologically, the predominant cell type in the pancreas is the acinar cell, accounting for approximately 80% of all the cells. Ductal epithelial cells constitute 10% to 15%, and islet cells constitute 1% to 2% of all the cells. A collagenous stroma is seen between these cells and carries the blood supply, nerves, and lymphatics to the pancreas.

The pancreas is supplied by the branches of the celiac axis and of the superior mesenteric artery (SMA). The superior pancreaticoduodenal arteries are branches of the gastroduodenal artery (GDA) and anastomose with the inferior pancreaticoduodenal arteries, which are branches of the SMA. The GDA arises from the common hepatic artery (CHA), a branch of the celiac axis (**Fig. 2**). In cases of celiac axis stenosis, enlarged pancreaticoduodenal arteries in the pancreatic head are seen on imaging and constitute a collateral pathway of blood supply from the SMA to the celiac axis (**Fig. 3**). The body and tail of the pancreas are supplied by branches of the splenic artery. The dorsal pancreatic artery typically arises from the splenic artery (but can have variable origin) and supplies the body and tail of the pancreas.[5] It has a course posterior to the pancreas. The pancreatica magna artery is the largest branch of the splenic artery and courses from left to right along the body and tail of the pancreas. Multiple small branches are given off from the splenic artery and also supply the body and tail.

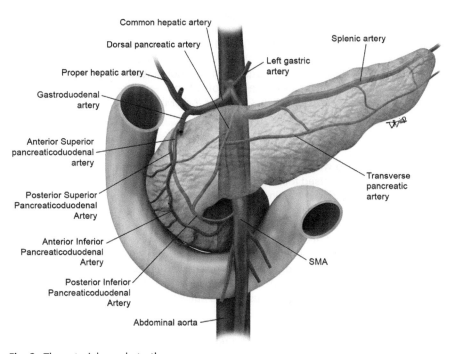

Fig. 2. The arterial supply to the pancreas.

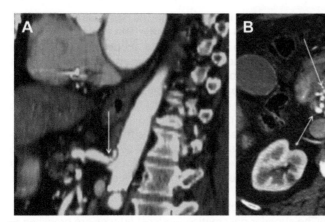

Fig. 3. (A) Sagittal planar reformatted image depicting median arcuate syndrome with narrowing of the celiac trunk (*arrow*). (B) Axial computed tomography image demonstrating arterial collaterals (*arrows*) via the pancreaticoduodenal arcade caused by celiac artery stenosis.

Michels described the vascular anatomy involving the celiac axis and SMA. This classic arterial anatomy has been seen in only 55% to 60% of patients.[6] The most common vascular variants are the replaced right hepatic artery arising from the SMA occurring in 11% (Michels type III anatomy) and the replaced left hepatic artery arising from the left gastric artery occurring in 10% of patients (Michels type II anatomy). Accurately identifying and reporting vascular variants is crucial in patients who are being considered for surgery as the presence of the variant anatomy can change the surgical plan.[7]

The venous drainage of the pancreas follows the arteries. Four major pancreaticoduodenal veins drain the head of the pancreas and empty into the gastrocolic branch of the superior mesenteric vein (SMV), portal vein, or jejunal branch of the SMV. Numerous veins also drain directly into the splenic vein.[8] The SMV and the splenic veins join posterior to the neck of the pancreas to form the portal vein. The inferior mesenteric vein may enter at this confluence in one-third of patients, enter the splenic vein close to this confluence in one-third of patients, or enter the SMV in one-third of patients.

TECHNIQUE
Ultrasound

In patients presenting with nonspecific abdominal pain, weight loss, or jaundice, the imaging modality often used for evaluation is ultrasound (US). At the authors' institution, patients are asked to be fasting for at least 4 hours before the procedure. A complete transabdominal US using a curved transducer is performed to include imaging of the liver, gallbladder, common duct, pancreas, spleen, kidneys, and vascular structures, such as the aorta and its branches, portal vein, and SMV.

US is widely available, reasonable, and does not use radiation. However, US is limited by being operator dependent and dependent on the body habitus of patients and because pancreatic masses can be obscured by overlying bowel gas. Despite this, US is frequently the initial imaging modality used because of the patients' presenting symptoms.

Computed Tomography

Multidetector row computed tomography (MDCT) is perhaps the most widely used modality in the staging of pancreatic neoplasms. The initial evaluation and follow-up in patients being considered for surgery is done using a pancreas protocol technique. At the authors' institution, this involves precontrast imaging from the dome of the liver to cover the entire liver reconstructed to 2.5-mm slice thickness images for review. Following this, a total of 125 mL of iodinated contrast is administered at a rate of 3 to 5 mL/s. Using bolus tracking, imaging is performed 10 seconds after a Hounsfield unit value of 100 is reached in the aorta at the level of the celiac axis. Scanning is performed from the dome of the liver to the iliac crests. This postcontrast sequence is referred to as the *pancreatic phase* or *late arterial phase* of imaging. *Portal venous phase* imaging is performed at a delay of 20 seconds from the pancreatic phase. Delayed images are obtained at a 15-second delay after the portal venous phase. Water is used as negative oral contrast. The images are reconstructed to 2.5-mm slice thickness for imaging review and at 0.625- or 1.25-mm slice thickness to create coronal and sagittal reformatted images.

Magnetic Resonance Imaging

The usual magnetic resonance imaging (MRI) examination at the authors' institution consists of axial T1 in and out of phase images; axial T2 fast spin echo with fat saturation sequence; axial dynamic 3-dimensional (3D) spoiled gradient echo sequence with fat saturation using parallel imaging obtained at 0, 20, 60, 120, and 180 seconds following the start of gadolinium-based intravenous (IV) contrast administration; delayed axial 3D spoiled gradient echo sequence with fat saturation at 5 minutes following contrast administration; diffusion sequence with b values of 0, 500, and 800; axial fast imaging using steady-state acquisition with fat saturation; and 3D MR cholangiopancreatography (MRCP) for cystic pancreatic lesions.

MRI is more expensive and less available when compared with CT. MRI is typically used as a problem-solving tool when CT cannot identify or characterize the pancreatic mass or a liver lesion in a patient with a pancreatic mass, in young patients especially for follow-up (to avoid repeated radiation exposure), and in patients who cannot receive iodinated IV contrast.

Octreotide or Somatostatin Receptor Scintigraphy (SRS)

Indium 111–labeled octreotide (a somatostatin analogue) can be used in the imaging of PanNETs. PanNETs that have a high expression of somatostatin receptors 2 and 5 can be detected by octreotide imaging. Octreotide imaging is obtained at 4 and 24 hours after the administration of the labeled octreotide. In addition to planar imaging, single-photon emission CT is performed on each patient to improve sensitivity.

Positron Emission Tomography–CT

Positron emission tomography (PET)-CT scans are obtained with patients fasting for 6 hours. The scans are performed on a dedicated 8-, 16-, or 64-MDCT scanner. The PET-CT scans are acquired approximately 1 hour after the administration of 8 to 12 mCi (296–444 MBq) of fluorine 18 (^{18}F) fluorodeoxyglucose (FDG). Blood glucose levels of less than or equal to 150 mg/dL are accepted for the purpose of the study. The scans are obtained with patients in a supine position and with the arms being extended above the patients' chest. The images are acquired from the skull base through the pelvis. The CT scans are obtained without oral or IV contrast agents and are reconstructed at 3-mm slice thickness images. These images are used for attenuation correction and also for diagnostic purposes.

PET-CT is more expensive and less available than CT. However, in patients with clinical suspicion of recurrent or progressive disease and the absence of imaging findings on CT, PET-CT can be used for further evaluation.

Gallium 68–Labeled PET Imaging

Using the concept of SRS, gallium 68 (^{68}Ga)–labeled somatostatin analogues are used as PET-CT tracers and have been shown in recent studies to have superior sensitivity and specificity. The advantages include shorter imaging time (45–90 minutes), easier availability of results, easier availability of tracer, and improved sensitivity and spatial resolution. The Gallium labeled somatostatin analogs include 68 gallium tetraazacy-clododecane tetraacetic acid–octreotate, which is predominantly a somatostatin receptor 2 analogue; 68 gallium DOTA Nal3-octreotide, a somatostatin receptor 2, 3 and 5 analogue; and 68 gallium DOTA Phe1 Tyr 3 octreotide, a somatostatin receptor 2 and 5 analogue.

Endoscopic US

Endoscopic US (EUS) combines US technology with endoscopy. A small US probe is attached at the tip of the endoscope and can be used to evaluate pancreatic lesions. A combination of radial and curvilinear arrays is used to obtain images. EUS allows for the real-time evaluation of pancreatic lesions and for fine-needle aspiration (FNA) when tissue diagnosis is needed.

The disadvantages are that EUS is invasive and operator dependent. However, the sensitivity of EUS is superior to MDCT; EUS-guided FNA can be performed to obtain tissue diagnosis.

PANCREATIC NEOPLASMS
PDAC

Epidemiology
PDAC is the fourth leading cause of cancer-related deaths in the United States and second only to colorectal cancer as a cause of gastrointestinal cancer–related deaths. In the United States, approximately 46,000 patients are diagnosed with PDAC annually.[1] The risk of developing pancreatic cancer increases with age. Almost all patients are older than 45 years. The incidence is greater in men than women (1.3–1.0) and is also more common in African Americans than Caucasians.

Risk factors
Smoking is a known reversible cause of increased risk of PDAC and has been shown to increase the risk by at least 1.5 times.[9–11] Studies have also shown that patients who are markedly overweight have an increased risk of pancreatic cancer. Lack of physical activity may also contribute to this increased risk in these patients.[12,13] Diets high in red meat and fat have also been linked to a higher risk of pancreatic cancer.[14,15] Patients with chronic pancreatitis have been shown to have an increase risk of PDAC.[16]

Hereditary and familial risk factors
Hereditary pancreatitis These patients often present with chronic pancreatitis before 20 years of age (**Table 1**). A consensus committee recommended screening for pancreatic cancer in patients with hereditary pancreatitis starting at 40 years of age.[17]

BRCA mutations Patients have been shown to have an increased risk of PDAC.[18] These patients also have an increased risk of breast, ovarian, fallopian tube, peritoneal, and prostate cancer.

Peutz-Jeghers syndrome This syndrome is an autosomal dominant syndrome with an increased risk of PDAC.[19,20] These patients also have an increased risk of small intestinal, gastric, esophageal, and gynecologic cancers.

Table 1 Hereditary risk factors for PDAC		
Syndrome	Gene	Chromosome Location
Hereditary breast/ovarian cancer	BRCA 2/BRCA 1	13q
Familial atypical multiple mole melanoma syndrome	CDKN2 A	9p
Peutz-Jeghers syndrome	STK 11	19p
Familial adenomatous polyposis	APC	5q
Hereditary nonpolyposis colon cancer syndrome	DNA mismatch genes	2p, 3p, 7p
Hereditary pancreatitis	PRSS 1/SPINK 1	5q, 7q

Familial atypical multiple mole melanoma syndrome Patients present with multiple nevi (usually more than 50), cutaneous and ocular melanomas, and pancreatic cancers.[21] Patients with familial atypical multiple mole melanoma syndrome have an increased risk of brain and nervous system, bladder cancers and sarcomas.

Hereditary nonpolyposis colon cancer or Lynch syndrome These patients have an increased risk for colorectal, endometrial, ovarian, gastric, small bowel, and pancreatic cancers.[22]

Familial pancreatic cancer Patients with multiple first- and second-degree relatives with pancreatic cancer without a known genetic defect are at an increased risk for PDAC. The risk is associated with the number of first-degree relatives with PDAC.[23,24]

Imaging appearance
US PDAC has an ill-defined, hypoechoic, hypovascular solid appearance on US (**Fig. 4**). PDAC can cause common bile duct (CBD) and pancreatic duct (PD) obstruction called the *double duct sign*. Imaging with Doppler will allow for identifying the relationship to celiac axis, SMA, portal vein, and SMV. Sensitivities between 83% and 88% have been reported.[25,26]

MDCT PDAC has an ill-defined low-attenuation appearance on CT (**Figs. 5** and **6**). The margins of the tumor are often difficult to perceive. There is periarterial extension seen.

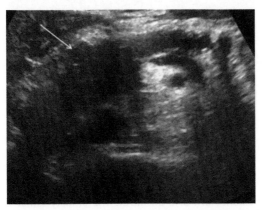

Fig. 4. Imaging appearance of PDAC on US. The arrow points to the ill-defined, hypoechoic PDAC in the head of the pancreas causing pancreatic ductal dilatation.

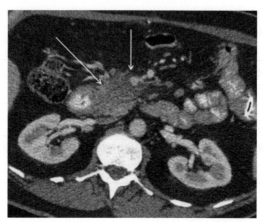

Fig. 5. Imaging appearance of PDAC on MDCT. The arrows point to the ill-defined, low-attenuation mass, which infiltrates around the superior mesenteric vessels.

The primary tumor is best seen on the pancreatic phase of imaging because of the increased enhancement of surrounding normal pancreatic parenchyma and the primary tumor being highlighted because of its low-attenuation appearance. The primary tumor can also occlude veins from mass effect with adjacent venous collaterals. Metastases to the nodes, liver, and peritoneum are the most common sites of spread. Small PDAC can be isoattenuating; in these instances, evaluation for secondary signs, such as duct dilatation, abrupt duct obstruction, venous obstruction, or contour abnormality, should be made.[27] The incidence of isoattenuating tumors varies, ranging from 11% to 27% based on the size of the PDAC.[27–29] The sensitivities of MDCT in the detection of PDAC vary based on the size of PDAC and typically range from 72% to 97% for all tumors.[30–32]

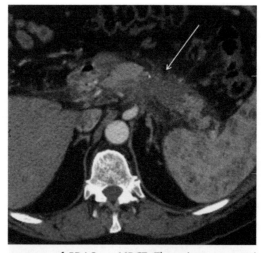

Fig. 6. Imaging appearance of PDAC on MDCT. The primary tumor is in the tail of the pancreas with infiltrative changes extending to abut the left adrenal gland and the celiac artery (*arrow*).

CT has a sensitivity of 94% for the assessment of vascular involvement.[33] A study by Lu and colleagues[34] showed that surface involvement of the vessel by the tumor on CT correlated with the likelihood of invasion. Fifty percent to 75% contiguity with the vessel was associated with an 88% likelihood of invasion, and greater than 75% contiguity was associated with 100% invasion.

Currently standardized terminology to reflect the extent of vascular involvement has come into place. Vascular involvement of less than or equal to 180° of the circumference[35] of the vessel is called *abutment* (**Fig. 7**). Vascular involvement of greater than 180° of the circumference of the vessel is called *encasement* (**Fig. 8**). This terminology has been incorporated into the treatment planning as discussed under "Staging."

MRI PDAC has low T1 signal intensity and intermediate T2 signal intensity and demonstrates an enhancement pattern similar to MDCT (**Fig. 9**). During the dynamic contrast enhancement, the primary tumor is best seen on the pancreatic phase of imaging because of the increased enhancement of surrounding normal pancreatic parenchyma and the primary tumor being highlighted because of its low signal intensity. Diffusion-weighted imaging may be of value in these tumors.[36,37] However, diffusion-weighted imaging has shown variability in PDAC,[38] with 38 tumors of 80 being hyperintense, 12 isointense, and 4 hypointense to the pancreas.

PET-CT PET-CT has a limited role in the staging of PDAC (**Fig. 10**) when the disease is operable.[39] The reported sensitivity and specificity are 46% to 71% and 63% to 100%, respectively.[40] However, PET-CT may have a role when CT is equivocal and IV contrast cannot be used, for patients with nondiagnostic biopsies and patients with metastatic disease to monitor therapy, and to detect recurrence.[41]

STAGING OF PDAC

The American Joint Committee on Cancer's (AJCC) seventh edition uses the TNM staging for PDAC. The TNM staging is shown in **Table 2**. However, in addition to this, PDAC is also staged by resectability criteria. These criteria are an evolving group of criteria. PDAC can be divided (**Table 3**) into resectable tumors (**Fig. 11**) (no metastatic disease and no vascular involvement), borderline resectable tumors (see

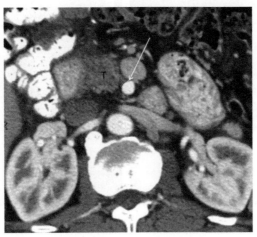

Fig. 7. PDAC (T) abutting the SMA (outlined by *red curve* involving less than 180° of the circumference of the SMA). The *arrow* points to the region of abutment of the SMA.

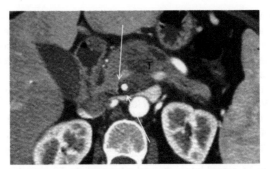

Fig. 8. PDAC (T) encasing the SMA (outlined by *red curve* involving more than 180° of the circumference of the SMA). This PDAC is locally advanced. The *arrows* point to the start and the end of the region of encasement of the SMA.

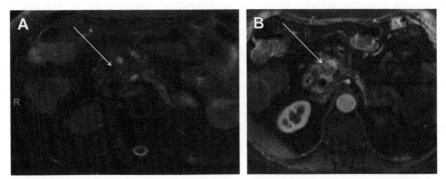

Fig. 9. (*A*) PDAC on MRI. PDAC in the head of the pancreas demonstrates low T2 signal intensity, which may be related to the presence of fibrous tissue. (*B*) PDAC on MRI. PDAC in the head of the pancreas demonstrates ill-defined margins and poor enhancement when compared with the rest of the pancreas. The *arrows* point to the PDAC.

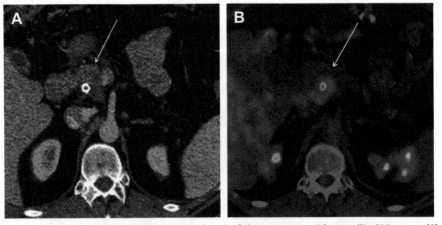

Fig. 10. (*A*) Poorly enhancing PDAC in the head of the pancreas with metallic CBD stent. (*B*) Low-level FDG uptake is seen in the PDAC in the head of the pancreas with adjacent metallic CBD stent, which may also contribute to FDG uptake from inflammation in this region. The *arrows* point to the PDAC.

Table 2
AJCC TNM staging

Stage	Description
Tx	Primary tumor cannot be assessed
T0	No evidence of primary tumor
Tis	Carcinoma in situ (rarely occurs)
T1	Tumor size ≤2 cm, not spread beyond the pancreas
T2	Tumor size >2 cm, not spread beyond the pancreas
T3	Tumor has extended beyond the pancreas but does not involve major blood vessels or nerves
T4	Tumor has extended beyond the pancreas and involves major blood vessels or nerves
Nx	Regional node involvement cannot be assessed
N0	Regional nodes not involved
N1	Regional node/nodes involved
M0	No distant metastases is present
M1	Distant metastases present

From AJCC: Exocrine and endocrine pancreas. In: Edge SB, Byrd DR, Compton CC, et al, editors. AJCC cancer staging manual. 7th edition. New York: Springer; 2010. p. 241–9; with permission.

Fig. 7),[35,42,43] locally advanced tumors (**Fig. 12**), and tumors with metastatic disease (**Fig. 13**). The borderline resectable criteria shown in **Table 3** are the MD Anderson criteria. These patients are treated with neoadjuvant chemotherapy and chemoradiation therapy. In the absence of progression, these patients are considered for surgery. Locally advanced tumors are those tumors with encasement of the celiac trunk or SMA and are not surgically resectable. As treatments for PDAC change, the borderline criteria will continue to change.

Table 3
Resectability criteria based on MD Anderson criteria

Resectable	Borderline Resectable	Locally Advanced	Metastatic Disease
No metastatic disease No vascular involvement	Short segment encasement of the CHA (type A) Abutment of the SMA (type A) Short segment occlusion of the SMV, SMV/PV confluence (type A) Indeterminate small liver or peritoneal nodules (type B) Associated comorbidities with borderline performance status (type C)	Encasing celiac trunk or SMA Venous encasement with poor surgical options	Metastatic disease at presentation

Abbreviation: PV, portal vein.

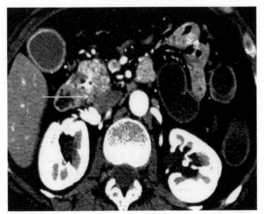

Fig. 11. Subtle, poorly enhancing PDAC in the head of the pancreas with adjacent CBD stent and artifact from this. This tumor is resectable and is separate from the major vessels. The *arrows* points to the PDAC.

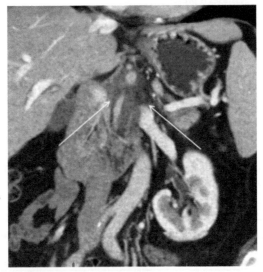

Fig. 12. Locally advanced PDAC encasing the SMA. The *arrows* point to the PDAC encasing the SMA seen in the coronal plane.

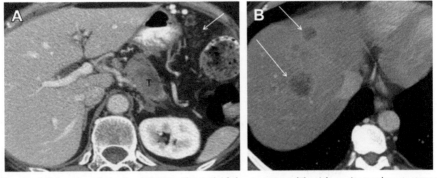

Fig. 13. (*A*) Poorly enhancing PDAC in the tail of the pancreas (T) with peritoneal metastases (*arrow*). (*B*) Low-attenuation liver metastases (*arrows*) in a patient with PDAC.

PanNETs
Epidemiology

PanNETs have an incidence of approximately 1 per 100,000 people per year and account for approximately 3% to 5% of all pancreatic tumors.[44] The incidence has increased 2 to 3 fold in the last 2 decades, with a prevalence of greater than 100,000 patients.[45] Most of PanNETs are sporadic. PanNETs arise from the pluripotent cells of the ductal epithelium[46] and not from the islet cells as previously thought. PanNETs stain positively for chromogranin and synaptophysin because of their shared histologic features with neuroendocrine tumors elsewhere in the body.

PanNETs are divided into functional tumors and nonfunctional tumors. Functional tumors produce a hormone with a clinically detectable syndrome. Nonfunctional tumors either do not produce a hormone or produce a hormone that is clinically silent. The most common functional tumors are insulinomas and gastrinomas. Other types include VIPoma, glucagonomas, and somatostatinomas. Currently, nonfunctional PanNETs account for 50% to 70% of all PanNETs.

Risk Factors

PanNETs can be seen with increased incidence in hereditary syndromes like in multiple endocrine neoplasia (MEN) I, von Hippel-Lindau (vHL), tuberous sclerosis, and neurofibromatosis type I.

MEN I

This disorder is an autosomal dominant inherited disorder. There is a mutation in the MEN I gene in 70% to 95% of patients with MEN I syndrome that is thought to be responsible for this disorder. MEN I syndrome has a high association with the occurrence of PanNETs. MEN I syndrome is characterized by the 3Ps, namely, parathyroid hyperplasia or tumors of the parathyroid, pituitary tumors, and PanNETs (Fig. 14). Other tumors are seen, such as carcinoid tumors and adrenocortical adenomas or carcinomas. More than 50% of patients present before 20 years of age. The leading causes of morbidity and mortality are related to PanNETs and carcinoid tumors.

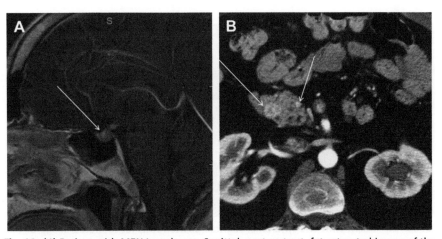

Fig. 14. (A) Patient with MEN I syndrome. Sagittal, postcontrast, fat-saturated image of the brain demonstrating a pituitary adenoma (arrow). (B) Patient with MEN I syndrome. PanNETs are hypervascular nodules seen in the head of the pancreas (arrows).

vHL syndrome

The vHL syndrome is an autosomal dominant inherited disorder characterized by a mutation in the vHL gene. The vHL gene codes for a vHL protein. This protein normally binds to the hypoxia inducible factor alpha (HIF α). When the vHL gene is mutated, the protein does not bind to HIF α, leading to the transcription of genes that code for growth factors, such as the vascular endothelial growth factor and the platelet-derived growth factor. The vHL syndrome is characterized by hemangioblastomas (which can occur in the retina and central nervous system), pheochromocytomas, renal cysts and renal cell carcinomas, pancreatic cysts (**Fig. 15**), pancreatic serous cystadenoma, and PanNETs. The leading cause of morbidity and mortality is renal cell carcinoma.

Tuberous sclerosis

Tuberous sclerosis is an autosomal dominant inherited disorder characterized by a mutation in the tuberous sclerosis complex genes 1 or 2. These genes code for the proteins hamartin and tuberin, which are tumor suppressor proteins. These patients often present with difficulty in learning. Patients with tuberous sclerosis can have giant cell astrocytomas, cortical tubers, subependymal nodules in the nervous system, facial angiofibromas, cardiac rhabdomyomas, cysts similar to lymphangioleiomyomatosis in the lungs, PanNETs (**Fig. 16**), renal cysts, angiomyolipomas of the kidneys, and rarely renal cell carcinomas.

Imaging

Insulinoma

Insulinoma is the most common functional PanNET and is characterized by inappropriately high insulin levels resulting in a hypoglycemic state. Patients can present with symptoms of hypoglycemia, such as with dizziness, excessive sweating, and unconsciousness. Patients may also present with neuroglycopenic symptoms, such as blurred vision, diplopia, confusion, and abnormal behavior.

Ninety percent of insulinomas are sporadic, and the remaining 10% are associated with MEN I syndrome. Ninety percent of insulinomas are solitary and small (less than 2 cm in size), and 90% of insulinomas are benign.[47] With complete surgical resection,

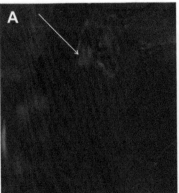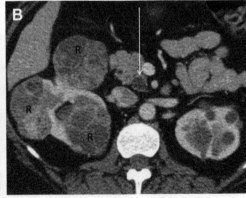

Fig. 15. (*A*) Patient with vHL syndrome. Sagittal, postcontrast, fat-saturated image of the spine demonstrates an enhancing hemangioblastoma within the spinal cord (*arrow*). A prior resection was attempted in this patient. (*B*) Patient with vHL syndrome. Axial CT depicts a cystic PanNET (*arrow*) and renal cell carcinomas (R).

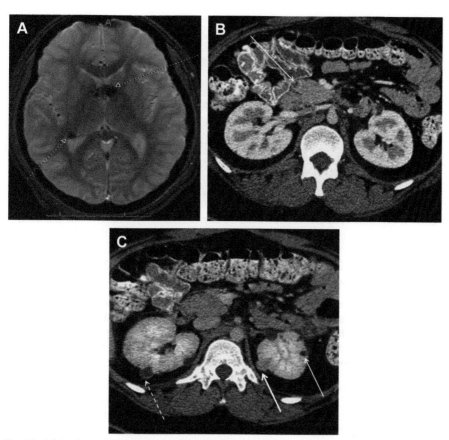

Fig. 16. (*A*) Patient with tuberous sclerosis. Axial MRI brain demonstrates calcified subepen-dymal nodules bilaterally (*arrows*). (*B*) Patient with tuberous sclerosis. Axial CT demonstrates a cystic PanNET with rim enhancement (*arrow*). (*C*) Patient with tuberous sclerosis. Spectrum of renal findings in tuberous sclerosis. Angiomyolipoma (*thin solid arrow*), renal cell carci-noma (*thick solid arrow*), and renal cyst (*dotted arrow*) are all seen in this patient.

a cure rate of greater than 95% is achieved.[48,49] Large insulinomas (>3 cm in size) may be associated with malignant behavior.

US Insulinomas appear as hypoechoic nodules within the pancreas on US. However, the sensitivity of transabdominal US is poor (9%–64%) because of the small size of insulinomas and their retroperitoneal location.[50]

Intraoperative US is of value to detect the primary insulinoma and its relation to the PD and also to look for additional insulinomas. Intraoperative US is associated with high sensitivity (**Fig. 17**).

MDCT Primary insulinomas are best seen on the pancreatic phase of enhancement as homogeneously enhancing nodules within the pancreas. Insulinomas are small, well-defined, and typically hypervascular tumors (**Fig. 18**). Additional sites of insulinomas within the pancreas may be found on CT, especially in patients with MEN I syndrome. The sensitivity of CT depends on the size of the insulinoma. As the size increases, there is increased sensitivity. Recent papers with the use of thin-section MDCT report

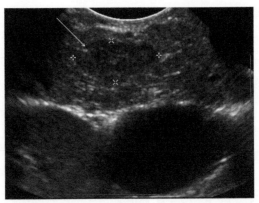

Fig. 17. Insulinoma seen on intraoperative US as a uniformly hypoechoic nodule (*arrow*).

higher sensitivities. One of the papers reports a sensitivity of 63.0% prospectively,[51] and another has a sensitivity as high as 94.4%.[52]

MRI As on CT, insulinomas appear as small, hypervascular, and homogenous tumors on MRI. Insulinomas are of intermediate to high T2 signal intensity. Papers have reported MRI sensitivities at around 90% to 92%.[53,54] MRI may be especially of value in young patients with MEN I requiring repeated imaging. MRI is noninvasive and without radiation risk.

Nuclear medicine imaging Insulinomas may express somatostatin receptor subtype 2 in 50% to 60% of the tumors; octreotide imaging, which uses a somatostatin analogue, is not sensitive in insulinoma detection. ^{68}Ga-labeled DOTA octreotide is not sensitive in insulinomas for the same reason.

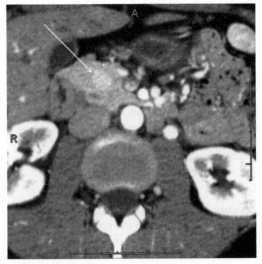

Fig. 18. Insulinoma on MDCT. A subtle and uniformly hypervascular pancreatic head nodule corresponds to the insulinoma (*arrow*).

Gastrinoma

Gastrinoma is the second most common functional PanNET and is characterized by inappropriately high levels of gastrin.[55] Because of the high levels of gastrin and gastric acid production, patients often have refractory peptic ulcer disease, reflux esophagitis, abdominal pain, diarrhea, and low gastric pH. Ninety percent of gastrinomas occur in the gastrinoma triangle, which is a triangle formed by the area between the cystic duct and CBD confluence, the junction of the second and third portions of the duodenum, and the junction of the neck and body of the pancreas. Twice as many gastrinomas occur in the duodenum as they do in the pancreas. The clinical syndrome associated with gastrinoma is known as *Zollinger Ellison syndrome*. Pancreatic gastrinomas tend to be larger in size (mean size is 3.8 cm).[56] More than 60% of gastrinomas are malignant at the time of presentation with lymph node and liver metastases. In 2% to 24% of patients, gastrinomas can have a site of origin other than the duodenum or the pancreas.

US Gastrinomas are larger than insulinomas and are hypoechoic and well defined on transabdominal US. A well-defined hyperechoic halo may be seen. Increased vascularity can be seen on Doppler images.[57] US may be of help in assessing gastrinomas because of their larger sizes. Limitations include retroperitoneal location, duodenal location (if a duodenal gastrinoma), and operator variability.

MDCT CT is typically the first line of imaging in PanNETs because of the availability and ability to detect metastatic disease in one imaging modality. MDCT has a wide range of sensitivities. As the size of the PanNET increases, the sensitivity increases.[58] In gastrinoma, because of the larger size of the tumor, there is higher sensitivity seen. The approximate sensitivity for PanNET with MDCT is reported to be between 63% and 94%.[52,59,60] The consensus statement states that the overall sensitivity of CT is approximately 82%, with a specificity of 92% in the detection of liver metastases.[60]

Gastrinomas are typically hypervascular tumors (**Fig. 19**). They may be homogeneous when small and heterogeneously enhancing when larger. It is thought that the enhancement is related to microvascular density.[61] They can show calcifications and central necrosis.[62] Occasionally, PanNETs may be isoattenuating or hypoattenuating to the rest of the pancreas; it is thought that this is related to poorer prognosis.[63,64]

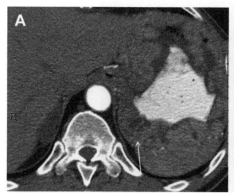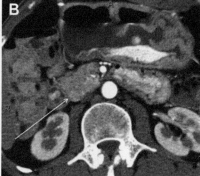

Fig. 19. (*A*) Gastrinoma on MDCT. Thickened gastric folds (*arrow*) from hypergastrinemia in this patient with a gastrinoma. (*B*) Gastrinoma on MDCT. Subtle hypervascular mass in the pancreatic head (*arrow*) corresponds to the gastrinoma.

Lymph node metastases are typically hypervascular with the short axis diameter of greater than 1 cm. Liver metastases can be homogeneously hypervascular or heterogeneously hypervascular in the early phase of enhancement and may demonstrate washout on the portal venous phase.

MRI Some studies have shown that MRI has an improved sensitivity when compared with CT in the detection of primary PanNETs,[53,65] with sensitivities up to 93%. Other studies have shown comparable sensitivities of CT and MRI in the detection of the primary tumor.[66] Studies have shown improved sensitivity of MRI when compared with CT in the detection of liver metastases.[66,67]

Gastrinomas are of low T1 signal intensity, intermediate to high T2 signal intensity, and demonstrate homogeneous or heterogeneous hypervascular enhancement based on their size. The liver metastases are low on T1, intermediate to high on T2, and demonstrate homogeneous or heterogeneous hypervascular enhancement.

Nuclear medicine imaging

Octreotide scan The sensitivity ranges from 75% to 100%, depending on the size of the gastrinoma.[68,69]

Gastrinomas appear as avid foci on octreotide imaging (**Fig. 20**), and octreotide imaging can be used to detect distant metastases. A limitation of octreotide is the poor spatial resolution, which can mask adjacent metastatic lymphadenopathy.

68-Ga-labeled PET Novel somatostatin analogues labeled with ^{68}Ga are being used as tracers for PET-CT imaging. Improved sensitivity in the detection of PanNETs has been shown over octreotide imaging, especially with improved spatial resolution.[70–72] An increased number of metastases have been shown in bones, soft tissue, and liver. In addition, ^{68}Ga-labeled imaging plays a role in planning peptide receptor radionuclide therapy.[73]

Nonfunctional PanNET

Nonfunctional PanNETs (NF PanNETs) are the most common type of PanNET, accounting for 50% to 70% of all PanNETs. Patients present with nonspecific symptoms, such as abdominal pain and weight loss, and occasionally may present with jaundice. Patients tend to present with larger tumors and more advanced disease.[74]

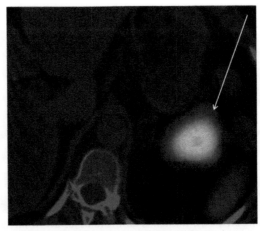

Fig. 20. Gastrinoma on octreotide imaging. A gastrinoma (*arrow*) is seen as an avid focus on octreotide imaging.

US

NF PanNETs are similar to gastrinomas and are hypoechoic and well defined on trans-abdominal US. A well-defined hyperechoic halo may be seen. Increased vascularity can be seen in the periphery on Doppler images.[57] These tumors tend to be heterogeneous with calcifications and cystic areas. Limitations include retroperitoneal location, overlying bowel gas, and operator variability.

MDCT

CT is typically the first line of imaging in all PanNETs and especially so in NF PanNETs. MDCT has a high sensitivity in NF PanNETs because of their larger sizes at presentation.[58] As previously stated, the estimated sensitivity for PanNET with MDCT is reported to be between 63% and 94%.[52,59,60] The consensus statement states that the overall sensitivity of CT is approximately 82%, with a specificity of 92% in the detection of liver metastases.[60]

NF PanNETs are typically heterogeneous tumors. They demonstrate heterogeneous enhancement (**Fig. 21**). They can show calcifications (20%–50%) and central necrosis.[62,75] NF PanNETs may be isoattenuating (**Fig. 22**) or hypoattenuating (**Fig. 23**) to the rest of the pancreas, and this is thought to be related to poorer prognosis.[63,64]

Lymph node metastases are typically hypervascular with the short axis diameter of greater than 1 cm. Liver metastases can be homogeneously hypervascular or heterogeneously hypervascular in the early phase of enhancement and may demonstrate washout on the portal venous phase.

MRI

As stated before, there is some controversy regarding CT versus MRI in PanNET detection. Some studies have shown that MRI has a superior sensitivity, with sensitivities up to 93%,[53,65] whereas other studies have shown comparable sensitivities of CT and MRI.[66] However, most studies have shown improved sensitivity of MRI when compared with CT in the detection of liver metastases.[66,67]

NF PanNETs are of low T1 signal intensity, intermediate to high T2 signal intensity, and demonstrate heterogeneous enhancement (**Fig. 24**). They can demonstrate hyperintense signal (more common) but also isointense or hypointense signal when compared with the rest of the pancreas. The liver metastases are low on T1, intermediate to high on T2, and demonstrate heterogeneous hypervascular enhancement.

A   **B**

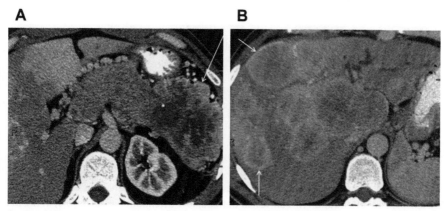

Fig. 21. (*A*) Hypervascular NF PanNET on MDCT. A large NF PanNET is seen in the tail of the pancreas (*arrow*) with heterogeneous enhancement. (*B*) NF PanNET on MDCT. Multiple, hypervascular liver metastases are seen (*arrows*).

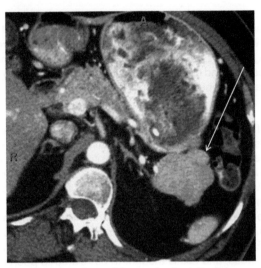

Fig. 22. Isoattenuating NF PanNET (*arrow*) is seen in the tail of the pancreas.

Nuclear medicine imaging

Octreotide scan The sensitivity ranges from 75% to 100% but is usually high in NF PanNET.[68,69] An important consideration is that NF PanNETs with a high proliferative index may not take up octreotide (see **Fig. 22**) and may demonstrate FDG uptake.[76]

NF PanNETs appear as avid foci on octreotide imaging, and octreotide imaging can be used to detect distant metastases. A limitation of octreotide is the poor spatial resolution, which can mask adjacent metastatic lymphadenopathy.

[18]F FDG PET-CT There is a limited role of FDG PET-CT in the imaging of pancreatic neuroendocrine tumors with high Ki 67 index (proliferation index). These tumors may not show octreotide uptake and are imaged with high sensitivity on ^{18}F FDG PET-CT.

[68]Ga-labeled PET Somatostatin analogues labeled with ^{68}Ga are being used for PET-CT imaging. Improved sensitivity in the detection of all PanNETs has been shown

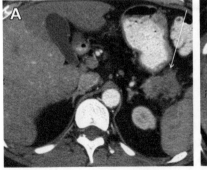
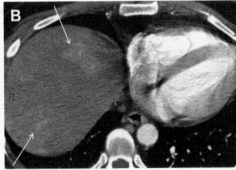

Fig. 23. (*A*) Low-attenuation NF PanNET. Ill-defined, low-attenuation mass (*arrow*) in the tail of the pancreas corresponds to an NF PanNET. (*B*) Multiple, hypervascular liver metastases (*arrows*) despite low-attenuation appearance to the primary tumor in the tail of the pancreas.

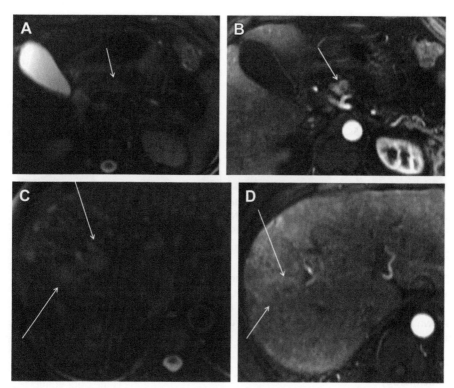

Fig. 24. (*A*) NF PanNET on MRI. T2 hyperintense NF PanNET is seen in the neck of the pancreas (*arrow*). (*B*) NF PanNET on MRI. Hypervascular NF PanNET is seen in the neck of the pancreas (*arrow*). (*C*) NF PanNET on MRI. T2 hyperintense liver metastases (*arrows*) are seen well. (*D*) NF PanNET on MRI. Poorly seen hypervascular liver metastases (*arrows*), better depicted on T2-weighted imaging.

over octreotide imaging, especially with improved spatial resolution.[70–72] An increased number of metastases have also been shown in bones, soft tissue, and liver. In addition, ^{68}Ga-labeled imaging plays a role in planning peptide receptor radionuclide therapy[73]; this modality may become the favored functional imaging in all PanNETs.

UNUSUAL APPEARANCE AND PATTERNS OF SPREAD PANNETS

PanNETs can be cystic in appearance in up to 17% of cases (**Fig. 25**).[55,77] These Pan-NETs can be completely cystic but demonstrate a hypervascular rim in 90% of cases.[55] These cystic tumors tend to be larger and more common than solid tumors in patients with MEN I.

NF PanNETs can cause venous tumor thrombus (**Fig. 26**) similar to renal cell carcinoma and hepatocellular carcinoma.[78–80] The venous tumor thrombi are seen as direct tumor extension into an adjacent vein with venous expansion and enhancing thrombus within the vein (the enhancement is similar to the PanNET).

NF PanNETs can also invade and grow into the main PD.[78]

Venous tumor thrombus and intraductal tumor are of importance because of the need for complete surgical resection. These areas may be missed before surgery, and knowledge of these is valuable in patients with NF PanNETs.

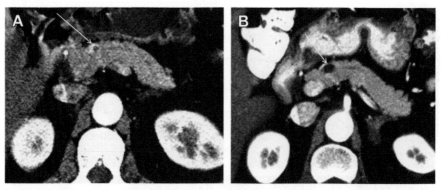

Fig. 25. (*A*) Cystic NF PanNET on MDCT. Cystic NF PanNET with rim enhancement (*arrow*) is seen. (*B*) Cystic NF PanNET on MDCT. Cystic NF PanNET (*arrow*) in the same patient after a period of 5 years. The rim enhancement is not as well seen and may be noted earlier.

STAGING

The staging system for PanNETs is the same as that for PDAC. This staging is shown on **Table 2**.

In addition, the AJCC and World Health Organization (WHO) have a grading system shown in **Tables 4** and **5**. This grading is useful in determining the proliferative index and prognosis in patients.

CYSTIC PANCREATIC LESIONS
Epidemiology

Incidental pancreatic cysts are diagnosed with increasing frequency because of the increased use of imaging. Pancreatic cysts may be detected in more than 2% of patients who undergo abdominal imaging for unrelated reasons.[81,82] Cystic lesions of the pancreas can be benign or malignant. Symptomatic cysts are associated with a higher rate of malignancy. Asymptomatic cysts may be benign, premalignant, or malignant. Pancreatic cystic neoplasms account for 10% to 15% of all pancreatic cysts and to less than 1% of primary pancreatic malignancies.[83] Primary cystic lesions of the pancreas include pseudocysts, lymphoepithelial cysts, serous cystadenomas, mucinous cystadenomas, and cystadenocarcinomas (mucinous cystic neoplasms

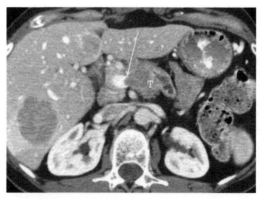

Fig. 26. NF PanNET with venous tumor thrombus. NF PanNET (T) is shown growing into the splenic portal venous confluence (*arrow*).

Table 4
AJCC grading of PanNETs

Grade	Mitotic Count	Ki 67 Index (%)
G1	<2	≤2
G2	2–20	3–20
G3	>20	>20

Adapted from Edge SB, Byrd DR, Compton CC, et al, editors. AJCC cancer staging manual. 7th edition. New York: Springer; 2010.

[MCN]), IPMN, and solid pseudopapillary epithelial neoplasms (SPENs) of the pancreas. Most cystic lesions are pancreatic pseudocysts, accounting for 70% of all pancreatic cysts.[84] Cystic tumors of the pancreas tend to occur in certain age groups. The SPENs typically occur in young women; the MCNs (resemble the MCN of the ovary) occur in middle-aged women; and the serous cystadenomas (SCA) occur in older women.[85] These respective cystic tumors have been called as the "daughter, mother and grandmother spectrum of cystic pancreatic neoplasms."[86] Both SPENs and SCAs can occur in men; they are more common in women.

Risk Factors

Pancreatitis is a risk factor for the formation of pseudocysts. Seventy-five percent to 85% of pseudocysts are seen in the setting of alcoholic or gall stone–related pancreatitis. In children, pseudocysts are most commonly seen in the setting of trauma.

SCAs are seen in vHL syndrome in 12% of patients.[87,88] Pancreatic cysts are seen in 7% to 10% of patients with autosomal dominant polycystic kidney disease.

Imaging

Pseudocysts

Pseudocysts are the most common cause of a cystic pancreatic lesion. Pseudocysts are used to refer to pancreatic and peripancreatic fluid collections that are present 4 weeks after an acute episode of pancreatitis. They have a well-defined fibrous wall. The symptoms of acute pancreatitis include abdominal pain, nausea, and vomiting.

Table 5
WHO grading of PanNETs

Differentiation	Grade	Mitotic Count	Ki 67 Index	WHO Category
Well differentiated	Low G1	<2	<3	Neuroendocrine tumor, grade 1
	Intermediate G2	2–20	3–20	Neuroendocrine tumor, grade 1
Poorly differentiated	High G3	>20	>20	Neuroendocrine carcinoma, grade 3, small cell
				Neuroendocrine carcinoma, grade 3, small cell

Adapted from Rindi G, Arnold R, Bosman FT, et al. Nomenclature and classification of neuroendocrine neoplasms of the digestive system. In: Bosman TF, Carneiro F, Hruban RH, et al, editors. WHO classification of tumours of the digestive system. 4th edition. Lyon (France): International Agency for Research on Cancer (IARC); 2010.

US

Pseudocysts are typically unilocular and well-defined anechoic or hypoechoic lesions within the pancreas. There are typically no mural nodules seen. They can have low-level echoes or may be hypoechoic because of the hemorrhage or proteinaceous content. They can communicate with the pancreatic duct. Limitations include retroperitoneal location, overlying bowel gas, and operator variability.

MDCT

Pseudocysts are well-defined low-attenuation (cystic) lesions within or adjacent to the pancreas. Their walls may initially appear irregular but become smooth and well defined over time (**Fig. 27**). Their walls are usually thin but may be thickened initially.[89] There can be a communication to the main pancreatic duct. If there is hemorrhage in a pseudocyst, this will be of high attenuation on the noncontrast CT. Pseudocysts can be locally aggressive with erosion of adjacent vessels and formation of pseudoaneurysms.[90] The most commonly involved arteries are the superior pancreaticoduodenal, gastroduodenal, and splenic arteries.

MRI

Pseudocysts can be of high T1 and high T2 signal intensity because of the presence of hemorrhage or proteinaceous content in the cysts. On the MRCP sequences, the communication with the pancreatic duct can be demonstrated. There is no internal enhancement seen. The wall of the pseudocyst can show enhancement.

EUS FNA

EUS FNA can be helpful in excluding cystic neoplasms of the pancreas. A high cyst fluid amylase (>250 IU/L) and a low cyst fluid carcinoembryonic antigen (CEA) (<200 ng/mL) are suggestive of a pseudocyst.[91]

SPEN

SPENs used to be clinically symptomatic. With the increased use of imaging, approximately 50% of SPENs are detected incidentally. These tumors are rare and account for only 1% to 2% of all exocrine pancreatic tumors. The common presenting symptoms include abdominal pain, nausea, vomiting, weight loss, and palpable abdominal mass.[92] These symptoms are typically seen in young women.[93,94] SPENs are usually of low malignant potential. These tumors are predominantly solid and develop cystic

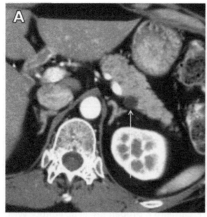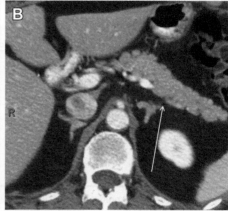

Fig. 27. (A) Pseudocyst (*arrow*) in the tail of the pancreas is a unilocular cystic lesion. (B) Pseudocyst has resolved with minimal changes from prior pseudocyst (*arrow*).

spaces when they degenerate. SPENs can be seen in older men with a more aggressive course. Abnormal nuclear position of beta catenin detected by immunohistochemistry is one of the ways to identify these neoplasms accurately. SPENs also express vimentin, CD 10, and neuron-specific enolase and show a loss of E-cadherin from the cytoplasmic membrane.[95]

US

These neoplasms can be divided into small neoplasms (<3 cm in size) and large neoplasms (>3 cm in size). When they are large, they are well-defined, hypoechoic masses that may have central anechoic areas from cystic degeneration. They can occasionally be completely cystic appearing. Calcifications may be present. When they are small, they can be ill-defined solid and hypoechoic masses.

MDCT

The large neoplasms are typically mixed solid and cystic neoplasms with calcifications (**Fig. 28**). Irregular peripheral calcifications can be seen in more than 65% of patients.[95,96] They demonstrate slow enhancement of the solid portions of the neoplasm.

When they are small, they are ill defined and more homogeneously solid with gradual enhancement.[97] Calcifications are also less common in smaller lesions.

Metastases have been reported in 5% to 15% of patients, with the most common sites being the liver, peritoneum, and nodes.[98–100]

MRI

SPENs can have a variable T1 and T2 signal intensity because of the cystic areas and hemorrhage (**Fig. 29**). They may have a low-signal-intensity T1 and T2 rim because of prior hemorrhage.[101,102] They follow the patterns of enhancement seen on CT.

As on CT, the smaller lesions are ill defined and more homogeneously solid with gradual enhancement.[97]

EUS FNA

SPENs may be completely solid (when small) and mixed solid and cystic (when large) in appearance. FNA helps in making the diagnosis due to the distinctive branching papillae with myxoid stroma of SPENs.[103]

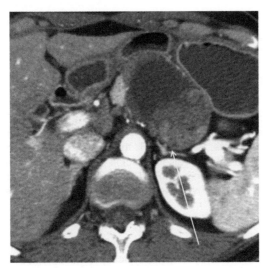

Fig. 28. SPEN (*arrow*) with mixed solid and cystic appearance on MDCT.

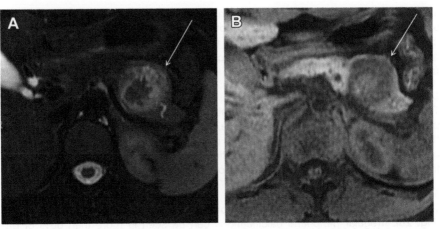

Fig. 29. (*A*) SPEN (*arrow*) with mixed T2 signal intensity. The central T2 hypointense area may correspond to hemorrhage or necrosis. (*B*) SPEN (*arrow*) with mixed T1 signal intensity. The central T1 hyperintense area may correspond to hemorrhage or necrosis.

MCNs

MCNs are mucin-producing neoplasms with an ovarian-type stroma.[104] Approximately 95% of MCNs occur in women. Only 2% to 5% are seen in men. Most MCNs occur in the body or tail of the pancreas. MCNs consist of mucinous cystadenomas, borderline MCN, and noninvasive and invasive mucinous cystadenocarcinomas.

US

Mucinous cystadenomas are typically cystic with less than 6 loculations and have cystic components, which may be larger than 2 cm in size. These lesions may have low-level echoes caused by mucinous content. MCNs can have peripheral calcifications and a thickened wall.[105] When there is a solid component or irregular wall, the possibility of a mucinous cystadenocarcinoma should be considered.

MDCT

Mucinous cystadenomas are typically cystic neoplasms with a few loculations. Peripheral calcifications can be seen in up to 15% of patients.[106,107] There can be enhancement of the wall of the mucinous cystadenoma. The presence of papillary projections, irregularly thickened wall, and calcifications should raise the possibility of mucinous cystadenocarcinomas (**Fig. 30**).

MRI

Mucinous cystadenomas demonstrate high T2 signal and variable T1 signal intensity based on the protein content of the cyst. There can be enhancement of the wall of the mucinous cystadenoma. Similar to CT, the presence of papillary projections and irregularly thickened wall should raise suspicion for mucinous cystadenocarcinomas. Calcifications are not well seen on MRI. The role of diffusion-weighted imaging and apparent diffusion coefficient remains controversial in the characterization of cystic pancreatic lesions.[108–110]

EUS FNA

The sensitivity and specificity of cyst fluid analysis is now approximately 57% to 94% and 85% to 97%.[111–113] The cyst fluid is typically low in amylase (<250 IU/L), high in CEA levels (>800 ng/mL), and can also have a high CA19-9 level when malignant.

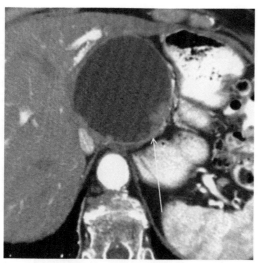

Fig. 30. Mucinous cystadenocarcinoma (*arrow*) with solid enhancing nodule in a large cystic lesion.

SCAs

SCAs are uncommon neoplasms accounting for 1% to 2% of all exocrine pancreatic tumors. More than 80% of these tumors occur in older women.[114] These tumors are typically benign. They tend to be asymptomatic and may be detected incidentally. They can produce symptoms with growth. As SCAs reach the 4 cm size, they may grow more rapidly (up to 2 cm per year); patients with SCAs can present with symptoms from mass effect of the pancreatic tumor.[115]

US

SCAs are cystic tumors with more than 6 loculations and have cystic components that are less than 2 cm in size. These cysts are separated by septations lined by epithelial cells. SCAs are well-defined lesions with a predominant solid hyperechoic appearance on US. This appearance is related to the septations and the smaller size of the cysts. If the cysts are larger, these can be seen as anechoic components within a predominantly hyperechoic solid mass. Calcifications are hyperechoic with posterior shadowing.

MDCT

SCAs are lobulated and cystic tumors on the noncontrast CT. They can demonstrate intense enhancement on the pancreatic parenchymal phase because of enhancement of the septations and appear as hypervascular masses (**Fig. 31**), especially when the cystic areas are small. When a definitive diagnosis cannot be made by CT, MRI may be of help in these patients. A central scar can be seen in up to 30% of patients. Coarse calcifications can be seen in the region of the central scar.

MRI

SCAs demonstrate high T2 signal intensity in the microcystic areas and have a characteristic appearance on T2-weighted images (see **Fig. 31**). The central scar and calcifications can be hypointense on T2-weighted sequences. They are usually hypointense on T1-weighted images. Comparable with CT, these lesions demonstrate intense early enhancement and can appear as hypervascular masses.

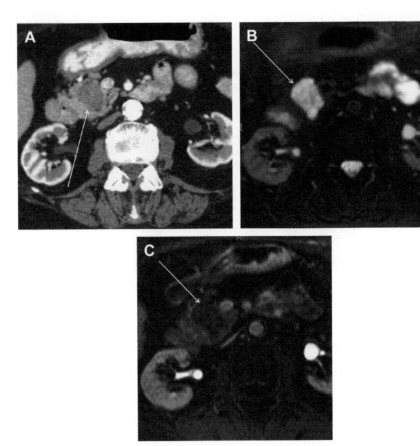

Fig. 31. (*A*) Serous cystadenoma. MDCT demonstrating an almost solid-appearing serous cystadenoma (*arrow*). (*B*) Serous cystadenoma. Serous cystadenoma (*arrow*) appears as a cluster of small cysts on T2-weighted imaging. (*C*) Serous cystadenoma. Serous cystadenoma (*arrow*) appears to be composed of multiple cysts on postcontrast images.

EUS FNA

EUS FNA can be useful in demonstrating the internal features of SCAs. Twenty percent to 50% of SCAs are positive for periodic acid Schiff reaction. The cyst fluid demonstrates serous fluid with low amylase (<250 IU/L), low CEA levels (<5 ng/mL), and low CA19-9 levels (<37 U/mL).

A variant of the SCA is the macrocystic SCA or oligocystic SCA. This entity consists of a cystic pancreatic lesion with cyst components approaching 1 to 2 cm in size. Sometimes the cyst components can be larger than 2 cm in size.[116–118] They can also contain fewer than 6 loculations and may be ill defined. Accurate differentiation from MCNs cannot be made in some instances based solely on imaging, and these lesions can be further evaluated with EUS FNA. These lesions also tend to be benign.

IPMNs

IPMNs are mucin-producing tumors arising from pancreatic ducts. They can be branch type, main duct type, or combined type, which involves both the branch duct and the main duct (**Figs. 32** and **33**). IPMNs can be divided into benign, borderline, and noninvasive or invasive mucinous adenocarcinomas. IPMNs can present with

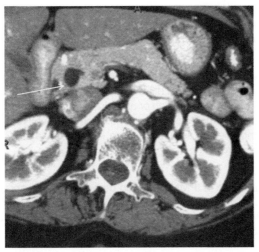

Fig. 32. Side branch IPMN (*arrow*) with a tail-like projection extending toward the main PD.

symptoms of abdominal pain and pancreatitis and can also be detected incidentally. There is a lack of ovarian-type stroma (that is seen in MCNs). IPMNs tend to affect older men more than women.

US

IPMNs can appear as areas of focal main pancreatic ductal dilatation in cases of the main duct type. In cases of the side branch type, US may demonstrate a multicystic pancreatic mass. The communication to the main pancreatic duct can be difficult to demonstrate on transabdominal imaging.

MDCT

Main duct IPMNs can present as sites of focal or diffuse main pancreatic ductal dilatation. The presence of enhancing irregular septations or nodules would suggest

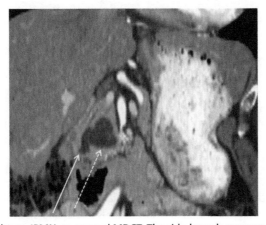

Fig. 33. Combined-type IPMN on coronal MDCT. The side-branch component (*dotted arrow*) in the head of the pancreas is seen. The main PD is also dilated (*solid arrow*), consistent with a combined-type IPMN.

mucinous adenocarcinoma (**Fig. 34**). In the branch duct–type IPMN, a unilocular small cystic mass or cluster of cysts can be seen. Communication with the main pancreatic duct may be seen on multiplanar reformats or curved planar reformats.

MRI

MRI and MRCP are of value in the characterization of IPMNs. Main duct IPMNs may present as focal or diffuse main duct dilatation. The side branch IPMN can appear as a T2 hyperintense unilocular cystic lesion or as a cluster of cysts in the pancreas close to the main duct. Communication can be demonstrated on the MRCP sequences. There can be enhancing nodules or septations seen in both types of IPMN suggestive of mucinous cystadenocarcinoma.

EUS FNA

EUS FNA is of great value in IPMNs and can demonstrate the communication to the main pancreatic duct and also the presence of papillary projections in the IPMN. It can also demonstrate the stringlike mucinous cystic fluid. IPMNs may have high amylase levels (>20,000 U/mL) and high CEA levels (>200 ng/mL).[119]

INTERNATIONAL CONSENSUS CRITERIA

There are evolving criteria for the prediction of malignancy in IPMNs based on imaging. The most recent international consensus guidelines from 2012 use the following criteria.

Pancreatic cysts of greater than 5 mm in diameter that communicate with the main pancreatic duct should be considered as branch duct IPMNs, with pseudocysts being in the differential diagnosis with a prior history of pancreatitis. Main duct IPMNs can be diagnosed in patients with a main duct greater than 5 mm with focal or diffuse dilatation without a cause to explain the ductal dilatation.

Features of high-risk stigmata on imaging include obstructive jaundice in patients with a cystic lesion of the pancreatic head, enhancing solid component, and a main pancreatic duct of 10 mm or greater in size. These patients should be resected.

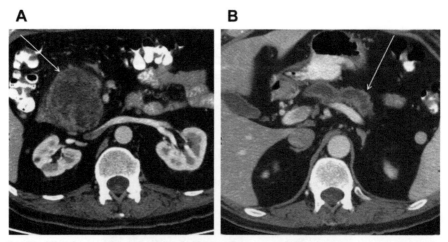

Fig. 34. (*A*) Adenocarcinoma arising in IPMN. There is a solid and cystic mass (*arrow*) in the head of the pancreas corresponding to the adenocarcinoma in this patient. (*B*) Adenocarcinoma arising in IPMN. There is main pancreatic ductal dilatation (*arrow*) from a main duct IPMN.

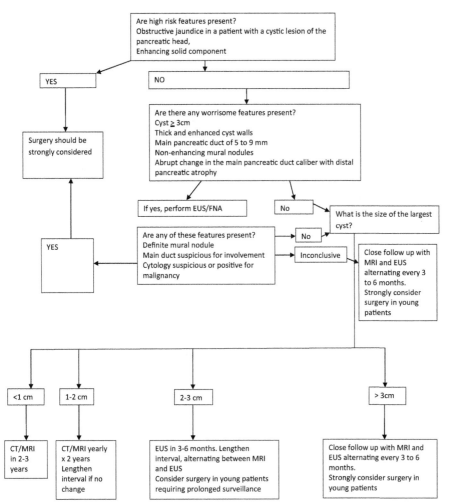

Fig. 35. Algorithm of International Consensus Criteria in Cystic Pancreatic Lesions. (*From* Tanaka M, Fernández-del Castillo C, Adsay V, et al. International consensus guidelines 2012 for the management of IPMN and MCN of the pancreas. Pancreatology 2012;12(3):183–97; with permission.)

Cysts with worrisome features on imaging include cysts that are 3 cm or greater, thick and enhanced cyst walls, main pancreatic duct of 5 to 9 mm, nonenhancing mural nodules, abrupt change in the main pancreatic duct caliber with distal pancreatic atrophy, and lymphadenopathy.[120,121] These patients should undergo evaluation with EUS FNA as demonstrated on **Fig. 35**.

SUMMARY

Pancreatic solid and cystic masses are being increasingly detected on routine imaging. Multimodality imaging plays an important role in the detection and characterization of these pancreatic masses. As resectability criteria continue to evolve, it is critical to obtain thin-section and high-quality imaging for accurate preoperative diagnosis. Management of pancreatic masses requires a multidisciplinary collaborative approach, with surgery being the definitive therapy in most solid masses.

REFERENCES

1. Siegel R, Ma J, Zou Z, et al. Cancer statistics, 2014. CA Cancer J Clin 2014;64: 9–29.
2. Porta M, Fabregat X, Malats N, et al. Exocrine pancreatic cancer: symptoms at presentation and their relation to tumour site and stage. Clin Transl Oncol 2005; 7:189–97.
3. Grutzmann R, Niedergethmann M, Pilarsky C, et al. Intraductal papillary mucinous tumors of the pancreas: biology, diagnosis, and treatment. Oncologist 2010;15:1294–309.
4. Vikram R, Balachandran A, Bhosale PR, et al. Pancreas: peritoneal reflections, ligamentous connections, and pathways of disease spread. Radiographics 2009;29:e34.
5. Witte B, Frober R, Linss W. Unusual blood supply to the pancreas by a dorsal pancreatic artery. Surg Radiol Anat 2001;23:197–200.
6. Winter TC 3rd, Nghiem HV, Freeny PC, et al. Hepatic arterial anatomy: demonstration of normal supply and vascular variants with three-dimensional CT angiography. Radiographics 1995;15:771–80.
7. Balachandran A, Darden DL, Tamm EP, et al. Arterial variants in pancreatic adenocarcinoma. Abdom Imaging 2008;33:214–21.
8. Mourad N, Zhang J, Rath AM, et al. The venous drainage of the pancreas. Surg Radiol Anat 1994;16:37–45.
9. Mack TM, Yu MC, Hanisch R, et al. Pancreas cancer and smoking, beverage consumption, and past medical history. J Natl Cancer Inst 1986;76:49–60.
10. Ghadirian P, Simard A, Baillargeon J. Tobacco, alcohol, and coffee and cancer of the pancreas. A population-based, case-control study in Quebec, Canada. Cancer 1991;67:2664–70.
11. Lynch SM, Vrieling A, Lubin JH, et al. Cigarette smoking and pancreatic cancer: a pooled analysis from the pancreatic cancer cohort consortium. Am J Epidemiol 2009;170:403–13.
12. Michaud DS, Giovannucci E, Willett WC, et al. Physical activity, obesity, height, and the risk of pancreatic cancer. JAMA 2001;286:921–9.
13. Arslan AA, Helzlsouer KJ, Kooperberg C, et al. Anthropometric measures, body mass index, and pancreatic cancer: a pooled analysis from the Pancreatic Cancer Cohort Consortium (PanScan). Arch Intern Med 2010;170:791–802.
14. Nothlings U, Wilkens LR, Murphy SP, et al. Meat and fat intake as risk factors for pancreatic cancer: the multiethnic cohort study. J Natl Cancer Inst 2005;97:1458–65.
15. Thiebaut AC, Jiao L, Silverman DT, et al. Dietary fatty acids and pancreatic cancer in the NIH-AARP diet and health study. J Natl Cancer Inst 2009;101:1001–11.
16. Lowenfels AB, Maisonneuve P, Cavallini G, et al. Pancreatitis and the risk of pancreatic cancer. International Pancreatitis Study Group. N Engl J Med 1993;328:1433–7.
17. Ulrich CD. Pancreatic cancer in hereditary pancreatitis: consensus guidelines for prevention, screening and treatment. Pancreatology 2001;1:416–22.
18. Iqbal J, Ragone A, Lubinski J, et al. The incidence of pancreatic cancer in BRCA1 and BRCA2 mutation carriers. Br J Cancer 2012;107:2005–9.
19. Giardiello FM, Brensinger JD, Tersmette AC, et al. Very high risk of cancer in familial Peutz-Jeghers syndrome. Gastroenterology 2000;119:1447–53.

20. Su GH, Hruban RH, Bansal RK, et al. Germline and somatic mutations of the STK11/LKB1 Peutz-Jeghers gene in pancreatic and biliary cancers. Am J Pathol 1999;154:1835–40.
21. Vasen HF, Gruis NA, Frants RR, et al. Risk of developing pancreatic cancer in families with familial atypical multiple mole melanoma associated with a specific 19 deletion of p16 (p16-Leiden). Int J Cancer 2000;87:809–11.
22. Kempers MJ, Kuiper RP, Ockeloen CW, et al. Risk of colorectal and endometrial cancers in EPCAM deletion-positive Lynch syndrome: a cohort study. Lancet Oncol 2011;12:49–55.
23. Tersmette AC, Petersen GM, Offerhaus GJ, et al. Increased risk of incident pancreatic cancer among first-degree relatives of patients with familial pancreatic cancer. Clin Cancer Res 2001;7:738–44.
24. Jacobs EJ, Chanock SJ, Fuchs CS, et al. Family history of cancer and risk of pancreatic cancer: a pooled analysis from the Pancreatic Cancer Cohort Consortium (PanScan). Int J Cancer 2010;127:1421–8.
25. Karlson BM, Ekbom A, Lindgren PG, et al. Abdominal US for diagnosis of pancreatic tumor: prospective cohort analysis. Radiology 1999;213:107–11.
26. Maringhini A, Ciambra M, Raimondo M, et al. Clinical presentation and ultrasonography in the diagnosis of pancreatic cancer. Pancreas 1993;8:146–50.
27. Yoon SH, Lee JM, Cho JY, et al. Small (</= 20 mm) pancreatic adenocarcinomas: analysis of enhancement patterns and secondary signs with multiphasic multidetector CT. Radiology 2011;259:442–52.
28. Ishigami K, Yoshimitsu K, Irie H, et al. Diagnostic value of the delayed phase image for iso-attenuating pancreatic carcinomas in the pancreatic parenchymal phase on multidetector computed tomography. Eur J Radiol 2009; 69:139–46.
29. Prokesch RW, Chow LC, Beaulieu CF, et al. Isoattenuating pancreatic adenocarcinoma at multi-detector row CT: secondary signs. Radiology 2002;224:764–8.
30. Bronstein YL, Loyer EM, Kaur H, et al. Detection of small pancreatic tumors with multiphasic helical CT. AJR Am J Roentgenol 2004;182:619–23.
31. Takakura K, Sumiyama K, Munakata K, et al. Clinical usefulness of diffusion-weighted MR imaging for detection of pancreatic cancer: comparison with enhanced multidetector-row CT. Abdom Imaging 2011;36:457–62.
32. DeWitt J, Devereaux B, Chriswell M, et al. Comparison of endoscopic ultrasonography and multidetector computed tomography for detecting and staging pancreatic cancer. Ann Intern Med 2004;141:753–63.
33. Karmazanovsky G, Fedorov V, Kubyshkin V, et al. Pancreatic head cancer: accuracy of CT in determination of resectability. Abdom Imaging 2005;30:488–500.
34. Lu DS, Reber HA, Krasny RM, et al. Local staging of pancreatic cancer: criteria for unresectability of major vessels as revealed by pancreatic-phase, thin-section helical CT. AJR Am J Roentgenol 1997;168:1439–43.
35. Katz MH, Pisters PW, Evans DB, et al. Borderline resectable pancreatic cancer: the importance of this emerging stage of disease. J Am Coll Surg 2008;206: 833–46 [discussion: 846–8].
36. Fattahi R, Balci NC, Perman WH, et al. Pancreatic diffusion-weighted imaging (DWI): comparison between mass-forming focal pancreatitis (FP), pancreatic cancer (PC), and normal pancreas. J Magn Reson Imaging 2009;29:350–6.
37. Balci NC, Perman WH, Saglam S, et al. Diffusion-weighted magnetic resonance imaging of the pancreas. Top Magn Reson Imaging 2009;20:43–7.
38. Fukukura Y, Takumi K, Kamimura K, et al. Pancreatic adenocarcinoma: variability of diffusion-weighted MR imaging findings. Radiology 2012;263:732–40.

39. Pappas SG, Christians KK, Tolat PP, et al. Staging chest computed tomography and positron emission tomography in patients with pancreatic adenocarcinoma: utility or futility? HPB (Oxford) 2014;16:70–4.

40. Kauhanen SP, Komar G, Seppanen MP, et al. A prospective diagnostic accuracy study of 18F-fluorodeoxyglucose positron emission tomography/computed tomography, multidetector row computed tomography, and magnetic resonance imaging in primary diagnosis and staging of pancreatic cancer. Ann Surg 2009;250:957–63.

41. Sahani DV, Bonaffini PA, Catalano OA, et al. State-of-the-art PET/CT of the pancreas: current role and emerging indications. Radiographics 2012;32: 1133–58 [discussion: 1158–60].

42. Varadhachary GR, Tamm EP, Abbruzzese JL, et al. Borderline resectable pancreatic cancer: definitions, management, and role of preoperative therapy. Ann Surg Oncol 2006;13:1035–46.

43. Varadhachary GR, Abbruzzese JL. Novel approaches to 'borderline resectable' pancreatic tumors. Oncology (Williston Park) 2008;22:1529–30.

44. Halfdanarson TR, Rubin J, Farnell MB, et al. Pancreatic endocrine neoplasms: epidemiology and prognosis of pancreatic endocrine tumors. Endocr Relat Cancer 2008;15:409–27.

45. Metz DC, Jensen RT. Gastrointestinal neuroendocrine tumors: pancreatic endocrine tumors. Gastroenterology 2008;135:1469–92.

46. Kloppel G. Tumour biology and histopathology of neuroendocrine tumours. Best Pract Res Clin Endocrinol Metab 2007;21:15–31.

47. Peplinski GR, Norton JA. Gastrointestinal endocrine cancers and nodal metastasis: biologic significance and therapeutic implications. Surg Oncol Clin N Am 1996;5:159–71.

48. Grant CS, van Heerden J, Charboneau JW, et al. Insulinoma. The value of intraoperative ultrasonography. Arch Surg 1988;123:843–8.

49. Hiramoto JS, Feldstein VA, LaBerge JM, et al. Intraoperative ultrasound and preoperative localization detects all occult insulinomas; discussion 1025-6. Arch Surg 2001;136:1020–5.

50. Tucker ON, Crotty PL, Conlon KC. The management of insulinoma. Br J Surg 2006;93:264–75.

51. Fidler JL, Fletcher JG, Reading CC, et al. Preoperative detection of pancreatic insulinomas on multiphasic helical CT. AJR Am J Roentgenol 2003;181:775–80.

52. Gouya H, Vignaux O, Augui J, et al. CT, endoscopic sonography, and a combined protocol for preoperative evaluation of pancreatic insulinomas. AJR Am J Roentgenol 2003;181:987–92.

53. Thoeni RF, Mueller-Lisse UG, Chan R, et al. Detection of small, functional islet cell tumors in the pancreas: selection of MR imaging sequences for optimal sensitivity. Radiology 2000;214:483–90.

54. Owen NJ, Sohaib SA, Peppercorn PD, et al. MRI of pancreatic neuroendocrine tumours. Br J Radiol 2001;74:968–73.

55. Lewis RB, Lattin GE Jr, Paal E. Pancreatic endocrine tumors: radiologic-clinico-pathologic correlation. Radiographics 2010;30:1445–64.

56. Jensen RT, Niederle B, Mitry E, et al. Gastrinoma (duodenal and pancreatic). Neuroendocrinology 2006;84:173–82.

57. D'Onofrio M, Mansueto G, Falconi M, et al. Neuroendocrine pancreatic tumor: value of contrast enhanced ultrasonography. Abdom Imaging 2004;29:246–58.

58. Boukhman MP, Karam JM, Shaver J, et al. Localization of insulinomas. Arch Surg 1999;134:818–22 [discussion: 822–3].

59. Rappeport ED, Hansen CP, Kjaer A, et al. Multidetector computed tomography and neuroendocrine pancreaticoduodenal tumors. Acta Radiol 2006;47: 248–56.
60. Sundin A, Vullierme MP, Kaltsas G, et al. ENETS consensus guidelines for the standards of care in neuroendocrine tumors: radiological examinations. Neuroendocrinology 2009;90:167–83.
61. Rodallec M, Vilgrain V, Couvelard A, et al. Endocrine pancreatic tumours and helical CT: contrast enhancement is correlated with microvascular density, histoprognostic factors and survival. Pancreatology 2006;6:77–85.
62. Poultsides GA, Huang LC, Chen Y, et al. Pancreatic neuroendocrine tumors: radiographic calcifications correlate with grade and metastasis. Ann Surg Oncol 2012;19:2295–303.
63. Worhunsky DJ, Krampitz GW, Poullos PD, et al. Pancreatic neuroendocrine tumours: hypoenhancement on arterial phase computed tomography predicts biological aggressiveness. HPB (Oxford) 2014;16:304–11.
64. Jang KM, Kim SH, Lee SJ, et al. The value of gadoxetic acid-enhanced and diffusion-weighted MRI for prediction of grading of pancreatic neuroendocrine tumors. Acta Radiol 2014;55:140–8.
65. Semelka RC, Custodio CM, Cem Balci N, et al. Neuroendocrine tumors of the pancreas: spectrum of appearances on MRI. J Magn Reson Imaging 2000; 11:141–8.
66. Dromain C, de Baere T, Baudin E, et al. MR imaging of hepatic metastases caused by neuroendocrine tumors: comparing four techniques. AJR Am J Roentgenol 2003;180:121–8.
67. Debray MP, Geoffroy O, Laissy JP, et al. Imaging appearances of metastases from neuroendocrine tumours of the pancreas. Br J Radiol 2001;74:1065–70.
68. Tamm EP, Kim EE, Ng CS. Imaging of neuroendocrine tumors. Hematol Oncol Clin North Am 2007;21:409–32, vii.
69. Miederer M, Weber MM, Fottner C. Molecular imaging of gastroenteropancreatic neuroendocrine tumors. Gastroenterol Clin North Am 2010;39:923–35.
70. Gabriel M, Decristoforo C, Kendler D, et al. 68Ga-DOTA-Tyr3-octreotide PET in neuroendocrine tumors: comparison with somatostatin receptor scintigraphy and CT. J Nucl Med 2007;48:508–18.
71. Schreiter NF, Brenner W, Nogami M, et al. Cost comparison of 111In-DTPA-octreotide scintigraphy and 68Ga-DOTATOC PET/CT for staging enteropancreatic neuroendocrine tumours. Eur J Nucl Med Mol Imaging 2012;39:72–82.
72. Kumar R, Sharma P, Garg P, et al. Role of (68)Ga-DOTATOC PET-CT in the diagnosis and staging of pancreatic neuroendocrine tumours. Eur Radiol 2011;21:2408–16.
73. Kaemmerer D, Peter L, Lupp A, et al. Molecular imaging with (6)(8)Ga-SSTR PET/CT and correlation to immunohistochemistry of somatostatin receptors in neuroendocrine tumours. Eur J Nucl Med Mol Imaging 2011;38:1659–68.
74. Falconi M, Plockinger U, Kwekkeboom DJ, et al. Well-differentiated pancreatic nonfunctioning tumors/carcinoma. Neuroendocrinology 2006;84:196–211.
75. Buetow PC, Parrino TV, Buck JL, et al. Islet cell tumors of the pancreas: pathologic-imaging correlation among size, necrosis and cysts, calcification, malignant behavior, and functional status. AJR Am J Roentgenol 1995;165:1175–9.
76. Binderup T, Knigge U, Loft A, et al. Functional imaging of neuroendocrine tumors: a head-to-head comparison of somatostatin receptor scintigraphy, 123I-MIBG scintigraphy, and 18F-FDG PET. J Nucl Med 2010;51:704–12.
77. Bordeianou L, Vagefi PA, Sahani D, et al. Cystic pancreatic endocrine neoplasms: a distinct tumor type? J Am Coll Surg 2008;206:1154–8.

78. Balachandran A, Tamm EP, Bhosale PR, et al. Venous tumor thrombus in nonfunctional pancreatic neuroendocrine tumors. AJR Am J Roentgenol 2012; 199:602–8.

79. Watase M, Sakon M, Monden M, et al. A case of splenic vein occlusion caused by the intravenous tumor thrombus of nonfunctioning islet cell carcinoma. Surg Today 1992;22:62–5.

80. Obuz F, Bora S, Sarioglu S. Malignant islet cell tumor of the pancreas associated with portal venous thrombus. Eur Radiol 2001;11:1642–4.

81. Laffan TA, Horton KM, Klein AP, et al. Prevalence of unsuspected pancreatic cysts on MDCT. AJR Am J Roentgenol 2008;191:802–7.

82. de Jong K, Nio CY, Hermans JJ, et al. High prevalence of pancreatic cysts detected by screening magnetic resonance imaging examinations. Clin Gastroenterol Hepatol 2010;8:806–11.

83. Warshaw AL, Rutledge PL. Cystic tumors mistaken for pancreatic pseudocysts. Ann Surg 1987;205:393–8.

84. Singhal D, Kakodkar R, Sud R, et al. Issues in management of pancreatic pseudocysts. JOP 2006;7:502–7.

85. Campbell F, Azadeh B. Cystic neoplasms of the exocrine pancreas. Histopathology 2008;52:539–51.

86. Mortelé KJ. Cystic pancreatic neoplasms: imaging features and management strategy. Semin Roentgenol 2013;48(3):253–63.

87. Neumann HP, Dinkel E, Brambs H, et al. Pancreatic lesions in the von Hippel-Lindau syndrome. Gastroenterology 1991;101:465–71.

88. Leung RS, Biswas SV, Duncan M, et al. Imaging features of von Hippel-Lindau disease. Radiographics 2008;28:65–79 [quiz: 323].

89. Kim YH, Saini S, Sahani D, et al. Imaging diagnosis of cystic pancreatic lesions: pseudocyst versus nonpseudocyst. Radiographics 2005;25:671–85.

90. Flati G, Salvatori F, Porowska B, et al. Severe hemorrhagic complications in pancreatitis. Ann Ital Chir 1995;66:233–7.

91. Park WG, Mascarenhas R, Palaez-Luna M, et al. Diagnostic performance of cyst fluid carcinoembryonic antigen and amylase in histologically confirmed pancreatic cysts. Pancreas 2011;40:42–5.

92. Romics L Jr, Olah A, Belagyi T, et al. Solid pseudopapillary neoplasm of the pancreas–proposed algorithms for diagnosis and surgical treatment. Langenbecks Arch Surg 2010;395:747–55.

93. Mao C, Guvendi M, Domenico DR, et al. Papillary cystic and solid tumors of the pancreas: a pancreatic embryonic tumor? Studies of three cases and cumulative review of the world's literature. Surgery 1995;118:821–8.

94. Buetow PC, Buck JL, Pantongrag-Brown L, et al. Solid and papillary epithelial neoplasm of the pancreas: imaging-pathologic correlation on 56 cases. Radiology 1996;199:707–11.

95. Ganeshan DM, Paulson E, Tamm EP, et al. Solid pseudo-papillary tumors of the pancreas: current update. Abdom Imaging 2013;38:1373–82.

96. Fasanella KE, McGrath K. Cystic lesions and intraductal neoplasms of the pancreas. Best Pract Res Clin Gastroenterol 2009;23:35–48.

97. Baek JH, Lee JM, Kim SH, et al. Small (<or = 3 cm) solid pseudopapillary tumors of the pancreas at multiphasic multidetector CT. Radiology 2010;257:97–106.

98. Tang LH, Aydin H, Brennan MF, et al. Clinically aggressive solid pseudopapillary tumors of the pancreas: a report of two cases with components of undifferentiated carcinoma and a comparative clinicopathologic analysis of 34 conventional cases. Am J Surg Pathol 2005;29:512–9.

99. Ng KH, Tan PH, Thng CH, et al. Solid pseudopapillary tumour of the pancreas. ANZ J Surg 2003;73:410–5.

100. Washington K. Solid-pseudopapillary tumor of the pancreas: challenges presented by an unusual pancreatic neoplasm. Ann Surg Oncol 2002;9:3–4.

101. Cantisani V, Mortele KJ, Levy A, et al. MR imaging features of solid pseudopapillary tumor of the pancreas in adult and pediatric patients. AJR Am J Roentgenol 2003;181:395–401.

102. Ohtomo K, Furui S, Onoue M, et al. Solid and papillary epithelial neoplasm of the pancreas: MR imaging and pathologic correlation. Radiology 1992;184:567–70.

103. Bardales RH, Centeno B, Mallery JS, et al. Endoscopic ultrasound-guided fine-needle aspiration cytology diagnosis of solid-pseudopapillary tumor of the pancreas: a rare neoplasm of elusive origin but characteristic cytomorphologic features. Am J Clin Pathol 2004;121:654–62.

104. Yamao K, Yanagisawa A, Takahashi K, et al. Clinicopathological features and prognosis of mucinous cystic neoplasm with ovarian-type stroma: a multi-institutional study of the Japan pancreas society. Pancreas 2011;40:67–71.

105. Sahani DV, Kambadakone A, Macari M, et al. Diagnosis and management of cystic pancreatic lesions. AJR Am J Roentgenol 2013;200:343–54.

106. Procacci C, Carbognin G, Accordini S, et al. CT features of malignant mucinous cystic tumors of the pancreas. Eur Radiol 2001;11:1626–30.

107. Chalian H, Tore HG, Miller FH, et al. CT attenuation of unilocular pancreatic cystic lesions to differentiate pseudocysts from mucin-containing cysts. JOP 2011;12:384–8.

108. Boraschi P, Donati F, Gigoni R, et al. Diffusion-weighted MRI in the characterization of cystic pancreatic lesions: usefulness of ADC values. Magn Reson Imaging 2010;28:1447–55.

109. Sandrasegaran K, Akisik FM, Patel AA, et al. Diffusion-weighted imaging in characterization of cystic pancreatic lesions. Clin Radiol 2011;66:808–14.

110. Wang Y, Miller FH, Chen ZE, et al. Diffusion-weighted MR imaging of solid and cystic lesions of the pancreas. Radiographics 2011;31:E47–64.

111. Bhutani MS, Gupta V, Guha S, et al. Pancreatic cyst fluid analysis–a review. J Gastrointestin Liver Dis 2011;20:175–80.

112. Yamashita Y, Namimoto T, Mitsuzaki K, et al. Mucin-producing tumor of the pancreas: diagnostic value of diffusion-weighted echo-planar MR imaging. Radiology 1998;208:605–9.

113. Sperti C, Pasquali C, Chierichetti F, et al. Value of 18-fluorodeoxyglucose positron emission tomography in the management of patients with cystic tumors of the pancreas. Ann Surg 2001;234:675–80.

114. Buck JL, Hayes WS. From the Archives of the AFIP. Microcystic adenoma of the pancreas. Radiographics 1990;10:313–22.

115. Dewhurst CE, Mortele KJ. Cystic tumors of the pancreas: imaging and management. Radiol Clin North Am 2012;50:467–86.

116. Khurana B, Mortele KJ, Glickman J, et al. Macrocystic serous adenoma of the pancreas: radiologic-pathologic correlation. AJR Am J Roentgenol 2003;181:119–23.

117. Kim SY, Lee JM, Kim SH, et al. Macrocystic neoplasms of the pancreas: CT differentiation of serous oligocystic adenoma from mucinous cystadenoma and intraductal papillary mucinous tumor. AJR Am J Roentgenol 2006;187:1192–8.

118. Cohen-Scali F, Vilgrain V, Brancatelli G, et al. Discrimination of unilocular macrocystic serous cystadenoma from pancreatic pseudocyst and mucinous cystadenoma with CT: initial observations. Radiology 2003;228:727–33.

119. Maire F, Voitot H, Aubert A, et al. Intraductal papillary mucinous neoplasms of the pancreas: performance of pancreatic fluid analysis for positive diagnosis and the prediction of malignancy. Am J Gastroenterol 2008;103:2871–7.

120. Bassi C, Crippa S, Salvia R. Intraductal papillary mucinous neoplasms (IPMNs): is it time to (sometimes) spare the knife? Gut 2008;57:287–9.

121. Tanaka M, Fernandez-del Castillo C, Adsay V, et al. International consensus guidelines 2012 for the management of IPMN and MCN of the pancreas. Pancreatology 2012;12:183–97.

Diagnostic Imaging of Hepatic Lesions in Adults

Ramit Lamba, MBBS, MD[a], Ghaneh Fananazapir, MD[a], Michael T. Corwin, MD[a], Vijay P. Khatri, MBChB, MBA[b],*

KEYWORDS

- Liver mass • Hepatocellular carcinoma • Magnetic resonance imaging
- Computed tomography

KEY POINTS

- Often multiple imaging modalities may be necessary to characterize liver lesions.
- Each modality has unique advantages and disadvantages.
- A knowledge of the common benign and malignant lesions observed in the liver is necessary for optimal differential diagnosis and subsequently management.
- Imaging is crucial along the entire trajectory of the management of patient with malignant lesions in the liver.
- A interdisciplinary team is requisite to obtain optimal oncologic outcomes.

INTRODUCTION

In patients without a known extrahepatic malignancy, a hepatic mass may be discovered incidentally on ultrasonography, computed tomography (CT) or magnetic resonance imaging (MRI). Metastatic disease should always be considered in the differential for a mass that does not meet imaging criteria for a simple cyst in a patient with known extrahepatic malignancy undergoing imaging surveillance. However, not infrequently these masses can represent an incidental benign mass such as a hemangioma or focal nodular hyperplasia (FNH). In patients with chronic liver disease or cirrhosis, a hepatic mass may be detected during imaging surveillance. Although hepatocellular carcinoma (HCC) is the leading differential for such masses, benign masses can occur in the cirrhotic liver, and nodules less than 2 cm in diameter in the cirrhotic liver frequently represent regenerating or dysplastic nodules.[1]

Disclosures/Grant Support/Financial Interest: None.
[a] Department of Radiology, University California, Davis Health System, Sacramento, CA, USA;
[b] Division of Surgical Oncology, Department of Surgery, University of California, Davis Comprehensive Cancer Center, University California, Davis Health System, 4501 X Street, Suite 3010D, Sacramento, CA 95817, USA
* Corresponding author.
E-mail address: vijay.khatri@ucdmc.ucdavis.edu

Surg Oncol Clin N Am 23 (2014) 789–820
http://dx.doi.org/10.1016/j.soc.2014.07.003
1055-3207/14/$ – see front matter © 2014 Elsevier Inc. All rights reserved.

Imaging, especially MRI and CT enhanced by contrast material, is instrumental in noninvasive characterization of a liver mass. The American College of Radiology (ACR) Appropriateness Criteria are evidence-based guidelines developed by experts in the field to guide referring physicians in choosing the most appropriate imaging test for a specific clinical condition.[2] Advances in MRI now allows rapid imaging and 3-dimensional acquisition, which, coupled with the soft-tissue contrast, renders MRI the imaging standard for noninvasive characterization of focal liver masses, also endorsed by the ACR.[3] The ACR Appropriateness Criteria guidelines for initial characterization of a focal liver lesion larger than 1 cm encountered in different clinical and imaging scenarios are summarized in **Table 1**. ^{18}F-Fluorodeoxyflucose (FDG) positron emission tomography (PET) combined with CT has an ancillary role in the evaluation of liver metastases if the primary tumor is FDG-avid.[4] Conventional catheter angiography and CT hepatic arteriography and portography, used historically, are no longer used for evaluation of liver masses. Technetium-99m (^{99m}Tc) sulfur colloid scan and ^{99m}Tc red blood cell (RBC) scintigraphy are rarely used for evaluation of liver masses. The choice of an imaging modality can vary significantly across institutions based on local radiologic expertise, availability of equipment, and the wishes and biases of treating physicians and radiologists.

Knowledge of the underlying key pathologic features and imaging findings of liver masses on MRI and CT allows characterization in most cases. Some masses, however, may exhibit overlapping and nonspecific radiologic features, and in such cases percutaneous image-guided biopsy may become necessary. This article discusses the typical gross morphologic and imaging features of malignant liver masses and certain benign liver masses that may mimic malignancy, preceded by a brief overview of the imaging techniques in current use.

MAGNETIC RESONANCE IMAGING

MRI has high sensitivity and specificity for both detection and characterization of benign and malignant focal liver masses. An important advantage of MRI over CT is the lack of ionizing radiation. However, disadvantages include greater cost, longer imaging times, and higher frequency of suboptimal imaging caused by motion artifacts, particularly in patients who cannot perform adequate breath-holding (15–20 seconds).

Of the variety of different protocols that exist for imaging the liver with MRI, a group of core pulse sequences are routinely obtained. The first of these is most often a set of T2-weighted images. Fluid is hyperintense on T2-weighted imaging, allowing for identification of cysts and cystic masses. Other lesions such as hemangiomas are typically markedly intense (slightly less so than cysts) on T2-weighted images. Both benign and malignant solid tumors may be mildly to moderately hyperintense, but T2-weighted imaging alone is neither highly sensitive nor specific in characterizing focal liver lesions. All liver protocols should also include T1-weighted "in and out of phase" imaging. These sequences are used to identify tissues with internal microscopic fat; which can be seen in some hepatic masses such as hepatocellular adenomas and HCCs. The mainstay of liver imaging with MRI is dynamic contrast-enhanced fat-saturated T1-weighted imaging using a gadolinium chelate. Conventional extracellular gadolinium-based contrast agents are analogous to iodinated contrast used in CT, and lesions will follow similar enhancement patterns on both modalities. First, precontrast images are acquired, which provide information regarding T1 characteristics of lesions (internal hemorrhage showing increased signal intensity) and serve as a baseline to evaluate for contrast enhancement. Following this, at least 3 dynamic acquisitions are obtained in the arterial, portal venous, and equilibrium phases after intravenous injection of a gadolinium-based contrast agent. A 10- to 20-minute delayed postcontrast image may also be obtained to evaluate a slowly filling hemangioma or for delayed enhancement in a mass. Magnetic resonance cholangio-pancreatography (MRCP) may sometimes be used to evaluate segmental biliary ductal dilatation. Hepatic arterial phase imaging (on both MRI and CT) is especially important to determine whether a focal liver lesion is hypervascular. The differential diagnoses for a hypervascular liver mass are hemangioma, FNH, hepatocellular adenoma, HCC, fibrolamellar HCC, and a hypervascular metastatic lesion.

Recently there has been much interest in the use of the hepatobiliary contrast agent gadoxetic acid (Eovist/Primovist; Bayer Healthcare, Berlin, Germany) in evaluating focal liver lesions.[5] Unlike conventional extracellular contrast agents, gadoxetic acid is transported into hepatocytes and subsequently excreted into the biliary system. This process is first evident at 2 to 3 minutes after contrast injection, with peak liver enhancement occurring between 15 and 20 minutes, the so-called hepatobiliary phase. The early dynamic images appear similar to those obtained with an extracellular agent. However, the normal liver becomes hyperintense at the hepatobiliary phase and any focal lesion that does not contain hepatocytes (metastases, cysts, hemangiomas, and so forth) will appear relatively hypointense. Lesions that contain normal hepatocytes, namely FNH, will appear hyperintense or isointense to surrounding liver.[6] A small percentage of HCCs and hepatic adenomas can also demonstrate uptake of the agent.[7–9] Gadoxetic acid–enhanced MRI has been shown to have higher sensitivity than CT and PET/CT in the detection of colorectal liver metastases.[10,11] It is also highly useful in distinguishing hepatocellular adenomas from FNH (both hypervascular lesions).[8,12] There is also interest in the use of hepatocellular agents for surveillance of small HCCs in the cirrhotic liver.[13] The literature suggests that the use of gadoxetic acid allows for more accurate identification of small, early HCCs and high-grade dysplastic nodules in comparison with conventional extracellular agents.[14,15] Disadvantages of MRI with gadoxetic acid include an increased incidence of dyspnea (and therefore respiratory motion artifact) immediately following injection, slightly less robust arterial phase, and decreased ability to evaluate for delayed enhancement (owing to hyperenhancement of the surrounding liver), a critical property of lesions such as hemangiomas and cholangiocarcinomas.[5,16,17] Superparamagnetic iron oxide particle–containing contrast agents, which are taken up selectively by the reticuloendothelial system, have been used sparingly in the past and are no longer in routine clinical use.

Diffusion-weighted imaging (DWI) has emerged as an important pulse sequence in liver MRI. DWI characterizes the amount of diffusion of water molecules within tissues. Lesions with high cellularity cause restricted diffusion of water molecules and therefore remain hyperintense on DWI pulse sequences. These sequences are T2-weighted and, hence, lesions with high signal intensity on T2-weighted images may also appear hyperintense on DWI. In the liver, this technique is most useful to identify the presence and number of focal liver lesions (ie, lesion detection). However, there is overlap between the amount of restricted diffusion seen in benign and malignant liver tumors; therefore, caution must be exercised when attempting to characterize focal liver lesions with DWI in isolation.[18,19] Along with fat-saturated T2-weighted imaging, it is one of the best sequences with which to identify lymph nodes.

MULTIDETECTOR COMPUTED TOMOGRAPHY

Given the high contrast and spatial resolution of multidetector CT (MDCT) and the ability to acquire isotropic data allowing routine multiplanar reformations in coronal and

Table 1
American College of Radiology Appropriateness Criteria for choosing an imaging study or procedure for the initial characterization of a liver lesion greater than 1 cm seen initially on US or CT (without or with contrast) or non-contrast-enhanced MRI

Clinical Variants	Lesion Initially Identified on US	Rating	Lesion Initially Identified on CT	Rating	Lesion Initially Identified on MRI Without Contrast	Rating	Lesion Initially Identified on US, CT, or MRI	Rating
Normal liver (no suspicion or evidence of extrahepatic malignancy or liver disease)	MRI abdomen without and with contrast (examination of choice)	8	MRI abdomen without and with contrast (if further characterization needed)	8	MRI abdomen without and with contrast (if further characterization needed)	8	Percutaneous biopsy liver (if lesion remains indeterminate after contrast-enhanced CT or MRI)	5
	CT abdomen without and with contrast (if not cystic on US)	7	US abdomen (decide cyst vs solid)	6	CT abdomen without and with contrast (if gadolinium contraindicated)	7		
					US abdomen (if CT contrast contraindicated)	6		
Known history of extrahepatic malignancy	MRI abdomen without and with contrast (if not cystic on US)	8	MRI abdomen without and with contrast (if further characterization needed)	8	MRI abdomen without and with contrast (if further characterization needed)	8	Percutaneous biopsy liver (if lesion remains indeterminate)	7
	CT abdomen without and with contrast	7	US abdomen (decide cyst vs solid)	7	CT abdomen without and with contrast (if gadolinium contraindicated)	7	FDG-PET/CT whole body (for complete staging if FDG-avid primary)	6
					US abdomen (decide cyst vs solid or confirm hemangioma)	6		

Clinical condition							
Known or suspected liver disease associated with a high risk of hepatocellular carcinoma (chronic hepatitis, cirrhosis, hemochromatosis, etc)	MRI abdomen without and with contrast (examination of choice for surveillance in young patient with hepatitis B or C) — 9	MRI abdomen without and with contrast (if CT not conclusive or following treatments) — 9	MRI abdomen without and with contrast (if further characterization needed) — 9	Percutaneous biopsy liver (if features are not typical) — 6			
	CT abdomen without and with contrast (if gadolinium contraindicated) — 7	US abdomen (decide cyst vs solid or to evaluate for biopsy or RFA) — 5	CT abdomen without and with contrast (if gadolinium contraindicated) — 7				
			US abdomen (to confirm cyst if lesion bright on T2) — 5				

Choices that are usually not appropriate are not included.

Rating scale: 1, 2, 3, usually not appropriate; 4, 5, 6, may be appropriate; 7, 8, 9, usually appropriate.

Abbreviations: CT, computed tomography; FDG-PET, ^{18}F-fluorodeoxyglucose positron emission tomography; MRI, magnetic resonance imaging; RFA, radiofrequency ablation; US, ultrasonography.

Adapted from Refs.[2-4]

sagittal planes, in addition to its high sensitivity, widespread access, and speed of imaging, CT is widely used for the detection of liver metastases following the diagnosis of a primary extrahepatic tumor and for the imaging surveillance of these metastases following treatment.[4] For the detection of metastasis, CT is performed only in the portal venous phase, typically acquired at 80 seconds following the start of the contrast injection. As with MRI, HCC surveillance using CT and characterization of an indeterminate liver lesion relies heavily on the dynamic appearance of the mass in arterial, portal venous, and equilibrium (delayed) phases of contrast enhancement. However, because CT uses ionizing radiation, there is concern for the risk of carcinogenesis, especially in younger patients. Multiphase liver imaging with CT thus has the downside of multiple exposures to ionizing radiation in a single examination. This fact, coupled with the superior sensitivity and specificity of MRI for characterization of liver lesions, relegates CT to the second-line modality.[3] It remains an excellent alternative for patients who are claustrophobic, unable to maintain a 15-second breath-hold, or with other contraindications that preclude MRI.

For multiphase CT, the authors perform a reduced-dose unenhanced scan followed by intravenous contrast-enhanced dynamic imaging in the late arterial, portal venous, and mid-equilibrium phases. The unenhanced phase can be helpful for the detection of acute intratumoral hemorrhage, which typically appears hyperattenuating to the liver. The arterial phase is acquired 8 seconds after a threshold of 175 Hounsfield units (HU) is reached in the upper abdominal aorta, using automated bolus-tracking software. The portal venous phase starts 50 seconds after the start of the arterial phase, and the equilibrium phase starts 150 seconds after the start of the arterial phase.

ULTRASONOGRAPHY

Ultrasonography is not a first-line modality for characterization of a liver mass, and is not recommended by the ACR Appropriateness Criteria for this role.[3] However, it can be a useful alternative for patients with renal insufficiency who are unable to receive contrast material on CT or MRI. It can also be helpful in confirming the cystic nature of a focal liver lesion or to confirm the diagnosis of a hemangioma seen incidentally on a portal-phase CT image or on unenhanced MRI.[3] With a few exceptions (eg, a hemangioma and simple cyst), imaging features of liver masses are generally nonspecific on ultrasonography. When a lesion is detected on a sonogram, further characterization is best performed using contrast-enhanced MRI.

The American Association for the Study of Liver Diseases (AASLD) recommends ultrasonography as the most appropriate screening modality for detection of HCC in patients at risk.[20] Ultrasonography has been reported to have a sensitivity of 65% to 80% and specificity greater than 90% when used for HCC screening.[20] However, the performance characteristics of ultrasonography have not been as well defined in nodular cirrhotic livers undergoing surveillance. Patients with advanced cirrhosis undergoing screening for HCC often demonstrate marked heterogeneity of the liver parenchyma, which leads to limited ability to detect lesions.

General advantages of ultrasonography include no exposure to ionizing radiation, relatively low cost, and widespread availability. Limitations include high operator dependency, limited beam penetration in morbidly obese patients, and limited acoustic windows in some patients because of overlying bowel gases and rib shadowing. Research performed outside the United States on second-generation ultrasonography contrast agents has demonstrated high accuracy in characterizing liver lesions, but to date these agents have not been approved for hepatic imaging in the United States.[21]

NUCLEAR MEDICINE

Nuclear medicine imaging has a limited role in the modern-day characterization of a primary liver mass. Scintigraphic studies uniformly suffer from a low spatial resolution. FDG-PET/CT is the most widely used nuclear medicine examination, predominantly used in the setting of metastatic disease with an FDG-avid primary tumor. However, the high background uptake of FDG in the liver can limit detection of some lesions. Although most liver lesions showing increased FDG uptake are malignant, occasionally nonneoplastic infectious and inflammatory processes and benign liver masses can show increased FDG uptake.[22] PET, however, has limited sensitivity for the detection of HCC (55%–64%), and even lower (18%) for cholangiocarcinoma.[22]

^{99m}Tc-labeled sulfur colloid may be used to distinguish between FNH and hepatocellular adenoma in patients for whom the glomerular filtration rate (GFR) precludes the use of CT or MRI contrast. Similarly, ^{99m}Tc RBC scans can be used for the diagnosis of a hemangioma if the GFR precludes the use of CT or MRI contrast. Finally, an ^{111}In octreoscan can be a useful adjunct for the diagnosis or follow-up of patients with liver metastases from a neuroendocrine primary.[3]

MALIGNANT LIVER MASSES
Hepatocellular Carcinoma

Imaging features
Grossly HCC can present as: (1) a single mass, which can be large or small (satellite nodules may be present around the mass); (2) multiple masses scattered throughout the liver; (3) confluent small lesions; or (4) diffuse infiltration in the liver.[23,24] Neoangiogenesis, characterized by formation of abnormal arterial supply, is an important trait of HCC. Large lesions tend to show central necrosis, and may contain intralesional microscopic or macroscopic fat.[24] A capsule can be present in 65% to 82% of large HCCs, although a capsule can also be seen in large regenerative and dysplastic nodules.[24] In general, HCCs associated with cirrhosis have a fibrous capsule, whereas those without cirrhosis are nonencapsulated. Venous invasion, particularly into the portal vein, is a characteristic of HCC, and the incidence of malignant portal vein thrombosis in association with HCC has been reported to range from 5% to 44%.[23–26] However, patients with cirrhosis can also develop benign portal vein thrombosis secondary to portal hypertension and venous stasis, with a reported prevalence of 0.65% to 15.8%.[23] A malignant thrombus is always contiguous with or directly in contact with a parenchymal tumor. Invasion into the hepatic veins or inferior vena cava can also occur, but is less common.

At present, ultrasonography and serum α-fetoprotein (AFP) are used to screen for HCC in cirrhotic patients.[20] However, in some studies the sensitivity of these tests has been shown to be only 50% to 60%.[23] If a lesion is seen on ultrasonography or the AFP level is higher than 20 ng/mL, further interrogation is warranted with a contrast material–enhanced MRI or CT scan. Large tumors in a cirrhotic liver, especially with vascular invasion, generally do not pose a diagnostic dilemma and can be readily diagnosed on CT. Unfortunately these tumors are associated with a poorer prognosis, and diagnosis must be focused on detection of small, potentially curable tumors. The detection of small tumors, defined as HCC measuring less than 2 cm, is challenging, however, especially on CT.[23] The diagnosis of small HCC in a cirrhotic liver is confounded by a spectrum of nonmalignant nodules that occur in cirrhotic liver, ranging from benign regenerative nodules to dysplastic nodules.[1,24,27]

On ultrasonography, tumors have variable echogenicity, and the most common appearance is that of a hypoechoic nodule (48%), followed by a mixed echogenicity nodule (25%).[28] Contrast-enhanced MRI has greater sensitivity than CT, which in turn has greater sensitivity than ultrasonography for the detection of HCC in a cirrhotic liver. Pooled estimates of 14 ultrasonography, 10 CT, and 9 MRI studies for the detection of HCC showed a respective sensitivity and specificity of 60% and 97% for ultrasonography, 68% and 93% for CT, and 81% and 85% for MRI.[29]

HCC has variable signal intensity on T1- and T2-weighted images, and the MRI signal may depend on the tumor size, grade, presence of intralesional fat, necrosis, or hemorrhage.[24] Larger tumors tend to show greater heterogeneity. In general, tumors are hypointense on T1-weighted images and show a moderately increased single intensity on T2-weighted images.[30] Sometimes tumors may be difficult to detect on T2-weighted images because of heterogeneity of the cirrhotic liver, which can obscure mildly hyperintense and isointense tumors. High signal intensity can be seen in some tumors on T1-weighted images and may be attributed to intralesional hemorrhage, fat, copper, or glycogen. Steatotic regions show loss of signal intensity on opposed-phase gradient-recalled echo images. Following contrast administration, on both CT and MRI the characteristic imaging feature of HCC is hyperenhancement (hypervascularity) during the arterial phase, with washout (tumor density or signal intensity lower than surrounding liver parenchyma) in the portal venous and equilibrium phases (**Figs. 1** and **2**).[23,24] In a patient with underlying cirrhosis, this combination of findings following contrast administration is considered diagnostic and sufficient to make the noninvasive diagnosis of an HCC. Washout of an arterially enhancing mass has a very high specificity for the diagnosis of HCC, with a reported sensitivity of 89% and specificity of 96%.[31] Small HCCs can be isointense on T1- and T2-weighted images, and detected only in the arterial phase.[30] On the delayed (equilibrium)-phase images, a thin enhancing rim (capsule) may be seen (see **Figs. 1B** and **2B**).[30] The arterial phase enhancement tends to be heterogeneous in large lesions and homogeneous in small lesions. The enhancing areas show washout in delayed phases. Large tumors may also occasionally predominantly show a pattern of intratumoral neovascularity in the arterial phase. Diffuse infiltrating tumors in a cirrhotic liver

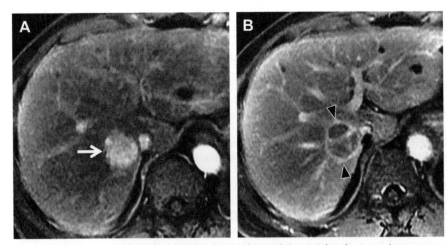

Fig. 1. Hepatocellular carcinoma. (*A*) Contrast-enhanced T1-weighted magnetic resonance imaging (MRI) in the arterial phase shows a well-circumscribed enhancing lesion in the right hepatic lobe (*arrow*). (*B*) Contrast-enhanced T1-weighted MRI in the delayed phase shows washout within the lesion with an enhancing capsule (*arrowheads*).

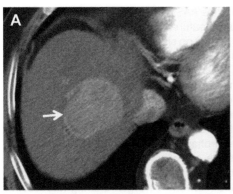
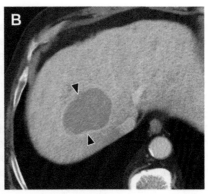

Fig. 2. Hepatocellular carcinoma. (*A*) Contrast-enhanced computed tomography (CT) in the arterial phase shows an enhancing lesion in the right hepatic lobe (*arrow*). (*B*) Contrast-enhanced CT in the delayed phase shows washout within the lesion and an enhancing capsule (*arrowheads*).

may be difficult to detect on unenhanced T1- or T2-weighted images, and can sometimes present a diagnostic challenge.[24]

On postgadolinium images, diffuse tumors show patchy enhancement in the arterial phase, but washout is seen in all tumors on the delayed postcontrast images.[32] Furthermore, they are frequently associated with portal venous tumor thrombosis and elevated serum AFP levels.[32] Subtraction of the unenhanced from the enhanced MR images is extremely helpful in assessing enhancement in nodules that have high signal intensity on unenhanced T1-weighted images. On gadoxetic acid–enhanced MRI the tumors typically show a low signal intensity in comparison with the surrounding nonneoplastic hepatic parenchyma in the hepatobiliary phase.[24] Malignant tumor thrombus typically shows increased signal intensity on T2-weighted images and expansion of the vein, compared with a low T2 signal intensity and near normal caliber of the vein in bland thrombosis.[33] Following contrast administration on CT and MRI, the presence of neovascularity or heterogeneous enhancement within the vein on the arterial-phase images is considered highly specific for tumor thrombosis (**Fig. 3**).[33]

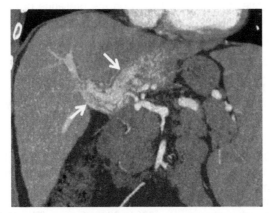

Fig. 3. Hepatocellular carcinoma with portal vein tumor thrombus. Contrast-enhanced CT in the arterial phase shows arterially enhancing thrombus within and expanding the portal vein (*arrows*).

Based on the current recommendation of the AASLD, biopsy is not needed if a mass greater than 2 cm in diameter shows classic features of HCC (hypervascularity in the arterial phase and washout in the venous phase) on either CT or MRI or when a mass 1 to 2 cm in diameter shows these features on both CT and MRI.[20,34] Therefore, imaging plays a crucial role in the diagnosis of HCC in cirrhotic livers. However, arterially enhancing nodules less than 2 cm in diameter are not uncommon in the cirrhotic liver. These nodules can pose a diagnostic challenge and dilemma, because most are benign and represent either regenerating and dysplastic nodules or arterioportal shunts, but those that represent small HCCs have a chance for curative treatment.[1,23,27] Nodules that show only arterial-phase enhancement and no washout in the portal venous or equilibrium phases are considered indeterminate and cannot be characterized as definite HCCs. Such nodules need closer follow-up imaging or, in challenging cases, biopsy.[23] The United Network for Organ Sharing has recently added rapid growth as a diagnostic criterion for HCC for nodules with a diameter greater than 1 cm at initial diagnosis and showing hyperenhancement in the late arterial phase, although this criterion should be used with great caution.[35] In cases of doubt, short-term follow-up imaging or biopsy may be considered. It is also important to distinguish such nodules from nontumorous peripheral or subcapsular wedge or geographic areas of arterial-phase hyperenhancement, referred to as transient hepatic density (on CT) or intensity (on MRI) differences.[1] Radiologic criteria favoring HCC are size larger than 2 cm, moderate hyperintensity on T2-weighted imaging (as opposed to dysplastic nodules, which are typically hypointense on T2), washout in the delayed phase, enhancing tumor capsule on delayed images, and rapid interval growth.[23]

Liver imaging reporting and data system

The Liver imaging reporting and data system (LI-RADS) was developed to standardize the terminology, interpretation, and reporting of HCC and other focal liver lesions in patients with cirrhosis or other risk factors for HCC. The latest version (v2013.1) applies to CT and MRI performed with extracellular contrast agents. Hepatobiliary contrast agents are expected to be incorporated into upcoming versions. Focal observations in the liver are assigned an LI-RADS category from 1 to 5, with increasing likelihood of being HCC (see **Fig. 2**). Importantly LI-RADS category 5 lesions are considered 100% certain to represent HCC, and this category is essentially equivalent to the Organ Procurement and Transplant Network class 5.[35] Observations are assigned to categories 3 through 5 based on the presence or absence of arterial hyperenhancement, size, and major criteria (washout appearance, capsule, and threshold growth), as shown in **Fig. 3**.

Fibrolamellar HCC

Fibrolamellar HCC is a rare primary liver tumor that predominantly occurs in young adults, with most cases occurring in patients without underlying hepatitis or cirrhosis.[36–38]

Imaging features

Fibrolamellar HCC typically presents as a large, well-circumscribed, lobulated solitary mass in a liver without cirrhosis, histologically characterized by the presence of fibrous strands in the tumor.[37] A central stellate scar has been reported in up to 71% of cases.[37] A capsule may be present, although it can be incomplete.[37] Focal calcifications are common and can be seen in 40% to 68% of cases (**Fig. 4**).[37,39] As opposed to conventional HCC, portal vein thrombosis is uncommon in fibrolamellar HCC and occurs in only 5% to 10% of cases.[36]

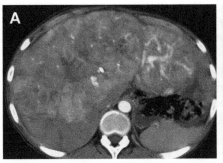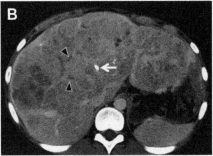

Fig. 4. Fibrolamellar hepatocellular carcinoma. (*A*) Contrast-enhanced CT in the arterial phase shows a large heterogeneously enhancing mass with a central scar largely replacing the liver, with arterially enhancing components. (*B*) Contrast-enhanced CT in the equilibrium phase shows an area of coarse calcification (*arrow*) and delayed enhancement within the central scar (*arrowheads*).

Owing to its rarity, there are only limited imaging reports of fibrolamellar HCC. On ultrasonography, echogenicity is variable and findings are nonspecific.[39] On noncontrast CT (NCCT) it presents as a large, well-defined, heterogeneous, predominantly hypoattenuating mass.[37] On MRI, fibrolamellar HCC is usually hypointense on T1-weighted images and hyperintense on T2-weighted images.[37] The fibrous central scar is typically hypointense on both T1- and T2-weighted images.[37,40] Calcification may be difficult to identify on MRI. On helical CT, after intravenous contrast administration, the tumor typically shows heterogeneous enhancement in the arterial phase (see **Fig. 4**A).[37] However, enhancement in the portal venous and delayed phases is variable. In the portal venous phase the tumor is isoattenuating to liver in 48% and hypoattenuating in 36%.[37] On delayed-phase CT images obtained at 10 to 20 minutes, the tumor generally appears hypoattenuating to the liver.[37] Earlier reports allude to lack of enhancement in the central scar,[40] but enhancement of the central scar in the delayed phase has been reported on both CT and MRI (see **Fig. 4**B).[37] The role of FDG-PET in fibrolamellar HCC has not been fully evaluated.

FNH is sometimes in the differential consideration for a mass with a central scar. The central scar in FNH is predominantly hyperintense on T2-weighted images, in contrast to the central scar in fibrolamellar HCC that is typically hypointense. Calcification is extremely rare in FNH, whereas it is frequently seen in fibrolamellar HCC. Following injection of hepatocellular-specific contrast agents, FNH typically shows uptake of contrast in the hepatobiliary phase as opposed to fibrolamellar HCC, which does not show any uptake.[5] Conventional HCC arising in a noncirrhotic liver may be difficult to differentiate from fibrolamellar HCC, especially if a central scar is absent. Calcifications can occasionally be seen in HCC arising in the noncirrhotic liver.[41] Intralesional fat does not occur in fibrolamellar HCC, contrary to its presence in some cases of conventional HCC.[37,41] The age of the patient, coexistence of viral hepatitis, and an elevated serum AFP level can be used as ancillary aids to make the diagnosis of a conventional HCC, but biopsy is needed for an accurate diagnosis.[41] A tumor without a prominent central scar may also be confused with intrahepatic (or peripheral) cholangiocarcinoma (ICC), although biliary obstruction is rare in the former.

Intrahepatic Cholangiocarcinoma

ICC is a malignant solid tumor arising from the epithelium of the intrahepatic bile ducts. Cholangiocarcinoma arising from the right and left hepatic ducts at or near their junction is considered an extrahepatic lesion (hilar cholangiocarcinoma or Klatskin tumor). ICC accounts for 10% of all cholangiocarcinomas, hilar cholangiocarcinoma accounts for 25%, and extrahepatic cholangiocarcinoma accounts for 65%.[42]

Imaging features

According to the classification of primary liver cancer proposed by the Liver Cancer Study Group of Japan, ICCs are classified into 3 types based on the gross appearance of tumor: mass-like (most common), periductal-infiltrating (resembles hilar or extrahepatic cholangiocarcinoma), and intraductal papillary mass (uncommon).[43]

Mass-like The usual gross appearance of mass-forming ICC is a large solid tumor, with irregular lobulated borders frequently with dense fibrous stranding in the central portion.[44] In one series, size of the tumors ranged from 1.2 to 17 cm.[45] Fibrous encapsulation is not seen.[25] Characteristically this malignancy has a large central core of fibrotic tissue relatively devoid of malignant cells, and most of the cancer cells are located on the tumor's periphery.[42] The tumor is not highly vascularized; hemorrhage, necrosis, and cystic degeneration are uncommon, as are calcifications.[42] Focal intrahepatic bile ductal dilatation is commonly seen around the tumor, reported in 52% of patients in one series with helical CT (**Fig. 5C**).[45] Masses abutting the liver capsule can result in capsular retraction, attributed to the fibrous nature of the tumor (see **Fig. 5A, B**). The incidence of capsular retraction has been reported to vary from 21% to 36%.[45,46] Satellite nodules around the tumor are common and can vary in size.[42,45,46] Invasion of portal or hepatic veins is uncommon. Portal thrombosis, when it does appear, is usually a result of secondary cholangitis and not tumor thrombosis.[42]

On ultrasonography, echogenicity of the tumor is variable and may be hypo-, iso-, or hyperechoic. However, the most common manifestation is that of a hypoechoic mass. Therefore, sonographically there are no specific features of mass-forming cholangiocarcinoma that distinguish it from the more common metastatic disease and HCC other than the fact that cholangiocarcinoma is more likely to be associated with dilated bile ducts and HCC primarily occurs in the cirrhotic liver. On NCCT, the tumor generally appears as a hypodense mass. All tumors are globally hypodense during the portal phase.[45] On MRI, the typical appearance of the tumor is a nonencapsulated mass that is hypointense on T1-weighted images and hyperintense on T2-weighted images.[42] Central hypointensity in the tumor reflective of fibrosis may be seen on T2-weighted images. This finding can also be seen occasionally in colorectal metastases, but is uncommon in other liver tumors.[47] On dynamic contrast-enhanced CT and MRI, most tumors show mild to moderate thin-rim–like or thick-band–like contrast enhancement around the tumor in hepatic arterial and portal venous phases, with progressive enhancement toward the central part of the tumor in the delayed phase (see **Fig. 5B**).[42,44–46,48,49] The entire mass may show enhancement on delayed-phase images obtained several minutes after contrast administration. In one series, tumor enhancement on delayed images was reported as 70%.[45] However, in some cases the tumor core may show no enhancement on delayed imaging, especially if central necrosis is present.[42,47] Hypovascular metastases, especially from adenocarcinoma of the gastrointestinal tract, may show an enhancement pattern similar to that of ICC. Absence of a possible primary site, and ancillary findings such as bile duct dilatation peripheral to the mass and capsular retraction, can be clues for differentiating mass-forming ICC from metastases.[44] In one series, intrahepatic bile duct dilatation was evident in 27 of 50 cases of cholangiocarcinoma but occurred in 1 of 34 hepatic colorectal metastases.[47] On gadoxetic acid–enhanced MRI the tumors are typically hypointense in the hepatobiliary phase. Lesion conspicuity is increased, and additional satellite nodules can be depicted in some patients in the hepatobiliary phase.[48,50]

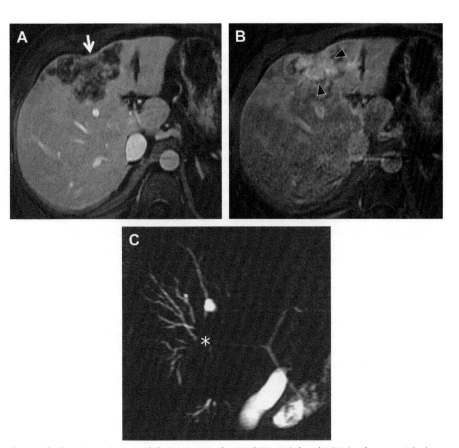

Fig. 5. Cholangiocarcinoma. (*A*) Contrast-enhanced T1-weighted MRI in the arterial phase shows a hypointense mass within segment IV of the left hepatic lobe with associated capsular retraction (*arrow*). (*B*) Contrast-enhanced T1-weighted MRI in the delayed phase shows increased enhancement of the mass (*arrowheads*). (*C*) Magnetic resonance cholangio-pancreatography in the coronal plane shows segmental biliary ductal dilatation peripheral to the mass (*asterisk*), which is not well seen on this sequence.

Periductal-infiltrating type Periductal-infiltrating ICC is radiologically and pathologi-cally identical to infiltrating hilar cholangiocarcinoma but has a different location (ie, peripheral to the secondary confluence). It grows along the bile ducts and causes irregular thickening and narrowing of the involved bile duct, eventually resulting in obstruction of ducts proximal to the tumor. In the later stage, the tumor may infiltrate the hepatic parenchyma and hepatic hilum.[42,44]

Intraductal-growing type Intraductal ICC is a low-grade malignancy that usually pre-sents as small, sessile, or polypoid masses, intraluminally within the bile ducts. It can produce mucus and occlude the bile ducts.[42,44]

Epithelioid Hemangioendothelioma

Epithelioid hemangioendothelioma (EH) is a rare vascular tumor of variable (usually low to intermediate grade) malignant potential.

Imaging features

Lesions vary in size from a few millimeters to several centimeters and are typically multifocal, involving both lobes.[25,51–54] Lesions are distributed predominantly in a peripheral subcapsular location, tend to coalesce, and often cause capsular retraction.[52,53,55–57] Calcification may be present in some lesions.[25,53,54,57] Portal thrombosis can occur.[55] Budd-Chiari syndrome can develop if the tumor invades hepatic veins.[58]

Ultrasonographic features are nonspecific and lesions have variable echogenicity, predominantly appearing as hypoechoic masses.[55,56] On NCCT, lesions are generally hypoattenuating.[53,56] On unenhanced T1-weighted MR images, lesions are typically hypointense relative to liver parenchyma and hyperintense on T2-weighted images.[53,55–57] Lesions can be heterogeneous on both T1 and T2, and show areas of hyperintensity indicating hemorrhage on T1-weighted images.[52,53] T2-weighted images frequently show target-like configuration of lesions (moderately hyperintense or low-signal peripheral rim and markedly hyperintense central region).[52,53,56] Following contrast enhancement, lesions typically show variable degrees of peripheral rim enhancement (target-like enhancement pattern) with central progression of enhancement on portal venous and delayed-phase images.[52,53,55,57–59] The tumor centers may be either enhanced or nonenhanced at delayed imaging.[58] Peripheral rim enhancement in some lesions may be discontinuous,[53] and central nodular enhancement can also occur.[51] A related sign, termed the lollipop sign, has been described on contrast-enhanced CT and MRI in cases of hepatic EH: a hepatic or portal vein tapering and terminating at or just within the edge of a well-defined peripherally enhancing (or nonenhancing) lesion.[59] Nuclear medicine is rarely used for the diagnosis of EH, but a few case reports in the literature describe high FDG uptake in most tumors on PET[58] while some lesions can have FDG uptake similar to that of the surrounding liver parenchyma.[52]

Thus, ultrasonography, CT, or MRI findings of multiple coalescent peripheral hepatic masses with capsular retraction along with a target-like appearance of the tumors on contrast-enhanced CT and MRI are highly suggestive of EH. Definitive diagnosis of hepatic EH requires a tumor biopsy. A positive result at immunohistochemical staining with antibodies to factor VIII, CD31, or CD34 helps confirm the diagnosis.[25,54]

The differential considerations for a subcapsular hepatic mass with capsular retraction include EH, peripheral cholangiocarcinoma, confluent foci of hepatic fibrosis (usually in the setting of advanced cirrhosis), previously treated metastatic lesions, and large atypical cavernous hemangioma.

Angiosarcoma

Angiosarcoma is a rare malignant tumor of vascular origin accounting for less than 2% of primary malignant liver tumors.[25,60,61]

Imaging features

The most common manifestation is of multifocal masses involving both lobes.[60–63] Other manifestations include a large focal solitary mass or diffuse tumor infiltration in the liver (least common).[62] Areas of hemorrhage, cystic degeneration, and necrosis can be present, and venous invasion can occur.[62,64,65] Spontaneous rupture has been reported in 15% to 27% of cases,[60,61,64] and angiosarcoma should be considered in the differential in patients presenting as such. Given the rarity of the diagnosis; most reports are limited to isolated case reports and small case series.

Radiologic findings are nonspecific and reflect the underlying gross alterations. On ultrasonography, therefore, the tumor has a variable nonspecific echogenicity. Acute hemorrhage in the tumor manifests as focal areas of increased echogenicity on ultra-sonography, increased attenuation on NCCT, and increased signal intensity on T1-weighted MRI.[62,63,65] Heterogeneous increased signal intensity is seen on T2-weighted images.[61–64] Following contrast administration, on both CT and MRI the tumor is generally hypoenhancing to liver and shows markedly heterogeneous enhancement, which is progressive on delayed-phase images with lack of central filling.[62–64] Foci of heterogeneous enhancement in tumor can persist in delayed phases.[62,63] Diffuse infiltrative tumor shows a heterogeneous appearance of the liver parenchyma on CT and MRI.[62] Angiosarcoma should be considered in patients presenting with this appearance. Data on PET are limited, with isolated case reports suggesting increased FDG uptake in angiosarcoma.[66,67]

The rarity of these tumors should be kept in mind before offering an imaging diagnosis. Given their vascular nature, biopsy has been previously reported to be associated with a high risk of hemorrhage,[61,64] although this was not observed in a later series of 9 patients undergoing biopsy.[62] In patients presenting with multiple masses, the leading differential consideration is still metastases. The diagnosis can be confused with cholangiocarcinoma if a large solitary mass is present.

Primary Lymphoma

Primary lymphoma of the liver is defined as an extranodal lymphoma arising in the liver with the bulk of the disease localized to this site. Contiguous lymph node involvement and distant spread may be seen. It is rare, and accounts for about 0.4% of all extra-nodal non-Hodgkin lymphomas and 0.016% of all non-Hodgkin lymphomas.[68] Primary lymphoma may manifest as a solitary or multiple masses.[25,69] Diffuse infiltration with hepatomegaly has been reported.[25,68,70] When presenting as multiple masses, the primary differential is metastatic disease. It has been reported to occur in the setting of chronic liver disease, hepatitis C, and human immunodeficiency virus infection.[68] Imaging findings are nonspecific and mostly limited to case reports or small series. On ultrasonography, the masses are hypoechoic or anechoic[68–70]; they are typically hypovascular on contrast-enhanced CT (**Fig. 6**), hypointense on T1-weighted images, and hyperintense on T2-weighted images.[69,70] Rim enhancement

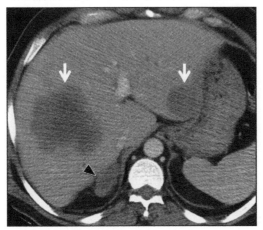

Fig. 6. Lymphoma. Contrast-enhanced CT in the portal venous phase shows well-circumscribed hypodense masses within the right and left hepatic lobes (*arrows*) with involvement of the right adrenal gland (*arrowhead*).

may be seen on CT or MRI following contrast injection.[70] Portal branches may be seen coursing through the tumor, a finding uncommon in other liver tumors.[68,71] The diagnosis is typically made on biopsy.

In contrast to primary lymphoma, secondary liver infiltration is a frequent occurrence, present in 50% to 60% of cases of non-Hodgkin lymphoma. However, liver involvement in these patients is frequently occult and is diagnosed only on biopsy.[25]

Other Sarcomas

Other primary hepatic sarcomas such as leiomyosarcoma, malignant fibrous histiocytoma, localized malignant mesothelioma, and Kaposi sarcoma are extremely rare, and have been the subject of case reports. Because of the rarity of these tumors and the fact that their radiologic features are nonspecific, they are rarely diagnosed preoperatively.[72] Radiology reports of these tumors are limited, and generally show features of a hypovascular malignant tumor.[72] Kaposi sarcoma, however, involves the liver secondarily in 12% to 25% of fatal cases of AIDS, but is not known to contribute significantly to its morbidity or mortality.[25] Rare cases of embryonal sarcoma, usually a childhood tumor, have been reported in adults.[25]

Biliary Cystadenoma and Cystadenocarcinoma

Biliary cystadenoma (BCA) and biliary cystadenocarcinoma (BCAC) are rare cystic epithelial tumors arising from biliary structures proximal to the hilum of the liver. Biliary cystic tumors (BCTs), constitute less than 5% of all liver cysts.[73] BCA is seen almost exclusively in women, with BCAC appearing equally in men and women.[25,73] The average age of patients is 50 to 60 years.[25]

Imaging features

BCTs are generally solitary, typically multilocular, range in size from 5 to 15 cm in diameter, and commonly occur in the left lobe of the liver.[25,73–76] Cystadenomas are well defined by a fibrous capsule.[25] The lesions generally show thick irregular walls as opposed to simple hepatic cysts. Internal septations are typically seen, with some cases showing a "cyst within cyst" appearance.[73] Upstream bile duct dilatation is common, being reported in 83% (10 of 12) cases in one study (**Fig. 7**).[75] Usually BCTs do not communicate with the bile ducts, and calcifications are uncommon.[77]

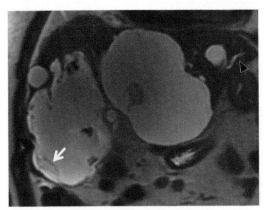

Fig. 7. Biliary cystadenoma. T2-weighted MRI in the coronal plane shows 2 large cystic masses with septations (*arrow*). Biliary ductal dilatation is noted in the left hepatic lobe (*arrowhead*).

Owing to their cystic nature, BCTs are anechoic on ultrasonography, show water density (<20 HU) on CT, and a homogeneous low-intensity T1 signal and high-intensity T2 signal on MRI.[73] The septations are better depicted on ultrasonography and MR than on CT. On T2-weighted images, including MRCP, septations are identified as linear low-signal intensity bands within high-intensity cysts (see **Fig. 7**).[74] The internal fluid within the tumors can show varied signal intensity on T1- and T2-weighted images attributable to difference in protein concentration.[74] The septations and mural nodules enhance following contrast administration on CT and MRI. MRCP is excellent in depicting upstream biliary dilatation. In the era of modern-day MRI, endoscopic retrograde cholangiopancreatography plays no role in the evaluation of BCTs. Although BCAC is more likely to contain mural or septal nodules and papillary projections, these features are not pathognomonic for BCAC.[73] BCA and BCAC thus cannot be reliably differentiated on imaging, so all such lesions are considered surgical. Discrimination between BCA and BCAC is of little practical importance because the treatment for suspected BCTs is complete surgical excision. The role of PET in separating BCA from BCAC is not known.[73] Cyst fluid aspiration and analysis does not have a role in distinguishing between a BCT and an atypical simple cyst.[76]

Cystic liver lesions are common. Fortunately, most cystic liver lesions are simple cysts; these occur commonly, are typically discovered incidentally, and are benign, rarely symptomatic, and generally left alone. On the other hand, because BCTs may be malignant, complete excision by surgery is warranted. Therefore, accurate differentiation of BCTs from large simple cysts is crucial for appropriate management. Cysts without internal septae or papillary projection are most likely simple hepatic cysts, and the presence of a septum and septal thickening are important predictors of BCTs in comparison with simple hepatic cysts.[77] Unfortunately, simple cysts can be large in size and septations can be seen in them.[75] In a comparison of 12 surgically resected, pathologically proven BCTs (8 BCAs and 4 BCACs) and 13 simple hepatic cysts, the presence of upstream bile duct dilatation had the highest specificity (100%) for the differentiation of BCTs from simple cysts, followed by perilesional transient hepatic attenuation differences (84.6%), lesion location in the left lobe (76.9%), and presence of a single as opposed to multiple cysts (69.2%).[75] Size has not been found to be a factor in differentiating BCTs from simple cysts.[75] Whereas most BCTs were located in the left lobe, most simple hepatic cysts were located in the right hepatic lobe (76.9%, 10 of 13).[75] BCTs tend to be solitary whereas simple hepatic cysts tend to be multiple. An increase of serum alkaline phosphatase has also been associated with BCTs.[76] Echinococcal cyst and liver abscess are the 2 other cystic liver lesions most likely to be confused with a BCT. Echinococcal cysts can present as a cyst with internal debris or a cyst with daughter cysts within it (**Fig. 8**). Liver abscesses typically have a septated or multilocular appearance, but the walls are much more irregular and thicker than those seen with BCTs. The combination of imaging characteristics, clinical presentation, history of nonresidence in an endemic area, and serologic analysis or culture of cyst contents can aid in making an accurate diagnosis. Other complex cystic lesions of the liver include a posttraumatic intrahepatic hematoma or biloma, undifferentiated (embryonal) sarcoma (a tumor primarily seen in children), primary or metastatic "cystic" necrotic neoplasm, and biliary intraductal papillary mucinous neoplasm.[73]

Hepatic Metastases

In the United States, metastasis is by far the most common malignancy of the liver, and should always be the first consideration when confronted with multiple noncystic liver lesions in any patient or a single noncystic lesion in a patient with known cancer

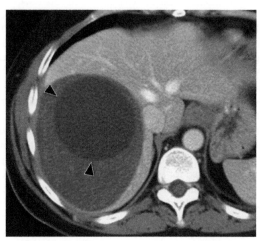

Fig. 8. Echinococcal cyst. Contrast-enhanced CT in the portal venous phase shows a well-circumscribed "cyst within a cyst" within the right hepatic lobe, with the inner cyst showing a lower-density component (*arrowheads*).

elsewhere. However, in most instances (80%), small lesions (<1 cm) do not represent metastatic disease even in patients a known malignancy.[78] The appearance of a new lesion in the liver in a patient with a history of cancer strongly suggests hepatic metastases. Colon, stomach, pancreas, breast, and lung are the most common primary sites.

Ultrasonography has low sensitivity for detecting metastatic disease, with sensitivities ranging from 40% to 77%, and less than 20% sensitivity for lesions smaller than 1 cm.[79] Sensitivity can be increased by using contrast-enhanced ultrasonography (CEUS), but CEUS agents are currently not approved in the United States. With ultrasonography, metastases can be hypoechoic, hyperechoic, cystic, or diffuse. There are no specific features of metastatic lesions, although multiplicity of lesions is suggestive. The depiction of a hypoechoic halo around a lesion (the target sign) is considered a classic feature of metastatic disease. However, the hypoechoic halo has also been described with HCC, adenomas, FNH, lymphoma, hemangiomas, and fungal microabscesses.[80]

In the United States, CT is the most widely used imaging modality for screening the abdomen and pelvis for metastatic disease. In addition to evaluating the liver, extrahepatic metastases can be evaluated during the same examination. CT also remains the most widely used examination for surveillance for metastatic disease after treatment of the primary neoplasm. On unenhanced CT, metastases typically appear hypodense unless there is intralesional hemorrhage or calcification (eg, melanoma, mucinous metastases). Although lesions vary widely in size and shape, most metastases are hypovascular (relative to enhancing normal hepatic parenchyma) and are hence best seen in the portal venous phase, which shows peak parenchymal enhancement. Peripheral rim enhancement can be seen. Necrotic and cystic areas can be seen in larger tumors. However, certain metastatic lesions show marked arterial-phase enhancement and are, hence, also depicted in the arterial phase. These lesions are relatively uncommon and include metastases from (but not limited to) neuroendocrine tumors (chiefly from the pancreas and small bowel), clear cell renal cell carcinoma, thyroid carcinoma, choriocarcinoma, and melanoma (**Fig. 9**).[81] Biphasic contrast-enhanced hepatic CT with imaging of the liver obtained in the arterial phase followed by imaging of the abdomen and pelvis in the portal venous phase

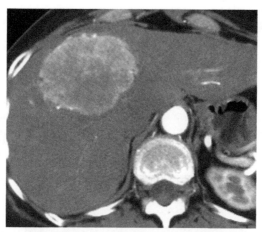

Fig. 9. Hypervascular metastasis from a gastrointestinal carcinoid. Contrast-enhanced CT in the arterial phase shows a well-circumscribed, avidly enhancing hepatic lesion.

should be considered for metastatic surveillance of these patients. Based on their experience, the authors strongly recommend this approach for surveillance of neuro-endocrine tumors because they can sometimes "blend in" on the portal-phase images, with failure to detect some hypervascular metastases in the portal phase also reported in a prior study.[82]

On MRI, metastases are typically hypointense on T1-weighted images. However, intralesional melanin and hemorrhage can appear hyperintense on T1-weighted images. Metastases show various degrees of hyperintensity on T2-weighted images and restricted diffusion on DWI. Postcontrast imaging characteristics are similar to those described by CT, but offer superior characterization and hence greater specificity for diagnosis of a given liver lesion, because benign lesions can coexist in the liver with metastatic disease. Following gadoxetic acid–enhanced MRI, contrast uptake by hepatocytes in the hepatobiliary phase provides excellent contrast between the liver parenchyma and metastatic lesions, with metastases typically appearing hypointense in this phase (**Fig. 10**). In a study comparing unenhanced and enhanced PET/CT and gadolinium-enhanced MRI for detection of colorectal metastases, gadolinium-enhanced MRI showed the highest detection rate (73.6%, 90.9%, and 95.4%, respectively).[83] In several studies, gadoxetic acid–enhanced MRI has been shown to have the highest sensitivity of current modalities in use for the detection of hepatic metastases, with a recent meta-analysis reporting sensitivity of 93% for detection of liver metastases.[84] MRI using hepatobiliary agents should thus be considered before surgery if metastasectomy is being planned.[17]

PET/CT is being increasingly used for the staging of tumors and detection of metastatic disease, and has the advantage of detecting extrahepatic metastases in the body. A limitation of FDG-PET, however, is that it may fail to show small (<1 cm) liver metastases.[4] PET/CT has been shown to have high sensitivity and specificity for the presence of liver metastases in patients with colorectal cancer.[85]

BENIGN LIVER MASSES
Hemangioma

A hemangioma is composed of blood-filled spaces lined by endothelium with fibrous septations. These lesions are the most common benign tumor of the liver, with a

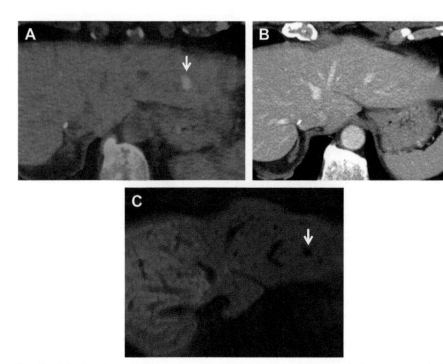

Fig. 10. Colonic adenocarcinoma metastasis. (A) Fused positron emission tomography/CT shows a small focus of hypermetabolic activity within the left hepatic lobe (arrow). (B) Contrast-enhanced CT in the portal venous phase fails to show a correlating lesion in the left hepatic lobe. (C) Contrast-enhanced T1-weighted MRI using a hepatocellular contrast agent in a 20-minute delayed phase clearly shows the concordant metastatic focus as an area of hypointensity within the left hepatic lobe (arrow).

prevalence of up to 20%, and a female to male ratio of from 2:1 to 5:1.[86] Hemangiomas are typically solitary but are multiple in 10% of cases. Most are asymptomatic and, as such, are discovered incidentally on imaging. Most are smaller than 3 cm in diameter.

Imaging features
On ultrasonography, hemangiomas are classically well-defined, hyperechoic lesions, which exhibit posterior acoustic enhancement. Even though these lesions are vascular in origin, they do not typically show vascular flow on color or power Doppler images, as the blood flow within these lesions is too slow to detect. If classic imaging findings are seen and the patient is at low risk for hepatic malignancy, ultrasonography can be sufficient for diagnosis.[79] However, if there are atypical features or the patient has an increased risk for hepatic malignancy, further evaluation with MRI should be considered. On CT, hemangiomas are hypodense on noncontrast images when compared with background liver. After delivery of contrast, hemangiomas typically exhibit peripheral, nodular, interrupted enhancement, with enhancing areas demonstrating the same attenuation as the aorta. On subsequent phases of contrast delivery, there is persistent centripetal filling of contrast.

MRI is the most useful modality for characterizing hemangiomas, with sensitivity and specificity of 98% and 99%, respectively.[87,88] On T1-weighted images, hemangiomas are classically hypointense to background liver. On T2-weighted images these lesions are markedly hyperintense, sometimes approaching the signal intensity of cerebrospinal fluid. The enhancement characteristics on MRI are analogous to those seen on postcontrast CT images (**Fig. 11**).

Focal Nodular Hyperplasia

The second most common benign liver lesion is FNH. Grossly FNHs typically have lobulated contours with a central scar and radiating fibrous septae. The central scar is composed of malformed vascular structures. Histologically, FNH is composed of nodular regions of hyperplastic parenchyma of essentially normal hepatocytes arranged in plates 1 to 2 cells thick. FNH is much more common in women, with a female to male ratio of 8:1.[89]

Imaging features

On ultrasonography, FNH is often not well visualized and can be hypo-, iso-, or hyper-echoic. A large central scar can make the lesion more conspicuous and is often hyper-echoic.[90] On unenhanced CT, FNH is generally hypodense or isodense to the remainder of the liver parenchyma. The lesion shows intense enhancement on arterial-phase images, with the lesion becoming more isodense to the normal liver parenchyma on portal venous and delayed-phase imaging. The central scar can show increasing enhancement on the more delayed images.

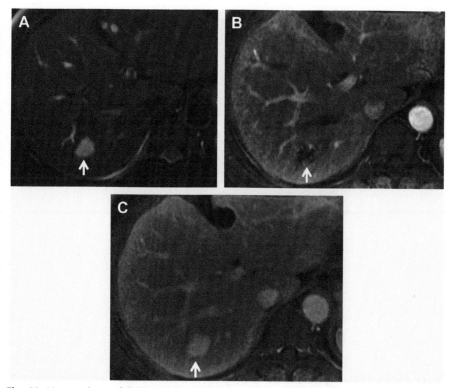

Fig. 11. Hemangioma. (*A*) T2-weighted MRI shows a markedly hyperintense lesion within the right hepatic lobe (*arrow*). (*B*) Contrast-enhanced T1-weighted MRI in the arterial phase shows a lesion with peripheral interrupted nodular enhancement (*arrow*). (*C*) Contrast-enhanced T1-weighted MRI in the delayed phase shows eventual complete filling of the lesion with contrast (*arrow*).

MRI is superior for detection and characterization of FNH in comparison with ultrasonography or CT. On T1-weighted images, FNH is isointense to mildly hypointense. On T2-weighted images it is isointense to mildly hyperintense. The central scar is generally hypointense on T1-weighted images and hyperintense on T2-weighted images. FNH shows the same enhancement pattern on MRI as on CT. Hepatobiliary contrast agents play an important role in confidently diagnosing FNH, especially when trying to distinguish between FNH and adenoma. FNH typically shows uptake of these agents and therefore appears hyperintense or isointense to normal liver in the hepatobiliary phase (**Fig. 12**).

Hepatocellular Adenoma

Hepatic adenomas are uncommon tumors of hepatocellular origin, with the main predisposing risk factor being long-term use of oral contraceptives, although steroid use and type I glycogen storage disease are also known risk factors.[79] These lesions are divided into 4 major subtypes: inflammatory, TCF1 mutated (steatotic), β-catenin mutated, and unclassified. The imaging appearances vary depending on the subtype. The risks of malignant degeneration and spontaneous hemorrhage are increased in inflammatory and β-catenin mutated subtypes, whereas these risks are low in steatotic adenomas. Hepatic adenomas are typically solitary, although multiple adenomas can

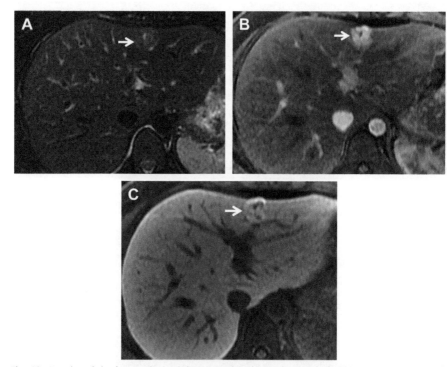

Fig. 12. Focal nodular hyperplasia. (*A*) T2-weighted MRI shows a subtle lesion within the left hepatic lobe (*arrow*) with a small central area of hyperintensity, representing the central scar. (*B*) Contrast-enhanced T1-weighted MRI in the arterial phase shows intense arterial enhancement of the lesion, with a central hypointense central scar (*arrow*). (*C*) Contrast-enhanced T1-weighted MRI using a hepatocellular contrast agent in a 20-minute delayed phase shows retained contrast within the lesion (*arrow*).

be present. Histologically, adenomas are composed of large plates of cells that resemble normal hepatocytes separated by sinusoids, which provide its arterial supply. Hepatic adenomas are not perfused by the portal vein, and are characterized by a lack of bile ducts and a paucity of and nonfunctioning Kupffer cells. The hepatocytes in an adenoma contain larger depositions of lipid, and extracellular lipid accumulation can lead to gross fatty deposition.[91]

Imaging features

On ultrasonography, hepatic adenomas show a variable appearance, owing to different quantities of lipid content, hemorrhage, and calcifications. On B-mode ultrasonography they can appear hypo-, iso-, or hyperechoic depending on the components of the adenoma. Color Doppler can demonstrate nonspecific flow within the lesion.

On CT, unenhanced images can provide important clues that can help in the characterization of an adenoma, including depiction of areas of hemorrhage, intralesional fat, and calcification. Most adenomas are sharply marginated but nonlobulated.[91] Enhancement characteristics are affected by the composition of the lesion. Typically, TCF1-mutated adenomas show mild uniform arterial hyperenhancement often to a lesser extent than FNH, and are isodense to the background liver parenchyma on the portal venous phase and delayed-phase images. Inflammatory adenomas tend to show intense arterial enhancement that persists in more delayed phases, and β-catenin mutated subtypes can show arterial enhancement with washout, mimicking HCC.

On MRI, imaging characteristics also vary depending on the composition of the adenoma. On T1-weighted images, adenomas can show a hyperintense signal owing to the presence of intralesional fat and/or hemorrhagic components. Use of fat-suppressed T1-weighted images in addition to opposed-phase imaging can help identify the presence of intralesional fat seen in TCF1-mutated adenomas, but this is rarely seen in other subtypes. Adenomas are typically mildly hyperintense on T2-weighted images compared with background liver; however, inflammatory adenomas can be markedly hyperintense. Postcontrast images have similar properties to those described on contrast-enhanced CT. Using hepatobiliary contrast agents increases the diagnostic confidence in distinguishing an adenoma from an FNH.[17] Because hepatic adenomas lack bile ducts, they do not demonstrate uptake of hepatobiliary contrast agents on delayed images and are therefore almost always hypointense (**Fig. 13**).

Hepatic Abscess

Abscesses are classified according to etiology as pyogenic (typically from *Clostridium* species and gram-negative bacteria), amebic (*Entamoeba histolytica*), and fungal (mostly from *Candida albicans*).[92] Clinical and serologic data can aid in differentiating a pyogenic from an amebic abscess. Fungal abscesses are typically multiple and smaller in size, and typically involve both the liver and spleen.

Imaging features

On ultrasonography, pyogenic and amebic abscesses are typically hypoechoic to anechoic with increased through-transmission. Air within the abscess can appear as echogenic specks. Classically, fungal abscesses are multiple small hyperechoic lesions with surrounding hypoechogenic rims.

On CT, pyogenic abscesses have irregular, sometimes shaggy margins, are hypodense on unenhanced images, and on postcontrast images show a hypoenhancing necrotic core and a thin rim of peripheral hyperemia (**Fig. 14**). The presence of air

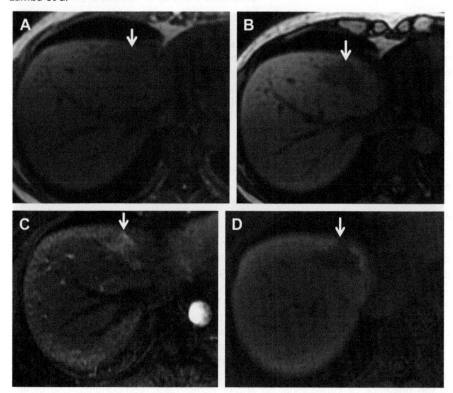

Fig. 13. Hepatic adenoma. (*A*) MRI in-phase image shows a subtle hypointense area within the left hepatic lobe (*arrow*). (*B*) MRI opposed-phase image shows decreased signal with respect to the in-phase image within the left hepatic lobe, consistent with intravoxel fat deposition (*arrow*). (*C*) Contrast-enhanced T1-weighted MRI in the arterial phase shows enhancement of the mass (*arrow*). (*D*) Contrast-enhanced T1-weighted MRI using a hepato-cellular contrast agent in a 20-minute delayed phase shows hypointensity corresponding with the lesion location (*arrow*).

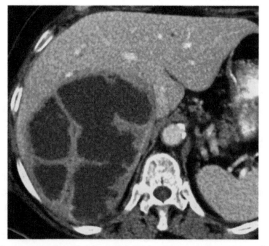

Fig. 14. Hepatic abscess. Contrast-enhanced CT in the portal venous phase shows a well-circumscribed predominantly low-density lesion with thick septations.

within this collection is useful, as this is rarely seen in amebic abscesses.[92] Multiple small hypodense lesions within the liver with some surrounding enhancement may indicate a diagnosis of fungal abscess, particularly if there is splenic involvement.

On MRI, abscesses are usually hypointense on T1-weighted images and hyperintense on T2-weighted images. Perilesional edema, manifesting as increased T2 signal surrounding the lesion, helps to distinguish an abscess from a benign cystic hepatic lesion. Postcontrast imaging characteristics are similar to those seen on CT. Fungal abscess can present as small foci of increased T2 signal throughout the liver and spleen.

Other Benign Masses

Hepatic angiomyolipomas (AMLs) are rare benign tumors composed of fat, smooth muscle, and vessels, classically seen in patients with tuberous sclerosis. There is marked variability in the amount of fat content of these lesions, and therefore the imaging characteristics vary. In a fat-containing lesion, central vascularity, as depicted on CT or MRI, has been proposed as a feature suggesting an AML (**Fig. 15**).[93] Their enhancement characteristics can mimic those of HCC and adenomas with arterial enhancement and delayed washout, thus sometimes requiring needle biopsy and/or surgical excision for definitive diagnosis.[94]

Solitary fibrous tumors usually involve the chest, but very rarely can involve the liver parenchyma. These tumors can be large, causing clinical symptoms from mass effect, are typically solitary and well circumscribed, and heterogeneously enhance on postcontrast CT and MRI studies. Imaging is not sufficient to make the diagnosis, and tissue sampling is required. Owing to their malignant potential and mass effect, these are usually surgically excised.[95]

Sarcoidosis has macroscopic hepatic manifestations in a small subset of patients. On postcontrast imaging, sarcoid granulomas usually appear as multiple small hypodense lesions on CT. The differential also includes metastatic disease, lymphoma, and fungal abscesses, for which biopsy may be required. Rarely, diffuse sarcoid granulomas within the liver can lead to a cirrhotic appearance.[96]

Hypervascular regenerative nodules are histopathologically similar to FNH, and are found in the setting of Budd-Chiari syndrome and autoimmune hepatitis with cirrhosis.[97] Imaging features can be indistinguishable from those of HCC, and may

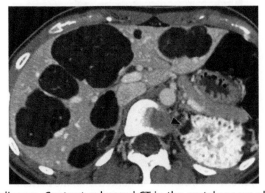

Fig. 15. Angiomyolipoma. Contrast-enhanced CT in the portal venous phase shows several predominantly fat-density hepatic lesions with internal vascularity. Numerous small angiomyolipomas are seen within the left kidney with a larger fat-containing angiomyolipoma medially (*arrowhead*).

require biopsy or close follow-up.[98] Hepatocellular contrast agents may be useful to help distinguish a regenerative nodule from a hepatocellular carcinoma, as regenerative nodules show contrast uptake in the hepatobiliary phase.

Pseudolesions Related to Fat Deposition

Hepatic steatosis is estimated to be present in 30% of the United States population and a larger percentage of obese patients.[99] Hepatic steatosis can be diffuse, geographic, or focal in its distribution. Focal steatosis or a focal area of fat sparing against the background of a steatotic liver, especially if round, can mimic a mass. Focal nodular steatosis appears as a homogeneous hyperechoic lesion on ultrasonography and can be commonly confused with a hemangioma. On CT, it appears as a hypodense mass on unenhanced images and is hypovascular compared with the background liver in all 3 contrast-enhanced phases. The lesion typically shows signal dropout on out-of-phase MR images, which, coupled with its triphasic hypovascularity, can generally be considered diagnostic (**Fig. 16**). Focal fatty sparing can pose more of a diagnostic dilemma. If there is a background of hepatic steatosis this diagnosis should be considered, although primary tumors and metastatic lesions can occur in a steatotic liver, and pose a diagnostic challenge.

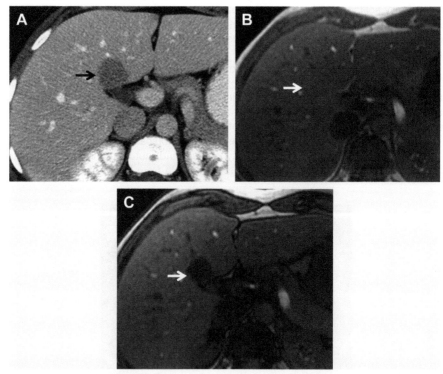

Fig. 16. Focal fatty infiltration. (*A*) Contrast-enhanced CT in the portal venous phase shows a well-circumscribed hypodense lesion within the left hepatic lobe (*arrow*). (*B*) MRI in-phase image shows relative isointensity of the area of concern with the background liver (*arrow*). (*C*) MRI opposed-phase image shows decreased signal with respect to the in-phase image, consistent with intravoxel fat deposition (*arrow*).

SUMMARY

The combination of the clinical presentation and imaging characteristics on contrast-enhanced CT or MRI allows noninvasive characterization of most liver lesions. MRI is the modality of choice for noninvasive characterization. When overlapping features exist, either imaging follow-up or percutaneous biopsy should be performed.

REFERENCES

1. Krinsky GA, Lee VS. MR imaging of cirrhotic nodules. Abdom Imaging 2000; 25(5):471–82.
2. ACR Appropriateness Criteria®; 1891 Preston White Dr Reston, VA 20191: American College of Radiology; November 2013 [April 6, 2014]. Available from: http://www.acr.org/quality-safety/appropriateness-criteria. Accessed on July 15, 2014.
3. ACR Appropriateness Criteria®: Liver lesion - initial characterization 1891 Preston White Dr Reston, VA 20191: American College of Radiology; 2010 [April 6, 2014]. Available from: http://www.acr.org/~/media/ACR/Documents/AppCriteria/Diagnostic/LiverLesionInitialCharacterization.pdf.
4. ACR Appropriateness Criteria®: Suspected liver metastases 1891 Preston White Dr Reston, VA 20191: American College of Radiology; 2011 [April 6, 2014]. Available from: http://www.acr.org/~/media/ACR/Documents/AppCriteria/Diagnostic/SuspectedLiverMetastases.pdf.
5. Ringe KI, Husarik DB, Sirlin CB, et al. Gadoxetate disodium-enhanced MRI of the liver: part 1, protocol optimization and lesion appearance in the noncirrhotic liver. AJR Am J Roentgenol 2010;195(1):13–28.
6. van Kessel CS, de Boer E, ten Kate FJ, et al. Focal nodular hyperplasia: hepatobiliary enhancement patterns on gadoxetic-acid contrast-enhanced MRI. Abdom Imaging 2013;38(3):490–501.
7. Goodwin MD, Dobson JE, Sirlin CB, et al. Diagnostic challenges and pitfalls in MR imaging with hepatocyte-specific contrast agents. Radiographics 2011; 31(6):1547–68.
8. Grazioli L, Bondioni MP, Haradome H, et al. Hepatocellular adenoma and focal nodular hyperplasia: value of gadoxetic acid-enhanced MR imaging in differential diagnosis. Radiology 2012;262(2):520–9.
9. Kitao A, Zen Y, Matsui O, et al. Hepatocellular carcinoma: signal intensity at gadoxetic acid-enhanced MR Imaging–correlation with molecular transporters and histopathologic features. Radiology 2010;256(3):817–26.
10. Muhi A, Ichikawa T, Motosugi U, et al. Diagnosis of colorectal hepatic metastases: comparison of contrast-enhanced CT, contrast-enhanced US, superparamagnetic iron oxide-enhanced MRI, and gadoxetic acid-enhanced MRI. J Magn Reson Imaging 2011;34(2):326–35.
11. Seo HJ, Kim MJ, Lee JD, et al. Gadoxetate disodium-enhanced magnetic resonance imaging versus contrast-enhanced ^{18}F-fluorodeoxyglucose positron emission tomography/computed tomography for the detection of colorectal liver metastases. Invest Radiol 2011;46(9):548–55.
12. Purysko AS, Remer EM, Coppa CP, et al. Characteristics and distinguishing features of hepatocellular adenoma and focal nodular hyperplasia on gadoxetate disodium-enhanced MRI. AJR Am J Roentgenol 2012;198(1):115–23.
13. Cruite I, Schroeder M, Merkle EM, et al. Gadoxetate disodium-enhanced MRI of the liver: part 2, protocol optimization and lesion appearance in the cirrhotic liver. AJR Am J Roentgenol 2010;195(1):29–41.

14. Motosugi U, Ichikawa T, Sou H, et al. Distinguishing hypervascular pseudole-sions of the liver from hypervascular hepatocellular carcinomas with gadoxetic acid-enhanced MR imaging. Radiology 2010;256(1):151–8.

15. Bartolozzi C, Battaglia V, Bargellini I, et al. Contrast-enhanced magnetic reso-nance imaging of 102 nodules in cirrhosis: correlation with histological findings on explanted livers. Abdom Imaging 2013;38(2):290–6.

16. Davenport MS, Viglianti BL, Al-Hawary MM, et al. Comparison of acute transient dyspnea after intravenous administration of gadoxetate disodium and gadoben-ate dimeglumine: effect on arterial phase image quality. Radiology 2013;266(2):452–61.

17. Zech CJ, Bartolozzi C, Bioulac-Sage P, et al. Consensus report of the Fifth Inter-national Forum for Liver MRI. AJR Am J Roentgenol 2013;201(1):97–107.

18. Qayyum A. Diffusion-weighted imaging in the abdomen and pelvis: concepts and applications. Radiographics 2009;29(6):1797–810.

19. Taouli B. Diffusion-weighted MR imaging for liver lesion characterization: a crit-ical look. Radiology 2012;262(2):378–80.

20. Bruix J, Sherman M, American Association for the Study of Liver Diseases. Man-agement of hepatocellular carcinoma: an update. Hepatology 2011;53(3):1020–2.

21. Correas J-M, Low G, Needleman L, et al. Contrast enhanced ultrasound in the detection of liver metastases: a prospective multi-centre dose testing study using a perfluorobutane microbubble contrast agent (NC100100). Eur Radiol 2011;21(8):1739–46.

22. Tan GJS, Berlangieri SU, Lee ST, et al. FDG PET/CT in the liver: lesions mimicking malignancies. Abdom Imaging 2014;39(1):187–95.

23. Willatt JM, Hussain HK, Adusumilli S, et al. MR Imaging of hepatocellular carci-noma in the cirrhotic liver: challenges and controversies. Radiology 2008;247(2):311–30.

24. Hanna RF, Aguirre DA, Kased N, et al. Cirrhosis-associated hepatocellular nod-ules: correlation of histopathologic and MR imaging features. Radiographics 2008;28(3):747–69.

25. Aaltonen LA, Hamilton SR, World Health Organization, International Agency for Research on Cancer. Pathology and genetics of tumours of the digestive sys-tem. Lyon (France); Oxford (United Kingdom): IARC Press; Oxford University Press (distributor); 2000. p. 314.

26. Llovet JM, Burroughs A, Bruix J. Hepatocellular carcinoma. Lancet 2003;362(9399):1907–17.

27. Freeny PC, Grossholz M, Kaakaji K, et al. Significance of hyperattenuating and contrast-enhancing hepatic nodules detected in the cirrhotic liver during arterial phase helical CT in pre-liver transplant patients: radiologic-histopathologic cor-relation of explanted livers. Abdom Imaging 2003;28(3):333–46.

28. Ignee A, Weiper D, Schuessler G, et al. Sonographic characterisation of hepa-tocellular carcinoma at time of diagnosis. Z Gastroenterol 2005;43(3):289–94.

29. Colli A, Fraquelli M, Casazza G, et al. Accuracy of ultrasonography, spiral CT, magnetic resonance, and alpha-fetoprotein in diagnosing hepatocellular carci-noma: a systematic review. Am J Gastroenterol 2006;101(3):513–23.

30. Kelekis NL, Semelka RC, Worawattanakul S, et al. Hepatocellular carcinoma in North America: a multiinstitutional study of appearance on T1-weighted, T2-weighted, and serial gadolinium-enhanced gradient-echo images. AJR Am J Roentgenol 1998;170(4):1005–13.

31. Marrero JA, Hussain HK, Nghiem HV, et al. Improving the prediction of hepatocellular carcinoma in cirrhotic patients with an arterially-enhancing liver mass. Liver Transpl 2005;11(3):281–9.

32. Kanematsu M, Semelka RC, Leonardou P, et al. Hepatocellular carcinoma of diffuse type: MR imaging findings and clinical manifestations. J Magn Reson Imaging 2003;18(2):189–95.

33. Tublin ME, Dodd GD 3rd, Baron RL. Benign and malignant portal vein thrombosis: differentiation by CT characteristics. AJR Am J Roentgenol 1997; 168(3):719–23.

34. Bruix J, Sherman M, American Association for the Study of Liver Disease Practice Guidelines Committee. Management of hepatocellular carcinoma. Hepatology 2005;42(5):1208–36.

35. Wald C, Russo MW, Heimbach JK, et al. New OPTN/UNOS policy for liver transplant allocation: standardization of liver imaging, diagnosis, classification, and reporting of hepatocellular carcinoma. Radiology 2013;266(2):376–82.

36. Ganeshan D, Szklaruk J, Kundra V, et al. Imaging features of fibrolamellar hepatocellular carcinoma. AJR Am J Roentgenol 2014;202(3):544–52.

37. Ichikawa T, Federle MP, Grazioli L, et al. Fibrolamellar hepatocellular carcinoma: imaging and pathologic findings in 31 recent cases. Radiology 1999;213(2): 352–61.

38. El-Serag HB, Davila JA. Is fibrolamellar carcinoma different from hepatocellular carcinoma? A US population-based study. Hepatology 2004;39(3):798–803.

39. Friedman AC, Lichtenstein JE, Goodman Z, et al. Fibrolamellar hepatocellular carcinoma. Radiology 1985;157(3):583–7.

40. Corrigan K, Semelka RC. Dynamic contrast-enhanced MR imaging of fibrolamellar hepatocellular carcinoma. Abdom Imaging 1995;20(2):122–5.

41. Brancatelli G, Federle MP, Grazioli L, et al. Hepatocellular carcinoma in noncirrhotic liver: CT, clinical, and pathologic findings in 39 U.S. residents. Radiology 2002;222(1):89–94.

42. Manfredi R, Barbaro B, Masselli G, et al. Magnetic resonance imaging of cholangiocarcinoma. Semin Liver Dis 2004;24(2):155–64.

43. Liver Cancer Study Group of Japan. The general rules for the clinical and pathological study of primary liver cancer. 4th edition. Tokyo: Kanehara; 2000.

44. Choi BI, Lee JM, Han JK. Imaging of intrahepatic and hilar cholangiocarcinoma. Abdom Imaging 2004;29(5):548–57.

45. Valls C, Guma A, Puig I, et al. Intrahepatic peripheral cholangiocarcinoma: CT evaluation. Abdom Imaging 2000;25(5):490–6.

46. Kim TK, Choi BI, Han JK, et al. Peripheral cholangiocarcinoma of the liver: two-phase spiral CT findings. Radiology 1997;204(2):539–43.

47. Maetani Y, Itoh K, Watanabe C, et al. MR imaging of intrahepatic cholangiocarcinoma with pathologic correlation. AJR Am J Roentgenol 2001;176(6): 1499–507.

48. Kang Y, Lee JM, Kim SH, et al. Intrahepatic mass-forming cholangiocarcinoma: enhancement patterns on gadoxetic acid-enhanced MR images. Radiology 2012;264(3):751–60.

49. Soyer P, Bluemke DA, Sibert A, et al. MR imaging of intrahepatic cholangiocarcinoma. Abdom Imaging 1995;20(2):126–30.

50. Peporte AR, Sommer WH, Nikolaou K, et al. Imaging features of intrahepatic cholangiocarcinoma in Gd-EOB-DTPA-enhanced MRI. Eur J Radiol 2013; 82(3):e101–6.

51. Mehrabi A, Kashfi A, Fonouni H, et al. Primary malignant hepatic epithelioid hemangioendothelioma: a comprehensive review of the literature with emphasis on the surgical therapy. Cancer 2006;107(9):2108–21.

52. Dong A, Dong H, Wang Y, et al. MRI and FDG PET/CT findings of hepatic epithelioid hemangioendothelioma. Clin Nucl Med 2013;38(2):e66–73.

53. Bruegel M, Muenzel D, Waldt S, et al. Hepatic epithelioid hemangioendothelioma: findings at CT and MRI including preliminary observations at diffusion-weighted echo-planar imaging. Abdom Imaging 2011;36(4):415–24.

54. Makhlouf HR, Ishak KG, Goodman ZD. Epithelioid hemangioendothelioma of the liver: a clinicopathologic study of 137 cases. Cancer 1999;85(3):562–82.

55. Amin S, Chung H, Jha R. Hepatic epithelioid hemangioendothelioma: MR imaging findings. Abdom Imaging 2011;36(4):407–14.

56. Miller WJ, Dodd GD 3rd, Federle MP, et al. Epithelioid hemangioendothelioma of the liver: imaging findings with pathologic correlation. AJR Am J Roentgenol 1992;159(1):53–7.

57. Lin J, Ji Y. CT and MRI diagnosis of hepatic epithelioid hemangioendothelioma. Hepatobiliary Pancreat Dis Int 2010;9(2):154–8.

58. Azzam RI, Alshak NS, Pham HP. AIRP best cases in radiologic-pathologic correlation: hepatic epithelioid hemangioendothelioma. Radiographics 2012;32(3):789–94.

59. Alomari AI. The lollipop sign: a new cross-sectional sign of hepatic epithelioid hemangioendothelioma. Eur J Radiol 2006;59(3):460–4.

60. Bioulac-Sage P, Laumonier H, Laurent C, et al. Benign and malignant vascular tumors of the liver in adults. Semin Liver Dis 2008;28(3):302–14.

61. Buetow PC, Buck JL, Ros PR, et al. Malignant vascular tumors of the liver: radiologic-pathologic correlation. Radiographics 1994;14(1):153–66 [quiz: 167–8].

62. Koyama T, Fletcher JG, Johnson CD, et al. Primary hepatic angiosarcoma: findings at CT and MR imaging. Radiology 2002;222(3):667–73.

63. Bruegel M, Muenzel D, Waldt S, et al. Hepatic angiosarcoma: cross-sectional imaging findings in seven patients with emphasis on dynamic contrast-enhanced and diffusion-weighted MRI. Abdom Imaging 2013;38(4):745–54.

64. Chung EM, Lattin GE Jr, Cube R, et al. From the archives of the AFIP: pediatric liver masses: radiologic-pathologic correlation. Part 2. Malignant tumors. Radiographics 2011;31(2):483–507.

65. Rademaker J, Widjaja A, Galanski M. Hepatic hemangiosarcoma: imaging findings and differential diagnosis. Eur Radiol 2000;10(1):129–33.

66. Oe A, Habu D, Kawabe J, et al. A case of diffuse hepatic angiosarcoma diagnosed by FDG-PET. Ann Nucl Med 2005;19(6):519–21.

67. Maeda T, Tateishi U, Hasegawa T, et al. Primary hepatic angiosarcoma on coregistered FDG PET and CT images. AJR Am J Roentgenol 2007;188(6):1615–7.

68. Mani H, Van Thiel DH. Mesenchymal tumors of the liver. Clin Liver Dis 2001;5(1):219–57, viii.

69. Gazelle GS, Lee MJ, Hahn PF, et al. US, CT, and MRI of primary and secondary liver lymphoma. J Comput Assist Tomogr 1994;18(3):412–5.

70. Maher MM, McDermott SR, Fenlon HM, et al. Imaging of primary non-Hodgkin's lymphoma of the liver. Clin Radiol 2001;56(4):295–301.

71. Avlonitis VS, Linos D. Primary hepatic lymphoma: a review. Eur J Surg 1999;165(8):725–9.

72. Kim KA, Kim KW, Park SH, et al. Unusual mesenchymal liver tumors in adults: radiologic-pathologic correlation. AJR Am J Roentgenol 2006;187(5):W481–9.

73. Soares KC, Arnaoutakis DJ, Kamel I, et al. Cystic neoplasms of the liver: biliary cystadenoma and cystadenocarcinoma. J Am Coll Surg 2014;218(1):119–28.

74. Lewin M, Mourra N, Honigman I, et al. Assessment of MRI and MRCP in diagnosis of biliary cystadenoma and cystadenocarcinoma. Eur Radiol 2006;16(2): 407–13.

75. Kim JY, Kim SH, Eun HW, et al. Differentiation between biliary cystic neoplasms and simple cysts of the liver: accuracy of CT. AJR Am J Roentgenol 2010;195(5): 1142–8.

76. Seo JK, Kim SH, Lee SH, et al. Appropriate diagnosis of biliary cystic tumors: comparison with atypical hepatic simple cysts. Eur J Gastroenterol Hepatol 2010;22(8):989–96.

77. Choi HK, Lee JK, Lee KH, et al. Differential diagnosis for intrahepatic biliary cystadenoma and hepatic simple cyst: significance of cystic fluid analysis and radiologic findings. J Clin Gastroenterol 2010;44(4):289–93.

78. Schwartz LH, Gandras EJ, Colangelo SM, et al. Prevalence and importance of small hepatic lesions found at CT in patients with cancer. Radiology 1999; 210(1):71–4.

79. Bartolotta TV, Taibbi A, Midiri M, et al. Focal liver lesions: contrast-enhanced ultrasound. Abdom Imaging 2009;34(2):193–209.

80. Harvey CJ, Albrecht T. Ultrasound of focal liver lesions. Eur Radiol 2001;11(9): 1578–93.

81. Silva AC, Evans JM, McCullough AE, et al. MR imaging of hypervascular liver masses: a review of current techniques. Radiographics 2009;29(2):385–402.

82. Oliver JH 3rd, Baron RL, Federle MP, et al. Hypervascular liver metastases: do unenhanced and hepatic arterial phase CT images affect tumor detection? Radiology 1997;205(3):709–15.

83. Cantwell CP, Setty BN, Holalkere N, et al. Liver lesion detection and characterization in patients with colorectal cancer: a comparison of low radiation dose non-enhanced PET/CT, contrast-enhanced PET/CT, and liver MRI. J Comput Assist Tomogr 2008;32(5):738–44.

84. Chen L, Zhang J, Zhang L, et al. Meta-analysis of gadoxetic acid disodium (Gd-EOB-DTPA)-enhanced magnetic resonance imaging for the detection of liver metastases. PLoS One 2012;7(11):e48681.

85. Chen LB, Tong JL, Song HZ, et al. (18)F-DG PET/CT in detection of recurrence and metastasis of colorectal cancer. World J Gastroenterol 2007;13(37):5025–9.

86. van Malenstein H, Maleux G, Monbaliu D, et al. Giant liver hemangioma: the role of female sex hormones and treatment. Eur J Gastroenterol Hepatol 2011;23(5): 438–43.

87. Szurowska E, Nowicki T, Izycka-Swieszewska E, et al. Is hepatotropic contrast enhanced MR a more effective method in differential diagnosis of hemangioma than multi-phase CT and unenhanced MR? BMC Gastroenterol 2011;11(1):43.

88. Cristiano A, Dietrich A, Spina JC, et al. Focal nodular hyperplasia and hepatic adenoma: current diagnosis and management. Updates Surg 2014;66(1):9–21.

89. Terkivatan T, van den Bos IC, Hussain SM, et al. Focal nodular hyperplasia: lesion characteristics on state-of-the-art MRI including dynamic gadolinium-enhanced and superparamagnetic iron-oxide-uptake sequences in a prospective study. J Magn Reson Imaging 2006;24(4):864–72.

90. Piscaglia F, Lencioni R, Sagrini E, et al. Characterization of focal liver lesions with contrast-enhanced ultrasound. Ultrasound Med Biol 2010;36(4):531–50.

91. Grazioli L, Federle MP, Brancatelli G, et al. Hepatic adenomas: imaging and pathologic findings. Radiographics 2001;21(4):877–92.

92. Vachha B, Sun MR, Siewert B, et al. Cystic lesions of the liver. Am J Roentgenol 2011;196(4):W355–66.
93. Basaran C, Karcaaltincaba M, Akata D, et al. Fat-containing lesions of the liver: cross-sectional imaging findings with emphasis on MRI. Am J Roentgenol 2005; 184(4):1103–10.
94. Takayama Y, Moriura S, Nagata J, et al. Hepatic angiomyolipoma: radiologic and histopathologic correlation. Abdom Imaging 2002;27(2):180–3.
95. Nath DS, Rutzick AD, Sielaff TD. Solitary fibrous tumor of the liver. Am J Roentgenol 2006;187(2):W187–90.
96. Koyama T, Ueda H, Togashi K, et al. Radiologic manifestations of sarcoidosis in various organs. Radiographics 2004;24(1):87–104.
97. Matsui O, Kobayashi S, Gabata T, et al. Vascular diseases of the liver. In: Hamm B, editor. Abdominal imaging. Berlin: Springer; 2013. p. 1135–68.
98. Czaja AJ. Hepatocellular carcinoma and other malignancies in autoimmune hepatitis. Dig Dis Sci 2013;58(6):1459–76.
99. Browning JD, Szczepaniak LS, Dobbins R, et al. Prevalence of hepatic steatosis in an urban population in the United States: impact of ethnicity. Hepatology 2004;40(6):1387–95.

Primary Malignant Tumors of Peritoneal and Retroperitoneal Origin
Clinical and Imaging Features

Meghan G. Lubner, MD, J. Louis Hinshaw, MD,
Perry J. Pickhardt, MD*

KEYWORDS

- Peritoneal • Retroperitoneal • Malignancy • Computed tomography
- Magnetic resonance imaging • Liposarcoma • Leiomyosarcoma

KEY POINTS

- Primary peritoneal and retroperitoneal malignancies are less common than metastatic disease.
- A variety of tumor types can occur in the peritoneum and retroperitoneum, and establishing a diagnosis from imaging alone can be difficult. Demographic and clinical information taken in concert with imaging findings can help narrow the differential diagnosis.
- Papillary serous carcinoma, the most common primary tumor of the peritoneum, occurs almost exclusively in women and is often densely calcified, which can aid in diagnosis.
- Liposarcoma is the most common primary tumor of the retroperitoneum, followed by leiomyosarcoma, each having imaging features that can suggest or even make the diagnosis.
- Imaging is useful in detection, staging, guiding biopsy (most often with computed tomography or ultrasonography), and evaluating response to therapy.

INTRODUCTION

Peritoneal carcinomatosis is a relatively common manifestation of many organ-based malignancies, particularly of the gastrointestinal tract and ovaries. Similarly, metastatic retroperitoneal lymphadenopathy and direct extension from an organ-based primary tumor are also common findings at imaging evaluation. Primary tumors of peritoneal and retroperitoneal origin occur much less frequently, but are often first

The authors have nothing to disclose.
Department of Radiology, University of Wisconsin School of Medicine and Public Health, 600 Highland Avenue, Madison, WI 53792, USA
* Corresponding author. Department of Radiology, University of Wisconsin Hospital and Clinics, E3/311 Clinical Science Center, 600 Highland Avenue, Madison, WI 53792.
E-mail address: ppickhardt2@uwhealth.org

identified on cross-sectional radiologic imaging studies, such as computed tomography (CT), ultrasonography, or magnetic resonance (MR) imaging.[1]

Neoplastic involvement of the peritoneum and retroperitoneum generally manifest with an abnormal increase in soft tissue, which can appear infiltrative or tumorous and be associated with variable amounts of cystic change, calcification, macroscopic fat, enhancement, and surrounding fluid. However, because many nonneoplastic and metastatic processes demonstrate similar imaging findings, the appearance of many primary malignancies of the peritoneum and retroperitoneum is nonspecific.[2] As a result, even in the absence of a known organ-based primary malignancy, metastatic disease is often the first consideration when confronted with an abnormal soft-tissue process arising within the peritoneal or retroperitoneal space. However, primary malignancies should also be considered in this setting.[3]

This review presents the salient clinical and imaging features of several primary neoplasms (**Box 1**) arising from the tissue components that comprise the ligaments, mesenteries, and connective tissues of the peritoneal and retroperitoneal spaces. Combining the imaging features with the patient's relevant clinical information can often refine the differential diagnosis for peritoneal-based and retroperitoneal-based neoplasms. In addition to detection and characterization, cross-sectional imaging is useful for directing biopsy for tissue diagnosis.[1]

ANATOMIC CONSIDERATIONS

The visceral and parietal peritoneum encloses the large potential space referred to as the peritoneal cavity. Pathologic processes that gain access to the peritoneal cavity can disseminate throughout this space via the relatively unrestricted movement of fluid and cells. Pathologic processes can also be disseminated within the subperitoneal space, which lies deep to the surface lining of the visceral and parietal peritoneum, omentum, and the various peritoneal ligaments and mesenteries.[4] The subperitoneal space has both intraperitoneal and extraperitoneal components that

---

Box 1
Primary peritoneal and retroperitoneal malignancies

Primary Peritoneal Malignancies

  Mesothelioma

  Papillary serous carcinoma

  Desmoplastic small round cell tumor

  Malignant fibrous histiocytoma

  Liposarcoma

  Other mesenchymal tumors

Primary Retroperitoneal Malignancies

  Liposarcoma

  Leiomyosarcoma

  Malignant fibrous histiocytoma

  Other mesenchymal tumors

  Paraganglioma

  Extragonadal germ cell tumors

bridge the peritoneum and retroperitoneum, which can result in bidirectional spread of disease processes. This concept helps to explain the involvement of both the peritoneal and retroperitoneal space that is sometimes encountered.[1]

The retroperitoneal space is not defined by specific anatomic structures delineating its borders, but rather as the space posterior to the peritoneal cavity. Retroperitoneal structures may be defined as primary (ie, located within the retroperitoneum at the beginning of embryogenesis) or secondary (ie, initially suspended by a mesentery during early embryogenesis but subsequently migrated posteriorly and fused to become retroperitonealized). The extraperitoneal pelvis, including the presacral space, essentially represents the inferior continuation of the retroperitoneal space.[5] The retroperitoneum and extraperitoneal pelvis represent a crossroads for several organ systems, containing portions of the gastrointestinal and genitourinary tracts, in addition to major vascular structures. The retroperitoneum, however, also contains connective tissues, fat, and neural elements.[1,4]

This article focuses on primary malignancies arising directly from the supporting tissues of the peritoneal, subperitoneal, and retroperitoneal spaces, rather than tumors that arise from the organs contained within these spaces.

PRIMARY PERITONEAL MALIGNANCIES
Papillary Serous Carcinoma

Clinical features
Primary papillary serous carcinoma of the peritoneum is a relatively uncommon malignancy that predominantly affects postmenopausal women.[6,7] Because this tumor is histologically identical to serous ovarian papillary carcinoma and is clearly distinguishable only when the ovaries are either not involved or superficially involved, its incidence is underestimated.[6] Treatment generally consists of an abdominal hysterectomy, bilateral salpingo-oophorectomy, and debulking surgery, which are followed by combination chemotherapy. Despite these interventions, the prognosis is dismal.[6,8]

Imaging features
Cross-sectional imaging often shows extensive, multifocal involvement of the peritoneum, with omental caking, ascites, and, importantly, no associated primary ovarian mass (**Fig. 1**). Misclassification as primary ovarian cancer is common in the authors' experience, and peritoneal origin may be first suggested by the radiologist. As with primary ovarian primary tumors there is often extensive calcification within the peritoneal implants, which can be a useful CT finding for differentiating this tumor from peritoneal mesothelioma.[6,8]

Mesothelioma

Clinical features
Mesothelial cells line the body cavities, including the pleura, peritoneum, pericardium, and scrotum. Mesothelioma is a rare tumor, which arises from these cells and most frequently involves the pleural space. However, approximately 30% arise solely from the peritoneum.[9] There are benign, borderline, and malignant variants, but benign cystic mesothelioma is not related to malignant mesothelioma. Compared with the pleural form, malignant mesothelioma of the peritoneum is less often associated with asbestos exposure.[9] However, cases with both pleural and peritoneal involvement are usually asbestos-related. In general, malignant mesothelioma of the peritoneum is an aggressive tumor with a rapidly progressive clinical course and a universally poor prognosis. For untreated cases, median survival ranges from 5 to 12 months, with little improvement seen in patients receiving multimodality therapy.[10]

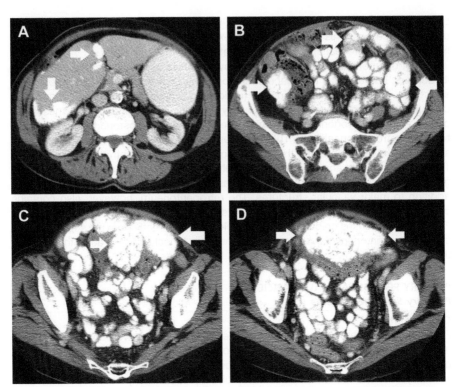

Fig. 1. Papillary serous carcinoma of the peritoneum. Contrast-enhanced computed tomography (CT) images (*A–D*) show densely calcified peritoneal implants (*arrows*) along the liver surface (*A*), in the paracolic gutters and anterior omentum (*B, C*), and in the pelvis (*D*) in this 75-year-old woman who presented with abdominal bloating. No ovarian tumor or involvement, which is a key part of making this diagnosis, was seen in this case (not shown).

Imaging features

The imaging features of peritoneal mesothelioma are variable.[3] The "dry" appearance consists of single or multiple peritoneal-based soft-tissue masses that may be large or confluent (**Fig. 2**). The "wet" appearance consists of peritoneal thickening that may be nodular and/or diffuse and is associated with peritoneal fluid (ascites) (**Fig. 3**). The tumor can be identified in any location within the omentum, mesentery, or peritoneal folds, and spreads along serosal surfaces. Scalloping, mass effect, or direct invasion of adjacent abdominal organs can be seen (see **Fig. 3A**). The most commonly involved organs are the colon and liver.[9] Calcification, either within the mass or associated with peritoneal plaques, is uncommon, and one should consider other causes in the setting of extensive calcification in a peritoneal-based tumor.

Desmoplastic Small Round Cell Tumor

Clinical features

Desmoplastic small round cell tumor is a rare, highly aggressive malignancy that has been relatively recently described.[11,12] It is a member of the family of lesions classified as small round blue cell tumors (lymphoma, neuroblastoma, rhabdomyosarcoma, Ewing sarcoma, neuroectodermic tumors), and is characterized by a recurrent specific chromosomal translocation and distinct immunohistochemical pattern (epithelial,

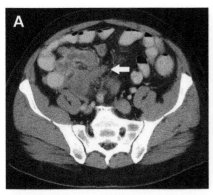

Fig. 2. Dry peritoneal mesothelioma. Contrast-enhanced axial CT images (*A, B*) show a lobulated, heterogeneous peritoneal mass (*arrows*) without associated ascites in this 63-year-old man who presented with fatigue, anemia, and abdominal pain.

mesenchymal, and neural markers).[12] It generally behaves like a soft-tissue sarcoma and has a predilection for primary peritoneal involvement, particularly in adolescent and young adult males. The disease tends to be rapidly progressive, and metastatic disease to the liver, lungs, lymph nodes, and bones are often present at diagnosis. Treatment is relatively ineffective, but attempted therapy often includes combination surgical debulking, chemotherapy, and radiation therapy.

Imaging features
The most common imaging appearance is that of multiple, bulky, rounded peritoneal-based masses (**Fig. 4**).[11] There can be associated ascites, and heterogeneous enhancement of the masses with areas of central necrosis is common. Contrast enhancement is often weak, likely because of the fibrous nature of the tumor.[12] The omentum and paravesical regions are often involved. Although the lesions are usually discrete, an infiltrative appearance is sometimes seen. Calcifications and lymphadenopathy are not usually present. These tumors are often ^{18}F-fluorodeoxyglucose avid, and positron emission tomography/CT can sometimes provide additional staging information.[13–15]

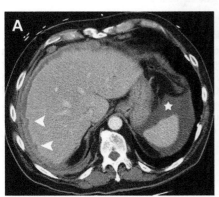
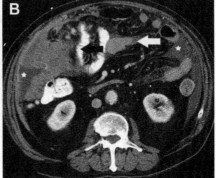

Fig. 3. Wet peritoneal mesothelioma. Contrast-enhanced axial CT images (*A, B*) show multifocal omental and peritoneal heterogeneous soft-tissue deposits (*arrows*) with associated ascites (*stars*). Note the scalloping along the liver surface (*arrowheads in A*).

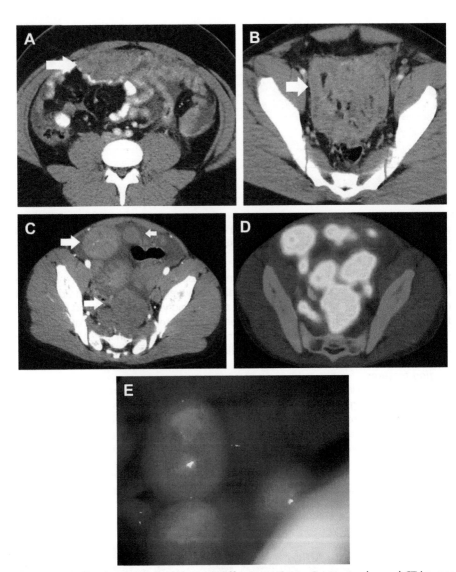

Fig. 4. Desmoplastic small cell tumor in 2 different patients. Contrast-enhanced CT images (*A, B*) in a young male patient show confluent, infiltrative soft tissue along the anterior omentum (*A*) and in the pelvis (*B*) (*arrows*) with associated small ascites. This appearance represents the infiltrative form of desmoplastic small cell tumor. Contrast-enhanced axial CT image (*C*) in a second young man shows ascites and multiple rounded heterogeneous peritoneal implants (*arrows*) that show ^{18}F-fluorodeoxyglucose avidity on PET (*D*), found at surgery (*E*) to represent desmoplastic small cell tumor.

Malignant Fibrous Histiocytoma

Clinical features

Primary sarcomas of the peritoneal/subperitoneal space, such as malignant fibrous histiocytoma (MFH) and liposarcoma, occur less frequently than their retroperitoneal counterparts.[16] These tumors are most frequently seen in adults and typically are fairly large at diagnosis.

MFH accounts for 20% to 24% of all soft-tissue sarcomas, most commonly arising in the extremities and retroperitoneum.[13,17] However, MFH is also reported to be the single most common primary peritoneal sarcoma.[16] It occurs more frequently in men, with a peak incidence in the fifth and sixth decades of life. The mass is often clinically silent until it is large, as it is usually painless. Constitutional symptoms such as fever, malaise, and weight loss can occur but are nonspecific. The only treatment is complete surgical resection, if possible. Metastatic disease most often involves the lungs, bone, and liver. Prognosis is related to tumor grade, size, and presence or absence of metastatic disease. Specifically, high-grade tumors and tumors larger than 10 cm have a poor outcome, with 10-year survival rates of less than 50%.[1,16,18]

Imaging features
Radiographically, MFH typically manifests as a large heterogeneous soft-tissue mass, as do most sarcomas. Biopsy is required to make a specific diagnosis. The mass is frequently lobulated with peripheral nodular enhancement, can have associated calcifications (in approximately 10%), and may demonstrate heterogeneity from central necrosis, hemorrhage, or myxoid degeneration (**Fig. 5**). Fatty components are not seen in MFH, and its presence would suggest liposarcoma.[13] The tumor may directly invade the abdominal musculature, but vascular invasion is rare.

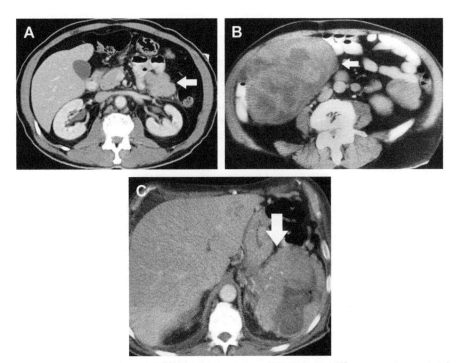

Fig. 5. Mesenteric malignant fibrous histiocytoma (MFH) in 3 different patients. Axial contrast-enhanced CT images in 3 different patients (*A–C*) show mesenteric mass lesions with variable, somewhat heterogeneous enhancement (*arrows*). The larger lesions (*B, C*) show areas of central necrosis.

Liposarcoma

Clinical features

Fat-containing tumors are common in general, and account for approximately half of all soft-tissue tumors in most surgical series.[19–21] However, most of these represent benign lipomas, and differentiating these tumors from liposarcoma is not a trivial matter.[21,22] Although liposarcoma is one of the most common primary retroperitoneal malignancies, primary peritoneal liposarcoma is relatively rare.[23] The clinical presentation is usually delayed because of the lack of associated symptoms. Ultimately the mass may become palpable, create symptoms related to mass effect on adjacent structures, be incidentally identified at the time of imaging. Treatment is surgical resection, with or without chemotherapy and radiotherapy. Prognosis is inversely related to differentiation of the tumor and directly related to completeness of resection.

Imaging features

When macroscopic fat is present, it is easily and confidently recognized on CT and MR imaging, and this observation significantly limits the differential diagnosis. If the mass is homogeneous, well defined, and consists almost entirely of fat with only minimal if any soft-tissue component, the diagnosis of a benign lipoma is almost certain. Liposarcomas are typically less well defined, have indistinct borders, and contain variable but increased amounts of soft tissue.[21–23] In fact, some poorly differentiated liposarcomas have no demonstrable fat on cross-sectional imaging and are therefore indistinguishable from other sarcomas (**Fig. 6**).

Other Malignant Mesenchymal Tumors

Clinical features

The remaining malignant mesenchymal tumors beyond MFH and liposarcoma essentially lack any distinguishing clinical or radiographic features. As a result, tissue biopsy or surgical resection is required for definitive diagnosis. However, malignant nerve sheath tumors and gastrointestinal stromal tumors (GIST) in the setting of neurofibromatosis type 1 (NF-1) can be an exception because the patient will often have clinical stigmata of NF-1 (eg, café-au-lait spots and cutaneous neurofibromas) or will already carry the diagnosis of NF-1.[24]

Peritoneal involvement by leiomyosarcoma and malignant GIST are most frequently due to metastatic spread from a primary gastrointestinal site, but primary peritoneal tumors can and do occur (**Fig. 7**).[25,26] In the past, high-risk GISTs were incorrectly classified as leiomyosarcomas (see section on retroperitoneal leiomyosarcomas). Fibrosarcoma of the mesentery and omentum in young patients can be difficult to differentiate from benign inflammatory pseudotumor (myofibroblastic tumor) at both imaging and pathologic evaluation.[27,28] Angiosarcoma can develop from the vascular elements of the subperitoneal space. Even synovial sarcomas can arise within the peritoneum, and these tumors can have associated dystrophic calcifications.[29]

Imaging features

Malignant nerve sheath tumors are often multifocal, and have a branching or coalescent appearance. These tumors are frequently of low attenuation on CT and have high signal on T2-weighted MR images. Consequently they are sometimes mistaken for cystic lesions. Frequently, there are associated nerve root lesions or other findings of NF-1. GIST should also be considered for peritoneal or retroperitoneal tumors in the setting of NF-1 (**Fig. 8**).

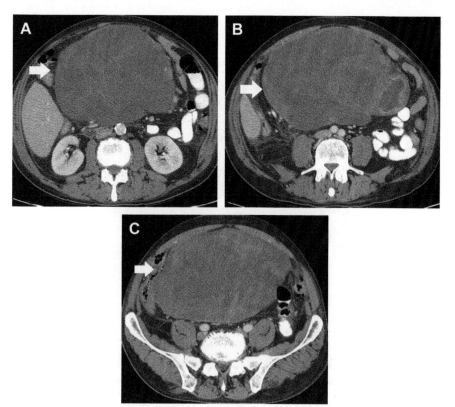

Fig. 6. (*A–C*) Peritoneal dedifferentiated liposarcoma in a 61-year-old man who presented with fatigue and anemia, found to have a large heterogeneous mesenteric mass without discernible macroscopic fat on contrast-enhanced CT (*arrows*). Surgical pathology demonstrated dedifferentiated liposarcoma with myxofibrosarcoma histology arising from the jejunal mesentery.

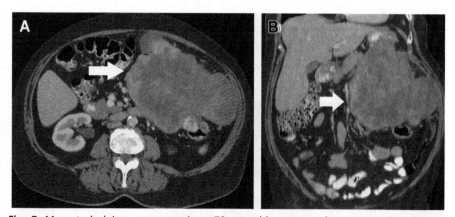

Fig. 7. Mesenteric leiomyosarcoma in a 70-year-old woman who presented with 2 to 3 months of abdominal bloating, found to have a large heterogeneous mesenteric mass (*arrows*) on axial (*A*) and coronal (*B*) contrast-enhanced CT images with central areas of low attenuation suggestive of necrosis. Preoperatively this was thought to arise from the stomach, but at surgery, this 27-cm lesion seemed adherent to and possibly arising from the transverse colonic mesentery/peritoneum, but clearly separate from the stomach. Surgical pathology demonstrated intermediate-grade leiomyosarcoma.

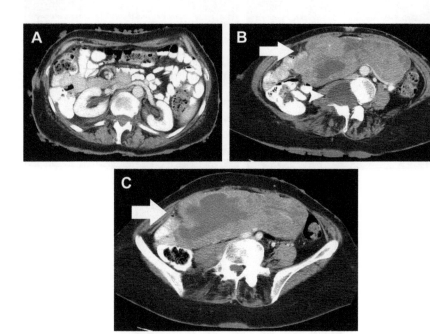

Fig. 8. Neurofibromatosis and gastrointestinal stromal tumor (GIST). Contrast-enhanced transverse CT images show numerous small skin lesions compatible with cutaneous neurofibromas (*A–C*), enlargement of a right lumbar neural foramen caused by lateral meningocele (*arrowhead in B*), and large heterogeneous mesenteric mass with central areas of necrosis or cystic change (*arrows in B, C*). This 56-year-old woman had a known diagnosis of neurofibromatosis type I, and surgical pathology on this heterogeneous mass confirmed GIST.

The remaining sarcomas are usually indistinguishable from each other on cross-sectional imaging, usually presenting as large soft-tissue masses. Synovial sarcomas may have associated dystrophic calcifications (**Fig. 9**), and angiosarcomas are typically hypervascular and may be associated with hemoperitoneum (**Fig. 10**), but these features are not always present, and significant overlap in imaging features exists (**Fig. 11**).[30]

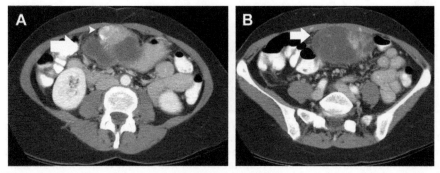

Fig. 9. Peritoneal synovial sarcoma. Contrast-enhanced CT images show a lobulated mixed solid and cystic mass lesion (*arrows in A, B*) in the gastrocolic ligament, with an anterior calcified nodule (*arrowhead in A*) found to represent synovial sarcoma.

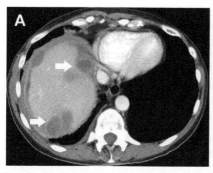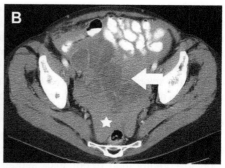

Fig. 10. Peritoneal angiosarcoma. Contrast-enhanced CT images (*A, B*) show low-attenuation, peripherally enhancing nodules in the pelvis and scalloping of the liver surface (*arrows in A, B*). Associated high-attenuation fluid is seen layering in the pelvis (*asterisk in B*), compatible with hemoperitoneum. This 67-year-old woman presented with several months of bloating and fatigue and was initially thought to have ovarian cancer with peritoneal carcinomatosis. However, surgical pathology demonstrated angiosarcoma implants on the uterus and ovary and throughout the peritoneum, with associated hemorrhage.

PRIMARY RETROPERITONEAL NEOPLASMS
Liposarcoma

Clinical features
As a group, sarcomas are the most common primary malignancies of the retroperitoneum. The 3 most common cell types include liposarcoma, leiomyosarcoma, and MFH. Beyond liposarcoma where the presence of fat usually provides a specific clue,[31,32] most of these malignant mesenchymal tumors arising within the retroperitoneum are difficult to differentiate on imaging or clinical grounds.

As with peritoneal fat-containing tumors, differentiating benign lipomas from liposarcomas can sometimes be extremely difficult.[21,22] Liposarcoma is one of the most common primary retroperitoneal malignancies.[33] The mass is often large at the time of

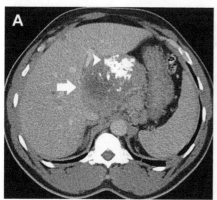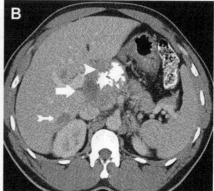

Fig. 11. Porta hepatis spindle cell sarcoma. Contrast-enhanced axial CT images of this 50-year-old man with abdominal pain show a heterogeneously enhancing mass (*arrows in A, B*) in the porta hepatis containing central necrosis and dystrophic calcifications (*arrowheads*). Although this has features similar to those of synovial sarcoma (see **Fig. 9**), this tumor was a high-grade spindle cell sarcoma. Note the low-attenuation metastatic lesion in the right hepatic lobe (*arrow with tail in B*).

diagnosis owing to the lack of associated clinical manifestations. The treatment is surgical resection, with the decision to administer additional chemotherapy and radiotherapy made on a case-by-case basis.[34] According to the 2002 World Health Organization histologic classification, liposarcoma is divided into 5 subtypes: well differentiated, dedifferentiated, myxoid, pleomorphic, and mixed.[33] Other variants have been described, including the sclerosing variant of well-differentiated liposarcoma.[35] Prognosis is related to the grade and subtype of the tumor and completeness of resection.[36]

Imaging features

A well-defined, homogeneous fatty mass is likely to represent a benign lipoma. However, characteristics that are associated with a higher risk of liposarcoma include a lesion size greater than 10 cm, thick septations, globular and/or nodular nonadipose regions, and a relative proportion of fat less than 75% (**Figs. 12** and **13**).[21–23,33,37] Note that thin septations are seen in both benign and malignant lesions and are not predictive. There is also significant overlap in both the imaging and histologic findings of lipomas and well-differentiated liposarcomas.[21]

Leiomyosarcoma

Clinical features

Leiomyosarcoma is the second most common primary retroperitoneal tumor in adults.[38] Most retroperitoneal leiomyosarcomas occur in women, usually in the fifth or sixth decade of life. The retroperitoneum represents the most common primary

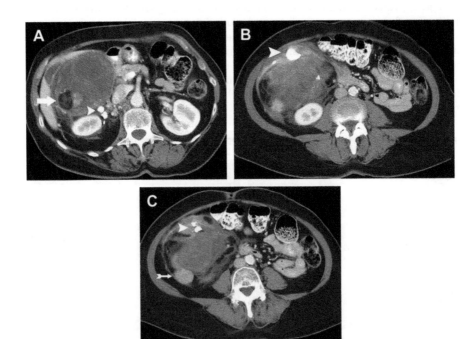

Fig. 12. Retroperitoneal liposarcoma. Contrast-enhanced axial CT images (*A–C*) show a heterogeneous mass likely arising from the anterior pararenal space in this 75-year-old woman. This lesion shows a lobule of macroscopic fat (*arrow in A*), dystrophic calcifications (*arrowheads, A–C*), low-attenuation fluid attenuation and soft-tissue nodules (*arrow with tail in C*). Surgical pathology demonstrated grade 2 dedifferentiated liposarcoma.

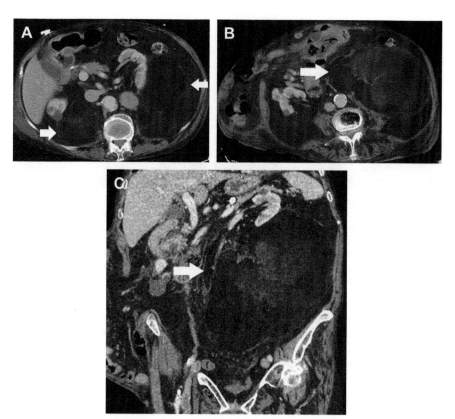

Fig. 13. Bilateral retroperitoneal liposarcomas. This 86-year-old woman with abdominal pain and distention was found to have bilateral fat containing masses on axial (*A, B*) and coronal (*C*) CT (*arrows*). Both lesions, larger on the left than on the right, contain a large amount of macroscopic fat with associated soft tissue, compatible with liposarcoma.

site of origin, followed by the uterus.[39] A significant number of these tumors arise from or involve the inferior vena cava (IVC).[38] Patients most commonly present with a large abdominal mass; however, tumors with an intravascular component may present with symptoms relating to venous compromise or thrombosis. The lungs are the most frequent site of metastatic involvement.[40] Treatment is difficult because surgical resection is often limited by the size and extent of the mass, while adjuvant chemotherapy and radiation therapy are relatively ineffective.[41]

Until recently, many GISTs were incorrectly classified as smooth muscle tumors (leiomyomas and leiomyosarcomas), but recent advances in immunohistochemistry and electron microscopy have shown that these tumors are indeed unique.[26,42] By comparison, true retroperitoneal GISTs are extremely rare and, although primary peritoneal origin is more common, it is still rare in comparison with a primary gastrointestinal tract origin.

Imaging features

Three major growth patterns of leiomyosarcoma can be seen at imaging: extravascular (most common, roughly 60% of cases), completely intravascular (least common, 5% of cases), and combined extravascular and intravascular (35% of cases) (**Figs. 14–16**).[38] Ultrasonography and angiography (by CT, MR, or conventional means) may be

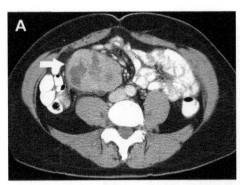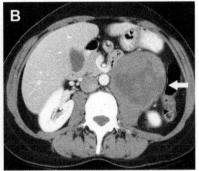

Fig. 14. Two different patients with retroperitoneal leiomyosarcoma. Contrast-enhanced axial CT image (*A*) shows a right retroperitoneal mass that is predominantly solid with small cystic or necrotic spaces, separate from the inferior vena cava (IVC) in an extravascular growth pattern, found to be a retroperitoneal leiomyosarcoma (*arrow, A*). Contrast-enhanced CT in a second patient (*B*) shows a round, heterogeneous left para-aortic mass with central low attenuation, also with an extravascular growth pattern (*arrow, B*), found to be retroperitoneal leiomyosarcoma.

useful in cases with an intravascular component (**Fig. 17**). Although involvement of the IVC is suggestive of leiomyosarcoma, other sarcomas can secondarily invade this structure, reducing the specificity of this finding somewhat. CT findings that may be suggestive of involvement of the IVC include imperceptible IVC and luminal tumor in IVC.[43]

Malignant Fibrous Histiocytoma

Clinical features

An MFH contains both fibroblastic and histiocytic cells in various proportions. Pleomorphic is the most common histologic subtype, but there are also myxoid, giant cell, inflammatory, and angiomatoid subtypes.[13,16,17] MFH generally presents in the fifth and sixth decades, and the most common symptoms are fever, malaise, and weight loss. Metastatic disease most frequently involves the lungs, but osseous and hepatic metastases are sometimes seen. Treatment is surgical resection and, although the risk of local recurrence is directly related to completeness of resection, the overall prognosis is more closely related to tumor grade (low, intermediate, or high), tumor size, and the presence of metastases.[13,34,41]

Imaging features

MFH usually manifests as a large, heterogeneous, soft-tissue mass on cross-sectional imaging (**Fig. 18**). The tumor heterogeneity is related to a combination of central necrosis, hemorrhage, and myxoid degeneration (variable). Enhancement is variable, but often nodular and peripheral. Calcifications are seen in approximately 10% of patients, but no fatty component or vascular invasion should be present.[13] MFH is frequently locally aggressive and often invades adjacent structures.

Other Malignant Mesenchymal Tumors

Clinical features

Similar to peritoneal sarcomas, retroperitoneal sarcomas generally lack distinguishing features. However, there are some characteristics that may be helpful in differentiating the various subtypes. As previously discussed, malignant nerve sheath tumors and

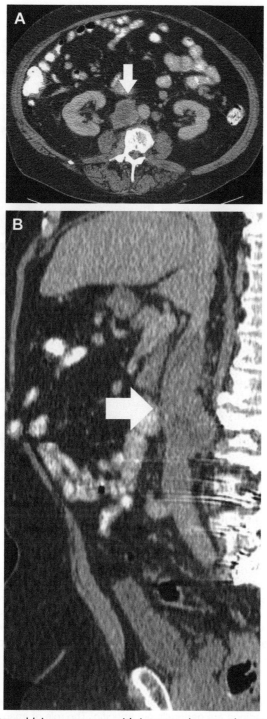

Fig. 15. Retroperitoneal leiomyosarcoma with intravascular growth pattern. Axial (*A*) and sagittal (*B*) contrast-enhanced CT images of the abdomen of this 70-year-old man who presented with vascular congestion show a focal mass lesion within the infrarenal IVC (*arrows*) expanding the lumen and demonstrating heterogeneous enhancement. Surgical pathology demonstrated leiomyosarcoma.

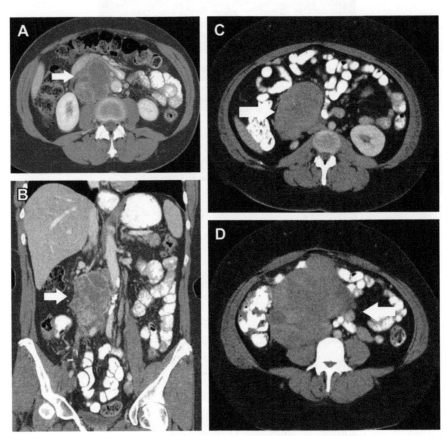

Fig. 16. Retroperitoneal leiomyosarcoma with both intravascular and extravascular growth patterns in 2 different patients. Axial (A) and coronal (B) contrast-enhanced CT images show a heterogeneous mass involving the IVC (arrows) but also extending out into the retroperitoneum, displacing the duodenum anteriorly. Axial contrast-enhanced CT images (C, D) in a second patient show a similar heterogeneous retroperitoneal mass (arrows) involving the IVC and extending out into the adjacent retroperitoneum.

GISTs are associated with NF-1, although primary retroperitoneal GISTs are rare. Fibrosarcoma is another rare retroperitoneal tumor, which can have variable biological behavior. Inflammatory fibrosarcoma can be difficult to distinguish from benign myofibroblastic tumor (inflammatory pseudotumor) in young patients; this malignancy can be locally aggressive and has the potential for metastasis.[27,28] Angiosarcoma, rhabdomyosarcoma, and hemangiopericytoma are rare, aggressive neoplasms that have an extremely poor prognosis (**Fig. 19**).

Imaging features
Most of these sarcomas manifest as large, heterogeneous, locally invasive masses, and the imaging findings are generally nonspecific. The role of imaging is to evaluate for the extent of disease, direct and guide percutaneous biopsy, and assess the response to therapy. Malignant nerve sheath tumors in the setting of NF-1 often have a branching, plexiform morphology, with low attenuation on CT and high signal on T2-weighted MR imaging that can mimic a cystic appearance.[44]

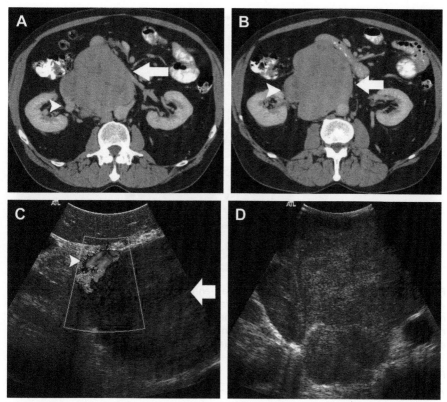

Fig. 17. Retroperitoneal leiomyosarcoma. Axial CT images (*A, B*) of this 61-year-old man with vague back and abdominal pain show a retroperitoneal mass (*arrows*) that abuts the IVC just below the level of the renal veins (*arrowhead in A*), but clearly involves the IVC more inferiorly (*arrowhead in B*). This appearance is confirmed with ultrasonography, which also shows the mass (*arrow in C*) and the adjacent IVC (*arrowhead in C*) on color Doppler superiorly, with tumor filling the expected location of the IVC inferiorly (*D*).

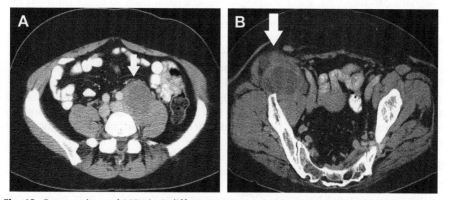

Fig. 18. Retroperitoneal MFH in 2 different patients. Axial contrast-enhanced CT image (*A*) shows a heterogeneous retroperitoneal mass lesion (*arrow*) in a 53-year-old woman who presented with leg weakness, found to have a pleomorphic type MFH. CT image of a second patient (*B*) shows a central low-attenuation mass (*arrow*) in the extraperitoneal space of the right pelvis.

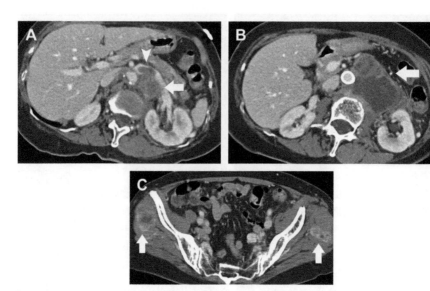

Fig. 19. Retroperitoneal angiosarcoma. Contrast-enhanced CT images (*A–C*) of a 73-year-old woman with abdominal pain and low-grade fevers, treated for presumed mycotic pseudoaneurysm of the aorta, show a growing peripherally enhancing mass abutting the aorta (*arrows in A, B*). Note the associated thrombus in the left renal vein (*arrowhead in A*) and the enhancing muscular metastases in the pelvis (*arrows in C*).

Paragangliomas

Clinical features

Paragangliomas arise from neuroendocrine cells derived from the embryologic neural crest. These tumors can occur anywhere along the sympathetic chain, and can be adrenal (ie, pheochromocytoma) or extra-adrenal in origin.[45,46] Paragangliomas, or extra-adrenal pheochromocytomas, can be hormonally active, secreting catecholamines, which can result in labile hypertension, palpitations, sweating, and headaches. Most paragangliomas are benign, but up to 10% metastasize and display malignant behavior (**Fig. 20**). Paragangliomas are most likely to occur between the ages or 30 and 45 years.[47]

Imaging features

Other than a characteristic location adjacent to the aorta (including the organ of Zuckerkandl), there are no imaging specific features for extra-adrenal paragangliomas. These tumors are often hypervascular, can be solitary or multifocal, and are often homogeneous in appearance (**Fig. 21**), although malignant lesions tend to be larger and demonstrate areas of central necrosis (see **Fig. 20**).[48–50] Associated calcifications are present in about 15% of cases. Local invasion or distant metastases are diagnostic of malignancy.

Germ Cell Tumors

Clinical features

Extragonadal germ cell tumors (EGGCT) represent approximately 5% of all germ cell tumors and are characterized by a midline location extending from the pineal gland to the coccyx.[51,52] Approximately 20% to 40% of EGGCTs are seminomas, with nonseminomatous germ cell tumors (eg, embryonal carcinoma, yolk-sac tumor, choriocarcinoma, teratoma, or combined) representing the remaining 60% to 80%.

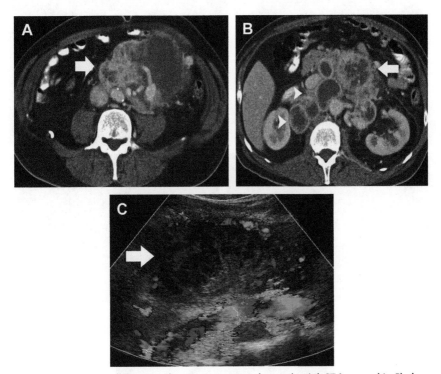

Fig. 20. Retroperitoneal paraganglioma. Contrast-enhanced axial CT images (*A, B*) show a peripherally enhancing tumor with prominent neovasculature along the left para-aortic position (*arrows*) in this 52-year-old man presenting with back pain and weight loss of 50 lb (22.7 kg) over the last 5 months. Note the necrotic-appearing associated retroperitoneal lymph nodes (*arrowheads in B*). Color Doppler ultrasonography (*C*) also shows this peripherally vascular, centrally necrotic mass (*arrow*). Percutaneous biopsy was performed using ultrasound guidance, and surgical pathology demonstrated paraganglioma.

Most of these tumors occur in the mediastinum, but the second most common site of involvement is the retroperitoneum (30%–40%). Because metastatic retroperitoneal involvement from a testicular primary germ cell tumor is much more common than a primary EGGCT, males should undergo testicular ultrasonography to exclude this possibility.[52]

The most common clinical symptoms from retroperitoneal EGGCT include a palpable abdominal mass, abdominal or back pain, and weight loss. Most EGGCTs occur in men. Treatment generally includes primary chemotherapy, followed by surgical resection of any significant residual mass. Although controversial, any residual mass measuring greater than 3 cm is usually resected and, if residual disease is identified in the pathologic specimen, further chemotherapy is given.[51,52] Although generally treated like a metastatic gonadal germ cell tumor, the prognosis of primary retroperitoneal EGGCT is somewhat worse but still favorable overall. Negative prognostic factors include nonseminomatous histology, elevated tumor markers at the time of diagnosis, and the presence of metastatic disease.

Imaging features

The cross-sectional imaging appearance of these tumors varies according to the underlying tissue type. Teratomas often have a markedly heterogeneous appearance

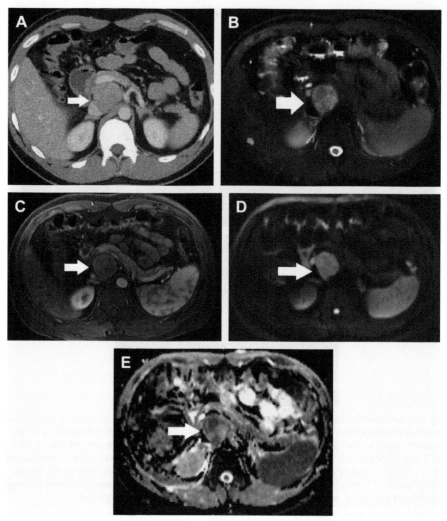

Fig. 21. Retroperitoneal paraganglioma. Contrast-enhanced CT (*A*) shows a heterogeneous round lesion abutting the IVC (*arrow*) in this 40-year-old man with right lower quadrant pain. The lesion is also shown (*arrows*) on T2-weighted magnetic resonance (MR) image (*B*) with increased signal and heterogeneous contrast enhancement (*C*), and restricted diffusion (*D, E*).

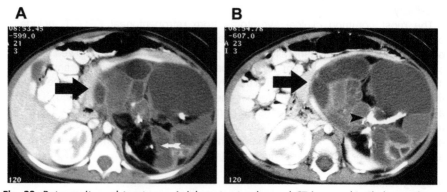

Fig. 22. Retroperitoneal teratoma. Axial contrast-enhanced CT images (*A, B*) show a large left retroperitoneal mass (*arrows*) containing fat (*arrow with tail in A*) and calcification (*arrowhead in B*), compatible with teratoma.

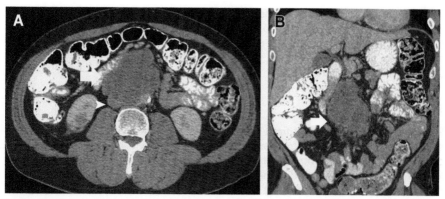

Fig. 23. Retroperitoneal germ cell tumor. Axial (*A*) and coronal (*B*) contrast-enhanced CT images of a 56-year-old man with abdominal pain show a low-attenuation retroperitoneal mass (*arrows*) abutting but not invading the IVC (*arrowhead in A*). Surgical pathology demonstrated a high-grade large cell tumor of germ cell origin.

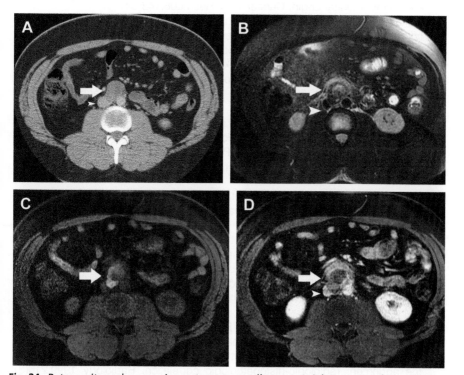

Fig. 24. Retroperitoneal nonseminomatous germ cell tumor. Axial contrast-enhanced CT image (*A*) shows a low-attenuation retroperitoneal lesion (*arrow in A–D*), abutting but not invading the IVC (*arrowhead in A, B*). T2-weighted MR image (*B*) shows heterogeneously increased T2 signal, and T1-weighted precontrast MR image (*C*) shows high signal intensity, possibly related to blood products or proteinaceous debris. A rim of enhancement is seen around the lesion on the postcontrast image (*D*). The mass effect on the IVC without invasion is shown once again (*arrowhead in D*).

attributable to varying combinations of soft tissue, calcification, fat, and fluid (**Fig. 22**). By contrast, seminomas tend to be large, homogeneous, lobulated soft-tissue masses. Nonseminomatous germ cell tumors are often very irregular in morphology and heterogeneous in appearance, with variable amounts of necrosis and hemorrhage (**Figs. 23** and **24**).

SUMMARY

Primary malignancies arising from the peritoneal, subperitoneal, and retroperitoneal spaces occur much less frequently than metastatic involvement from primary organ-based tumors or lymphoproliferative diseases. Nonetheless, these rare primary lesions should be considered in the absence of a known or suspected organ-based malignancy. Although establishing the specific histologic diagnosis on imaging can be difficult, cross-sectional imaging can be useful for detection, characterization, staging, directing biopsy, and evaluating the response to therapy.

REFERENCES

1. Hinshaw JL, Pickhardt PJ. Imaging of primary malignant tumors of peritoneal and retroperitoneal origin. Cancer Treat Res 2008;143:281–97.
2. Pickhardt PJ, Bhalla S. Unusual nonneoplastic peritoneal and subperitoneal conditions: CT findings. Radiographics 2005;25(3):719–30.
3. Pickhardt PJ, Bhalla S. Primary neoplasms of peritoneal and sub-peritoneal origin: CT findings. Radiographics 2005;25(4):983–95.
4. Pickhardt PJ. Peritoneum and retroperitoneum. In: Slone RM, Fisher AJ, Pickhardt PJ, et al, editors. Body CT: a practical approach. New York: McGraw-Hill; 2000. p. 159–77.
5. Hain KS, Pickhardt PJ, Lubner MG, et al. Presacral masses: multimodality imaging of a multidisciplinary space. Radiographics 2013;33(4):1145–67.
6. Altaras MM, Aviram R, Cohen I, et al. Primary peritoneal papillary serous adenocarcinoma: clinical and management aspects. Gynecol Oncol 1991;40(3):230–6.
7. Iavazzo C, Vorgias G, Katsoulis M, et al. Primary peritoneal serous papillary carcinoma: clinical and laboratory characteristics. Arch Gynecol Obstet 2008;278(1):53–6.
8. Demir MK, Unlu E, Genchellac H, et al. Primary serous papillary carcinoma of the retroperitoneum: magnetic resonance imaging findings with pathologic correlation. Australas Radiol 2007;51(Spec No):B71–3.
9. Busch JM, Kruskal JB, Wu B. Armed Forces Institute of Pathology. Best cases from the AFIP. Malignant peritoneal mesothelioma. Radiographics 2002;22(6):1511–5.
10. Loggie BW, Fleming RA, McQuellon RP, et al. Prospective trial for the treatment of malignant peritoneal mesothelioma. Am Surg 2001;67(10):999–1003.
11. Pickhardt PJ, Fisher AJ, Balfe DM, et al. Desmoplastic small round cell tumor of the abdomen: radiologic-histopathologic correlation. Radiology 1999;210(3):633–8.
12. Chouli M, Viala J, Dromain C, et al. Intra-abdominal desmoplastic small round cell tumors: CT findings and clinicopathological correlations in 13 cases. Eur J Radiol 2005;54(3):438–42.
13. Ros PR, Viamonte M Jr, Rywlin AM. Malignant fibrous histiocytoma: mesenchymal tumor of ubiquitous origin. AJR Am J Roentgenol 1984;142(4):753–9.

14. Zhang WD, Li CX, Liu QY, et al. CT, MRI, and FDG-PET/CT imaging findings of abdominopelvic desmoplastic small round cell tumors: correlation with histopathologic findings. Eur J Radiol 2011;80(2):269–73.
15. Pickhardt PJ. F-18 fluorodeoxyglucose positron emission tomographic imaging in desmoplastic small round cell tumor of the abdomen. Clin Nucl Med 1999; 24(9):693–4.
16. Bodner K, Bodner-Adler B, Mayerhofer S, et al. Malignant fibrous histiocytoma (MFH) of the mesentery: a case report. Anticancer Res 2002;22(2B): 1169–70.
17. Schaefer IM, Fletcher CD. Myxoid variant of so-called angiomatoid "malignant fibrous histiocytoma": clinicopathologic characterization in a series of 21 cases. Am J Surg Pathol 2014;38(6):816–23.
18. Ko SF, Ng SH, Lin JW, et al. Cystic malignant fibrous histiocytoma of the mesovarium. AJR Am J Roentgenol 2001;176(2):549–50.
19. Rydholm A, Berg NO. Size, site and clinical incidence of lipoma. Factors in the differential diagnosis of lipoma and sarcoma. Acta Orthop Scand 1983;54(6): 929–34.
20. Myhre-Jensen OA. consecutive 7-year series of 1331 benign soft tissue tumours. Clinicopathologic data. Comparison with sarcomas. Acta Orthop Scand 1981;52(3):287–93.
21. Gaskin CM, Helms CA. Lipomas, lipoma variants, and well-differentiated liposarcomas (atypical lipomas): results of MRI evaluations of 126 consecutive fatty masses. AJR Am J Roentgenol 2004;182(3):733–9.
22. Kransdorf MJ, Bancroft LW, Peterson JJ, et al. Imaging of fatty tumors: distinction of lipoma and well-differentiated liposarcoma. Radiology 2002;224(1): 99–104.
23. O'Regan KN, Jagannathan J, Krajewski K, et al. Imaging of liposarcoma: classification, patterns of tumor recurrence, and response to treatment. AJR Am J Roentgenol 2011;197(1):W37–43.
24. Sinha R, Verma R, Kong A. Mesenteric gastrointestinal stromal tumor in a patient with neurofibromatosis. AJR Am J Roentgenol 2004;183(6):1844–6.
25. Kim HC, Lee JM, Kim SH, et al. Primary gastrointestinal stromal tumors in the omentum and mesentery: CT findings and pathologic correlations. AJR Am J Roentgenol 2004;182(6):1463–7.
26. Sandrasegaran K, Rajesh A, Rydberg J, et al. Gastrointestinal stromal tumors: clinical, radiologic, and pathologic features. AJR Am J Roentgenol 2005; 184(3):803–11.
27. Patnana M, Sevrukov AB, Elsayes KM, et al. Inflammatory pseudotumor: the great mimicker. AJR Am J Roentgenol 2012;198(3):W217–27.
28. Meis JM, Enzinger FM. Inflammatory fibrosarcoma of the mesentery and retroperitoneum. A tumor closely simulating inflammatory pseudotumor. Am J Surg Pathol 1991;15(12):1146–56.
29. Ko SF, Chou FF, Huang CH, et al. Primary synovial sarcoma of the gastrocolic ligament. Br J Radiol 1998;71(844):438–40.
30. Bakri A, Shinagare AB, Krajewski KM, et al. Synovial sarcoma: imaging features of common and uncommon primary sites, metastatic patterns, and treatment response. AJR Am J Roentgenol 2012;199(2):W208–15.
31. Engelken JD, Ros PR. Retroperitoneal MR imaging. Magn Reson Imaging Clin N Am 1997;5(1):165–78.
32. Granstrom P, Unger E. MR imaging of the retroperitoneum. Magn Reson Imaging Clin N Am 1995;3(1):121–42.

33. Hong SH, Kim KA, Woo OH, et al. Dedifferentiated liposarcoma of retroperitoneum: spectrum of imaging findings in 15 patients. Clin Imaging 2010;34(3): 203–10.

34. Miah AB, Hannay J, Benson C, et al. Optimal management of primary retroperitoneal sarcoma: an update. Expert Rev Anticancer Ther 2014;14(5):565–79.

35. Bestic JM, Kransdorf MJ, White LM, et al. Sclerosing variant of well-differentiated liposarcoma: relative prevalence and spectrum of CT and MRI features. AJR Am J Roentgenol 2013;201(1):154–61.

36. Toulmonde M, Bonvalot S, Ray-Coquard I, et al. Retroperitoneal sarcomas: patterns of care in advanced stages, prognostic factors and focus on main histological subtypes: a multicenter analysis of the French Sarcoma Group. Ann Oncol 2014;25(3):730–4.

37. Song T, Shen J, Liang BL, et al. Retroperitoneal liposarcoma: MR characteristics and pathological correlative analysis. Abdom Imaging 2007;32(5):668–74.

38. Hartman DS, Hayes WS, Choyke PL, et al. From the archives of the AFIP. Leiomyosarcoma of the retroperitoneum and inferior vena cava: radiologic-pathologic correlation. Radiographics 1992;12(6):1203–20.

39. Clary BM, DeMatteo RP, Lewis JJ, et al. Gastrointestinal stromal tumors and leiomyosarcoma of the abdomen and retroperitoneum: a clinical comparison. Ann Surg Oncol 2001;8(4):290–9.

40. Sondak VK, Economou JS, Eilber FR. Soft tissue sarcomas of the extremity and retroperitoneum: advances in management. Adv Surg 1991;24:333–59.

41. Smith MJ, Ridgway PF, Catton CN, et al. Combined management of retroperitoneal sarcoma with dose intensification radiotherapy and resection: long-term results of a prospective trial. Radiother Oncol 2014;110(1):165–71.

42. Erlandson RA, Klimstra DS, Woodruff JM. Subclassification of gastrointestinal stromal tumors based on evaluation by electron microscopy and immunohistochemistry. Ultrastruct Pathol 1996;20(4):373–93.

43. Webb EM, Wang ZJ, Westphalen AC, et al. Can CT features differentiate between inferior vena cava leiomyosarcomas and primary retroperitoneal masses? AJR Am J Roentgenol 2013;200(1):205–9.

44. Matsuki K, Kakitsubata Y, Watanabe K, et al. Mesenteric plexiform neurofibroma associated with Recklinghausen's disease. Pediatr Radiol 1997;27(3): 255–6.

45. Melicow MM. One hundred cases of pheochromocytoma (107 tumors) at the Columbia-Presbyterian Medical Center, 1926-1976: a clinicopathological analysis. Cancer 1977;40(5):1987–2004.

46. Glenn F, Gray GF. Functional tumors of the organ of Zuckerkandl. Ann Surg 1976;183(5):578–86.

47. Hayes WS, Davidson AJ, Grimley PM, et al. Extraadrenal retroperitoneal paraganglioma: clinical, pathologic, and CT findings. AJR Am J Roentgenol 1990; 155(6):1247–50.

48. Balcombe J, Torigian DA, Kim W, et al. Cross-sectional imaging of paragangliomas of the aortic body and other thoracic branchiomeric paraganglia. AJR Am J Roentgenol 2007;188(4):1054–8.

49. Ingram M, Barber B, Bano G, et al. Radiologic appearance of hereditary adrenal and extraadrenal paraganglioma. AJR Am J Roentgenol 2011;197(4): W687–95.

50. Leung K, Stamm M, Raja A, et al. Pheochromocytoma: the range of appearances on ultrasound, CT, MRI, and functional imaging. AJR Am J Roentgenol 2013;200(2):370–8.

51. Nichols CR, Fox EP. Extragonadal and pediatric germ cell tumors. Hematol Oncol Clin North Am 1991;5(6):1189–209.
52. Shinagare AB, Jagannathan JP, Ramaiya NH, et al. Adult extragonadal germ cell tumors. AJR Am J Roentgenol 2010;195(4):W274–80.

Current Status of Imaging for Adrenal Gland Tumors

Julie H. Song, MD*, William W. Mayo-Smith, MD

KEYWORDS

- Adrenal • Adrenal mass • Adrenal tumor • Adrenal incidentaloma
- Hyperfunctioning adrenal mass

KEY POINTS

- Adrenal masses are common and mostly benign in patients without known malignancy.
- Most adrenal masses can be accurately characterized by contemporary computed tomography, magnetic resonance imaging, and positron emission tomography.
- Computed tomography and magnetic resonance imaging are excellent tools in the detection of clinically suspected hyperfunctioning adrenal mass.
- Appropriate utilization of imaging is important for optimal management, to separate benign inconsequential adrenal masses from those that require treatment.

The adrenal gland is a common site of disease and can harbor a wide range of pathology. Because of expanding clinical indications for cross-sectional imaging and improved spatial resolution of computed tomography (CT), magnetic resonance imaging (MRI) and ultrasound scan, adrenal masses are now frequently discovered incidentally. The prevalence of adrenal masses at CT is approximately 5%,[1–3] comparable to the estimated prevalence in the general population of 3% to 7%.[4–6] Most adrenal lesions are benign, most commonly nonfunctioning adenoma. However, the adrenal gland is also a common site of metastasis in oncologic patients. The adrenal gland can also be the source of hyperfunctioning tumors that require intervention and, more rarely, primary malignant neoplasms. Contemporary adrenal imaging is highly accurate in both the detection and characterization of adrenal masses. This article discusses the role of imaging in the evaluation of more common adrenal masses, with primary emphasis on CT and MRI.

PREIMAGING PLANNING
Normal Adrenal Gland

The adrenal glands are well visualized on abdominal CT and MRI. They are located anterosuperiorly to the kidneys within the perirenal space, enclosed by perirenal

The authors have nothing to disclose.
Department of Diagnostic Imaging, Rhode Island Hospital, Alpert School of Medicine, Brown University, 593 Eddy Street, Providence, RI 02903, USA
* Corresponding author.
E-mail address: jsong2@lifespan.org

fascia. The normal adrenal glands are homogeneous in density or signal, and have an inverted V or Y shape (**Fig. 1**). The arterial supply to the glands is via the superior, middle, and inferior adrenal arteries (branches of the inferior phrenic artery, aorta, and renal artery, respectively). The venous drainage of the adrenal glands is predominantly by the central vein, typically draining directly into the inferior vena cava on the right and the caudal path on the left into the left renal vein. The adrenal gland is composed of the adrenal cortex and medulla, 2 functioning units with different embryologic origin and endocrine functions. The adrenal cortex secretes cortisol, aldosterone, and androgen, and the adrenal medulla secretes epinephrine and norepinephrine.

Principles and Rationales for Imaging Studies

The selection of the optimal adrenal imaging modality depends on the reason for imaging, whether the test is for detection or characterization of an adrenal mass, as described in a later discussion. Other factors, such as contrast allergy, renal insufficiency, and radiation concern may also play a role in imaging modality selection.

Detection of an abnormality is finding the lesion, most commonly to assess for metastasis in patients with an established malignancy. In this setting of metastatic workup, contrast-enhanced CT is the most appropriate tool with positron emission tomography (PET) increasingly used in certain malignancies, such as lung cancer. Another important clinical scenario of adrenal mass detection is to localize a suspected hyperfunctioning tumor in a patient with biochemical evidence of hormonal excess. Either CT or MRI is used to localize most of the hyperfunctioning tumors, and occasionally metaiodobenzylguanidine scintigraphy may be necessary to localize a suspected pheochromocytoma.

Characterization of an abnormality is determining lesion histology using imaging. Certain adrenal masses have specific benign diagnostic features at detection, so that further workup is not warranted. However, adrenal masses often have a nonspecific appearance, especially at original contrast-enhanced CT performed for another reason. For these adrenal "incidentalomas," defined as adrenal masses detected incidentally on an imaging examination performed for other reasons, the imaging goal is to separate a benign mass, most commonly an adenoma, from a mass that requires treatment. CT and MRI are the most commonly used imaging tools in characterizing adrenal masses, with PET usually reserved for patients with known extra-adrenal malignancy. The imaging appearances on these studies reflect physiologic differences of

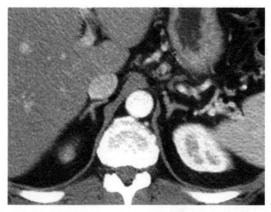

Fig. 1. Normal adrenal glands in 37-year-old man. Axial contrast-enhanced CT image shows normal adrenal glands in inverted Y configuration.

adenoma from malignant masses: intracytoplasmic lipid content, contrast washout pattern, and metabolic activity.

CT is highly accurate in diagnosing adenoma, because both lipid content and washout characteristics can be used, as discussed later. The main advantages of MRI over CT are in patients in whom iodinated contrast is contraindicated because of allergy or renal insufficiency or in young patients in whom radiation exposure is a concern. The premise behind PET imaging is that malignant tumors are usually glucose avid because of increased metabolic activity. Most metastatic adrenal masses show increased activity, whereas most benign adrenal lesions do not. The need for imaging-guided biopsy to diagnose an adrenal mass has decreased in recent years as advances in adrenal imaging now allow accurate characterization of most adrenal masses.[7] The imaging modalities used to characterize adrenal masses are summarized in **Table 1**.

DIAGNOSTIC IMAGING TECHNIQUES
CT

Most adrenal masses are well visualized on routine abdominal CT, typically reconstructed at 5-mm thickness. Dedicated adrenal CT is performed when necessary to further characterize a known adrenal mass. Adrenal CT is performed with the patient in supine position as follows:

- Unenhanced sections are acquired through the adrenal gland with image reconstruction at 2 to 3 mm in axial and coronal planes.
- An elliptical region of interest (ROI) is placed in an adrenal mass. If the density of the adrenal mass measures ≤10 Hounsfield units (HU), then it is a benign lipid-rich adenoma and the examination is complete.
- If the density of the adrenal mass measures greater than 10 HU, then contrast material is injected intravenously.
- The next data sets are acquired at 60 seconds and 15 minutes after the start of contrast injection using the same CT acquisition parameters.
- Density measurements are obtained of the adrenal mass on unenhanced, dynamic, and delayed imaging, and percentage of contrast washout is calculated using the formula further discussed below.

MRI

The principle MRI technique used in adrenal evaluation is chemical shift imaging (CS-MRI) obtained with in-phase and out-of-phase T1 gradient-recalled echo pulse sequences. CS-MRI exploits the different resonant frequencies of protons in fat and

Table 1		
Modality selection for adrenal mass characterization		
Imaging Procedure	**Rationale for Selection**	**Issues**
CT	Most widely available Diagnosis based on density or CT washout	Contrast allergy and renal insufficiency (when contrast is necessary for diagnosis) Radiation in young patients
MRI	Young patients and patients with renal insufficiency	MR incompatible device (eg, pacemaker)
PET	Mostly in patients with known cancer	Not recommended in patients without a known malignancy

water molecules, with fat protons resonating at a slower frequency. Thus, at a predetermined echo time when the protons in fat and water molecules are out of phase, the net effect is signal cancellation within a voxel compared with when the protons are in phase. Most adrenal adenomas containing sufficient amount of lipid, thus, lose signal on out of phase compared with in phase. The lipid-rich adrenal adenoma will appear dark on out-of-phase imaging. When an adrenal mass is not diagnostic of an adenoma at CS-MRI, T2-weighted sequence and gadolinium-based, contrast-enhanced series are obtained for further characterization of an adrenal mass.

PET

PET and PET-CT utilizing fluorine-18-2fluoro-2-deoxy-D-glucose (FDG) are primarily performed in oncologic patients. To achieve and optimize a diagnostic scan, patients need to refrain from significant exercise for 24 hours, and their glucose level has to be less than 200 mg/dL before PET. At total-body PET-CT, CT, and PET are acquired separately. First, the patient receives intravenous administration of the FDG radiopharmaceutical, and then 75 minutes later, a CT without intravenous iodinated contrast is obtained followed immediately by PET acquisition. After these acquisitions, the CT images are fused (coregistered) with the metabolic PET dataset, which provides accurate anatomic localization of abnormal PET activity and also allows adrenal CT density measurements. These factors improve diagnostic performance of adrenal characterization in oncology patients.

INTERPRETATION AND ASSESSMENT OF CLINICAL IMAGES
Adenoma

Adenomas are the most common adrenal lesion encountered in the general population, and most are not hyperfunctioning. Adenomas are typically well-defined, round, or oval masses of smooth margins and homogeneous density. One of the key diagnostic features of adenomas is the presence of intracellular lipid. Adrenal adenomas are composed of varying amount of intracytoplasmic lipid, and at unenhanced CT their density measurements are inversely related to the amount of lipid content.[8] Based on this principle, adenomas can be separated from malignant masses using unenhanced CT density measurements.[9,10] A threshold of 10 HU allowed adenoma to be diagnosed with 71% sensitivity and 98% specificity on a meta-analysis, and is the standard threshold used to diagnose a lipid-rich adenoma on CT (**Fig. 2**).[11]

The diagnosis of adenoma on CS-MRI also relies on the presence of intracytoplasmic lipid, which leads to signal loss of an adenoma on out-of-phase compared with in-phase images.[12,13] The signal loss can be quantified using signal intensity index with the diagnostic threshold at 16.5%.[14] However, simple visual analysis is as effective and simpler to use, thus, is more commonly used in clinical practice.[15] AT CS-MRI, an adenoma is diagnosed when an adrenal mass becomes dark on out-of-phase compared with in-phase images, using the spleen as the reference (**Fig. 3**). With CS-MRI, adenomas are differentiated from metastasis with sensitivity and specificity of 81% to 100% and 94% to 100%, respectively.[16,17]

Approximately 20% to 30% of adrenal adenomas are lipid poor and do not contain sufficient amount of lipid to be diagnosed based on the CT density measurement or at CS-MRI. However, after enhancement with intravenous contrast, adenomas lose contrast rapidly, whereas the washout of metastases is more prolonged.[18,19] Based on this physiologic difference, adenomas can be separated from nonadenomas by calculating contrast washout percentage at a delayed phase, optimally 15 minutes after contrast injection.[18] The absolute percentage of enhancement washout (APW) is

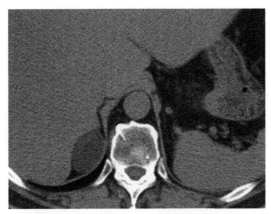

Fig. 2. Lipid-rich adenoma in 58-year-old man. Axial unenhanced CT image shows a well-defined 3.7-cm right adrenal mass with attenuation of −8 HU, diagnostic of a lipid-rich adenoma.

calculated using the following formula, and a value of 60% or greater is diagnostic of an adenoma (**Fig. 4**):

$$APW = \frac{(\text{enhanced HU}) - (15 \text{ min delayed HU})}{(\text{enhanced HU}) - (\text{unenhanced HU})} \times 100\%$$

In the absence of the initial unenhanced phase, a relative percentage washout (RPW) is calculated as follows, and a value of 40% or greater is diagnostic of an adenoma:

$$RPW = \frac{(\text{enhanced HU}) - (15 \text{ min delayed HU})}{(\text{enhanced HU})} \times 100\%$$

The accuracy of washout analysis has been confirmed on multiple studies.[20–23] In one study of 166 adrenal masses, the combined adrenal protocol was 96% accurate in distinguishing adenoma from nonadenoma.[22] Furthermore, the diagnostic accuracy is independent of lipid content.[20,21]

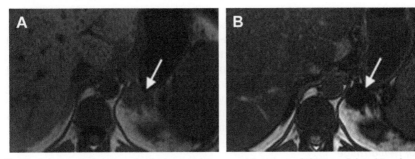

Fig. 3. A 1.7-cm left adrenal adenoma in 50-year-old woman. (*A*) T1-weighted in-phase MRI shows a left adrenal mass (*arrow*) that is hyperintense relative to the spleen. (*B*) T1-weighted out-of-phase MRI shows marked signal intensity loss relative to the spleen, diagnostic of an adenoma. Note also the presence of signal loss in the liver, reflecting steatosis.

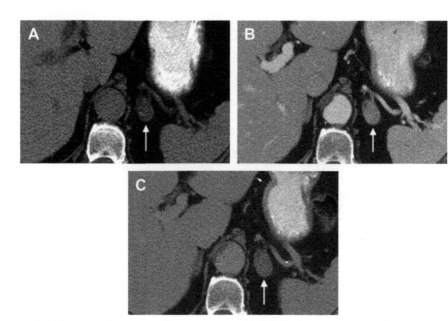

Fig. 4. Lipid-poor adenoma in 71-year-old woman. (*A*) Axial unenhanced CT image shows a 2.5-cm left adrenal mass (*arrow*) with attenuation of 16 HU. (*B*) On dynamic contrast-enhanced phase scan, adrenal mass enhances to 99 HU. (*C*) On 15-minute delayed scan, adrenal mass attenuation is 37 HU. APW and RPW are 75% and 63%, respectively, diagnostic of an adenoma.

Myelolipoma

Adrenal myelolipomas are benign tumors composed of mature fat and hematopoietic tissue. They are usually incidentally found asymptomatic masses, but large masses may rarely cause pain from spontaneous hemorrhage. With the widespread use of cross-sectional imaging, incidental detection of myelolipoma has increased.[3] On CT and MRI, these lesions are easily recognized because they contain macroscopic fat, although the amount of fat and soft tissue is variable (**Fig. 5**). Pseudocapsules are common and calcifications are present in 24% of adrenal myelolipomas.[24]

Cyst and Pseudocyst

Adrenal cysts and pseudocysts are uncommon benign lesions usually found incidentally. They are mostly asymptomatic. Adrenal cysts are well-defined homogeneous round masses of near-water attenuation (0 HUs at CT) and a thin wall. On MRI, adrenal cysts also follow the signal of water (dark on T1-weighted images, bright on T2-weighted image) (**Fig. 6**). Adrenal cysts do not internally enhance using CT or MRI intravenous contrast. The wall may contain thin calcification, and the thin wall may enhance with intravenous contrast.[25] Adrenal pseudocysts, which result from a previous episode of hemorrhage, may appear more complex with higher internal density, thicker walls, internal septations, and calcifications.[25]

Adrenal Hemorrhage

Adrenal hemorrhage can occur in the setting of trauma, anticoagulation, blood dyscrasia, sepsis, hypotension, renal vein thrombosis, and severe stress such as surgery. Trauma accounts for 80% of adrenal hemorrhage, which is usually unilateral,

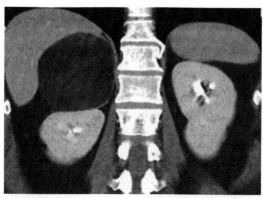

Fig. 5. Myelolipoma in 49-year-old man. Coronal reformatted contrast-enhanced CT image shows an 8.1-cm encapsulated right adrenal mass predominantly consisting of macroscopic fat.

typically on the right. Adrenal hemorrhage can rarely result in adrenal insufficiency (Addison's disease) if there is bilateral involvement. On CT, acute adrenal hematoma is round or oval with increased density of 50 to 90 HU on unenhanced CT (**Fig. 7**). The size and density of the mass decrease over time, and the mass usually resolves spontaneously or calcifies, although some may liquefy and persist as pseudocysts. On MRI, the appearance of hematoma is variable depending on the age of hematoma, but most commonly is bright on T1-weighted images and dark on T2-weighted images.

Pheochromocytoma

Pheochromocytoma is an uncommon, catecholamine-secreting tumor arising from the adrenal medulla. Ten percent of pheochromocytomas are bilateral, 10% are multiple, and 10% are associated with hereditary syndromes. Approximately 10% of pheochromocytomas are silent, although the number of incidentally discovered pheochromocytomas has been reported to be increasing.[26,27] Pheochromocytomas have variable imaging appearances.[28] On CT, small lesions are homogenous with soft tissue density (**Fig. 8**), but large masses are often heterogeneous and may contain areas of necrosis or hemorrhage. On MRI, pheochromocytomas have classically been described to be markedly hyperintense on T2-weighted images (**Fig. 9**); however,

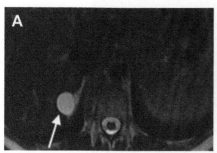
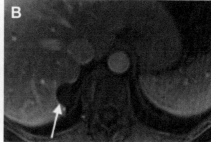

Fig. 6. Adrenal cyst in 50-year-old man. (*A*) Axial T2-weighted MRI shows a well-defined 1.8-cm right adrenal mass (*arrow*) of fluid signal. (*B*) Axial gadolinium-enhanced T1-weighted MRI shows the mass with fluid signal, imperceptible wall, and no enhancement.

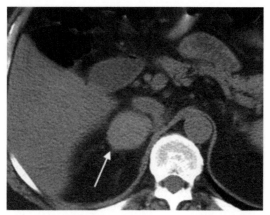

Fig. 7. Adrenal hemorrhage in 73-year-old man. Axial unenhanced CT image shows 4.2-cm right adrenal mass (*arrow*) with attenuation of 55 HU, consistent with acute hemorrhage.

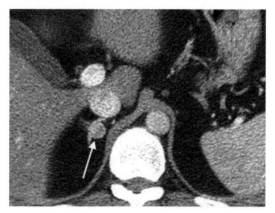

Fig. 8. Pheochromocytoma in 42-year-old man. Axial contrast-enhanced CT image shows a homogeneous 1.5-cm right adrenal mass (*arrow*) with avid enhancement.

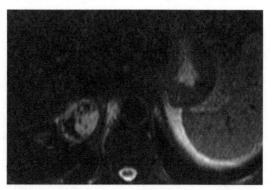

Fig. 9. Pheochromocytoma in 60-year-old man. Axial T2-weighted MR image shows a heterogeneous 4.5-cm right adrenal mass with a large area of marked hyperintensity.

more recent series found that these tumors can be moderately hyperintense or even hypointese.[17,29] Pheochromocytomas usually enhance avidly after contrast injection. Approximately 10% of pheochromocytomas are malignant, but there are no specific radiologic features to diagnose malignancy other than invasion of local structures or distant metastases.

Adrenocortical Carcinoma

Adrenocortical carcinoma is a very rare, primary malignant tumor arising from the adrenal cortex with prevalence of 1 to 2 patients per million population.[30] It can be aggressive and typically presents late with a large mass. Approximately 50% of the carcinomas are hormonally active, most commonly producing cortisol, and may lead to Cushing syndrome. On CT and MRI, an adrenocortical carcinoma is a large (usually >6 cm) heterogeneously enhancing mass. It is frequently associated with central necrosis and hemorrhage, and calcifications are present in 30% (**Fig. 10**).[31] Venous invasion into inferior vena cava is a common feature, often a diagnostic clue, and defining the superior extent of tumor thrombus is important for surgical planning to define the point for vascular control.

Metastasis

The adrenal glands are common sites of metastasis. At autopsy, adrenal metastases were found in 27% of patients with malignant epithelial tumors.[32] Most patients with adrenal metastasis have an established extra-adrenal malignancy, and the common primary malignancies include carcinomas of the lung, breast, pancreas, and gastrointestinal tract.[33] When an adrenal mass is detected in oncologic patients, the main dilemma is whether the mass is a metastasis or an incidental benign adenoma. The imaging features of adrenal metastasis are often nonspecific at routine contrast-enhanced CT or MRI. Heterogeneous density, necrosis, and irregular margin can be present in metastasis, especially when they are large. However, small metastatic masses may be homogeneous with smooth margin, and appear benign.[34] Thus, further characterization is often necessary using one of the imaging tools discussed above, especially if the adrenal gland is the only potential site of metastasis, as the diagnosis would likely alter the patient prognosis and treatment options. On unenhanced CT, the metastatic adrenal masses usually measure greater than 10 HU. At

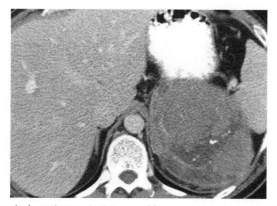

Fig. 10. Adrenocortical carcinoma in 39-year-old man. Axial contrast-enhanced CT image shows a 14-cm left adrenal mass with central heterogeneous attenuation and multiple punctuate calcifications.

CT washout analysis, metastatic masses usually show delayed washout with APW less than 60% and RPW less than 40%.[18,22] At MRI, most metastases are isointense to hypointense on T1-weighed sequence, usually hyperintense on T2-weighed sequence, and, most importantly, lack signal loss on opposed-phase at CS-MRI. At PET and PET-CT, most adrenal metastases are FDG-avid and show increased activity relative to the liver (**Fig. 11**). PET or PET-CT are found to differentiate benign from malignant adrenal masses in cancer patients with sensitivity from 93% to 100%.[35–38] Some benign lesions can show mildly increased uptake, and a recent meta-analysis reported specificity of PET to be at 91% in separating benign from malignant adrenal masses.[38]

OPTIONS/PATHWAYS FOR SURGICAL INTERVENTION
Hyperfunctioning Tumor

The search for a hyperfunctioning adrenal tumor is usually prompted by the clinical presentation of hormonal excess, which is confirmed by abnormal biochemical assay. The role of imaging is then primarily to detect the culprit mass, such as a cortisol-producing adenoma, an aldosteronoma, or a pheochromocytoma.

- Cortisol-producing adenomas, responsible for 20% of Cushing syndrome, are the most common cause of adrenocorticotropic hormone–independent Cushing syndrome. They are readily detected on CT, as they are typically larger than 2 cm.[17,39] These adenomas have similar CT appearance to that of nonfunctioning adenomas with abundant intracellular lipid causing a low-density adrenal mass.[8,39]
- Aldosterone-producing adenomas, which cause 80% of Conn's syndrome, are usually smaller than 2 cm with a significant portion less than 1 cm.[40,41] Occasionally, adrenal vein sampling may still be necessary to localize and lateralize the site of hypersecretion when CT findings are equivocal.[42]
- Once a pheochromocytoma is suspected clinically, the diagnosis is confirmed by elevated urine or plasma metanephrine levels. Ninety-eight percent of pheochromocytomas arise in the abdomen, mostly manifesting as adrenal masses, and they are readily localized on CT or MRI. Metaiodobenzylguanidine scintigraphy is highly accurate in diagnosing pheochromocytoma and is useful in those exceptional cases in which the mass is not identified on CT or MRI or in patients at risk of multiple pheochromocytoma and metastasis.[43,44]

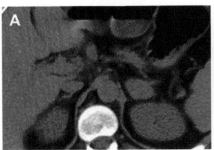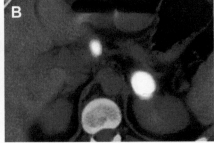

Fig. 11. Adrenal metastasis in 48-year-old man with lung cancer. (*A*) Axial unenhanced CT image shows a 3.2-cm left adrenal mass with attenuation of 32 HU. (*B*) Axial CT and PET co-registered image shows markedly increased FDG uptake in the left adrenal metastasis. Note also increased uptake in the metastatic lymph node.

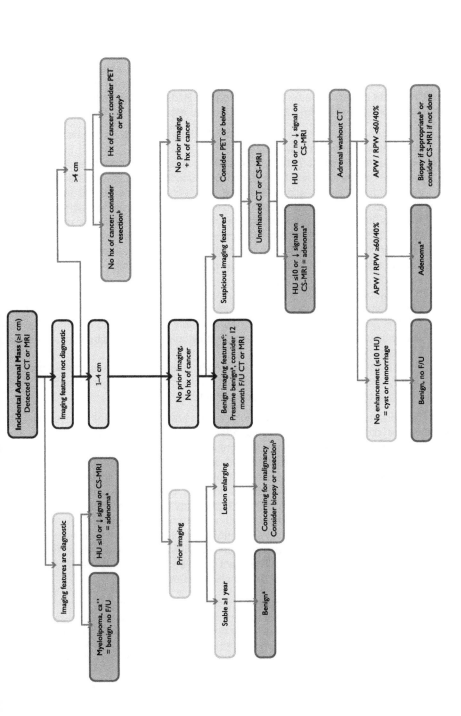

Incidental Adrenal Mass

Most incidentally detected adrenal masses are benign in patients without history of malignancy.[3] In these patients, an exhaustive workup is not indicated for most small (<4 cm) asymptomatic masses. Imaging features, lesion size, lesion stability, and patient history of malignancy are the primary factors that guide management of an incidental adrenal mass as they relate to risk of malignancy. An adrenal imaging flow chart from the white paper of the American College of Radiology Committee on Incidental Findings is presented in **Fig. 12**.[45] The suggested algorithm is as follows:

- If an adrenal mass of any size has a specific diagnostic feature of a benign lesion, no additional imaging is warranted.
- For an adrenal mass smaller than 4 cm with nondiagnostic features, if the mass has been stable for at least a year, no follow-up is necessary, as it is likely benign. An enlarging mass should be biopsied or resected to exclude malignancy.
- For an adrenal mass smaller than 4 cm with nondiagnostic but benign-appearing features, if there is no prior imaging and no cancer history, follow-up unenhanced CT or CS-MRI in 12 months may be considered. If there are suspicious features, unenhanced CT or CS-MRI should be considered and, if needed, adrenal CT with washout analysis. If these studies do not confirm a benign diagnosis, biopsy would be prudent.
- In oncologic patients, if the adrenal mass does not have specific benign diagnostic features and there is no prior imaging for comparison, unenhanced CT, CS-MRI, or PET should be performed, possibly proceeding to adrenal CT with washout analysis if needed. If none of these studies establish a benign diagnosis, then biopsy is appropriate.
- An adrenal mass larger than 4 cm is usually resected in patients without cancer history because of risk of adrenocortical carcinoma. In oncologic patients, PET or biopsy is recommended to exclude metastasis.

It is important to recognize that although recent advances in imaging have allowed noninvasive differentiation of adrenal adenomas from other adrenal lesions as described above, imaging cannot determine the functional status of an adrenal mass. Biochemical testing is required to determine if the adrenal mass is secreting excess hormones. Currently, most endocrinologists recommend screening biochemical assay for all incidental adrenal masses. However, because this approach would be costly, others recommend reserving full biochemical workup for those patients with clinical findings supportive of a hyperfunctioning tumor.[45] Subclinical hyperfunction of an incidental adrenal mass is a new entity in which an incidental adrenal mass is detected and a biochemical assessment shows slightly elevated levels of hormone, but the patient is not symptomatic. The exact prevalence and management of patients with subclinical adrenal hyperfunction are still debated.

Fig. 12. Recommended algorithm for management of incidental adrenal masses as proposed by American College of Radiology. [a] If patient has clinical sign or symptoms of adrenal hyperfunction, consider biochemical evaluation. [b] Consider biochemical testing to exclude pheochromocytoma. [c] Benign imaging features = homogeneous, low density, smooth margins. [d] Suspicious imaging features = heterogeneous, necrosis, irregular margins. APW, absolute percentage washout; CS-MRI, chemical shift MRI; F/U, follow-up; HU, Hounsfield unit; Hx, history; RPW, relative percentage washout; ↓, decrease. (*From* Berland LL, Silverman SG, Gore RM, et al. Managing incidental findings on abdominal CT: white paper of the American College of Radiology Incidental Findings Committee. J Am Coll Radiol 2010;7:764; with permission.)

SUMMARY

Adrenal glands can harbor a wide spectrum of pathology. Most incidental adrenal masses are benign in patients without malignancy, but in oncologic patients, adrenal glands are common sites of metastasis. Contemporary CT, MRI, and PET are excellent imaging tools in the detection and characterization of adrenal masses, and imaging findings alone can noninvasively diagnose most adrenal masses. The diagnosis of hyperfunctioning adrenal mass is made in conjunction with biochemical analysis. Appropriate utilization of imaging is important for optimal management of adrenal masses to separate benign inconsequential adrenal masses from those that require treatment.

REFERENCES

1. Kloos RT, Gross MD, Francis IR, et al. Incidentally discovered adrenal masses. Endocr Rev 1995;16:460–84.
2. Bovio S, Cataldi A, Reimondo G, et al. Prevalence of adrenal incidentaloma in a contemporary computerized tomography series. J Endocrinol Invest 2006;29: 298–302.
3. Song JH, Chaudhry FS, Mayo-Smith WW. The incidental adrenal mass on CT: prevalence of adrenal disease in 1,049 consecutive adrenal masses in patients with no known malignancy. AJR Am J Roentgenol 2008;190:1163–8.
4. NIH state-of-the-science statement on management of the clinically inapparent adrenal mass ("incidentaloma"). NIH Consens State Sci Statements 2002;19: 1–25.
5. Grumbach MM, Biller BM, Braunstein GD, et al. Management of the clinically inapparent adrenal mass ("incidentaloma"). NIH Conference. Ann Intern Med 2003;138:424–9.
6. Young WF Jr. The incidentally discovered adrenal mass. N Engl J Med 2007;356: 601–10.
7. Paulsen SD, Nghiem HV, Korobkin M, et al. Changing role of imaging-guided percutaneous biopsy of adrenal masses: evaluation of 50 adrenal biopsies. AJR Am J Roentgenol 2004;182:1033–7.
8. Korobkin M, Giordano TJ, Brodeur FJ, et al. Adrenal adenomas: relationship between histologic lipid and CT and MR findings. Radiology 1996;200:743–7.
9. Lee MJ, Hahn PF, Papanicolaou N, et al. Benign and malignant adrenal masses: CT distinction with attenuation coefficients, size and observer analysis. Radiology 1991;179:415–8.
10. Korobkin M, Brodeur FJ, Yutzy GG, et al. Differentiation of adrenal adenomas from nonadenomas using CT attenuation values. AJR Am J Roentgenol 1996; 166:531–6.
11. Boland GW, Lee MJ, Gazelle GS, et al. Characterization of adrenal masses using unenhanced CT: an analysis of the CT literature. AJR Am J Roentgenol 1998;171: 201–4.
12. Mitchell DG, Crovello M, Matteucci T, et al. Benign adrenocortical masses: diagnosis with chemical shift MR imaging. Radiology 1992;185:345–51.
13. Outwater EK, Siegelman ES, Radecki PD, et al. Distinction between benign and malignant adrenal masses: value of T1-weighted chemical-shift MR imaging. AJR Am J Roentgenol 1995;165:579–83.
14. Fujiyoshi F, Nakajo M, Fukukura Y, et al. Characterization of adrenal tumors by chemical shift fast low-angle shot MR imaging: comparison of four methods of quantitative evaluation. AJR Am J Roentgenol 2003;180:1649–57.

15. Mayo-Smith WW, Lee MJ, McNicholas MM, et al. Characterization of adrenal masses (<5cm) by use of chemical shift MR imaging: observer performance versus quantitative measures. AJR Am J Roentgenol 1995;165:91–5.

16. Boland GW, Blake MA, Hahn PF, et al. Incidental adrenal lesions: principles, techniques, and algorithms for imaging characterization. Radiology 2008;249: 756–75.

17. Mayo-Smith WW, Boland GW, Noto RB, et al. State-of-the-art adrenal imaging. Radiographics 2001;21:995–1012.

18. Korobkin M, Brodeur FJ, Francis IR, et al. CT time-attenuation washout curves of adrenal adenomas and nonadenomas. AJR Am J Roentgenol 1998;170:747–52.

19. Szolar DH, Kammerhuber FH. Adrenal adenomas and nonadenomas: assessment of washout at delayed contrast-enhanced CT. Radiology 1998;207:369–75.

20. Caoili EM, Korobkin M, Francis IR, et al. Delayed enhanced CT of lipid-poor adrenal adenomas. AJR Am J Roentgenol 2000;175:1411–5.

21. Peña CS, Boland GW, Hahn PF, et al. Characterization of indeterminate (lipid-poor) adrenal masses: use of washout characteristics at contrast-enhanced CT. Radiology 2000;217:798–802.

22. Caoili EM, Korobkin M, Francis IR, et al. Adrenal masses: characterization with combined unenhanced and delayed enhanced CT. Radiology 2002;222:629–33.

23. Blake MA, Kalra MK, Sweeney AT, et al. Distinguishing benign from malignant adrenal masses: multi-detector row CT protocol with 10-minute delay. Radiology 2006;238:578–85.

24. Kenney PJ, Wagner BJ, Rao P, et al. Myelolipoma: CT and pathologic features. Radiology 1998;208:87–95.

25. Rozenblit A, Morehouse HT, Amis ES. Cystic adrenal lesions: CT features. Radiology 1996;201:541–8.

26. Baguet JP, Hammer L, Mazzuco TL, et al. Circumstances of discovery of phaeochromoytoma: a retrospective study of 41 consecutive patients. Eur J Endocrinol 2004;150:681–6.

27. Motta-Ramirez GA, Remer EM, Herts BR, et al. Comparison of CT findings in symptomatic and incidentally discovered pheochromocytomas. AJR Am J Roentgenol 2005;185:684–8.

28. Blake MA, Kalra MK, Maher MM, et al. Pheochromocytoma: an imaging chameleon. Radiographics 2004;24:S87–9.

29. Jacques AE, Sahdev A, Sandrasagara M, et al. Adrenal phaeochromocytoma: correlation of MRI appearances with histology and function. Eur Radiol 2008; 18:2885–92.

30. Allolio B, Fassnacht M. Clinical review: adreno-cortial carcinoma-clinical update. J Clin Endocrinol Metab 2006;91:2027–37.

31. Bharwani N, Rockall AG, Sahdev A, et al. Adrenocortical carcinoma: the range of appearances on CT and MRI. AJR Am J Roentgenol 2011;196:W706–14.

32. Abrams HL, Spiro R, Goldstein N. Metastases in carcinoma: analysis of 1000 autopsied cases. Cancer 1950;3:74–85.

33. DeAtkine AB, Dunnick NR. The adrenal glands. Semin Oncol 1991;18:131–9.

34. Song JH, Grand DJ, Beland MD, et al. Morphologic features of 211 adrenal masses at initial contrast-enhanced CT: can we differentiate benign from malignant lesions using imaging features alone? AJR Am J Roentgenol 2013;201:1248–53.

35. Metser U, Miller E, Lerman H, et al. 18F-FDG PET-CT in the evaluation of adrenal masses. J Nucl Med 2006;47:32–7.

36. Kumar R, Xiu Y, Yu JQ, et al. 18F-FDG PET in evaluation of adrenal lesions in patients with lung cancer. J Nucl Med 2004;45:2058–62.

37. Chong S, Lee KS, Kim HY, et al. Integrated PET-CT for the characterization of adrenal gland lesions in cancer patients: diagnostic efficacy and interpretation pitfalls. Radiographics 2006;26:1811–26.

38. Boland GW, Dwamena BA, Sangwaiya MJ, et al. Characterization of adrenal masses by using FDG PET: a systematic review and meta-analysis of diagnostic test performance. Radiology 2011;259:117–26.

39. Rockall AG, Babar SA, Sohaib SA, et al. CT and MR imaging of the adrenal glands in ACTH-independent cushing syndrome. Radiographics 2004;24: 435–52.

40. Dunnick NR, Leight GS Jr, Roubidoux MA, et al. CT in the diagnosis of primary aldosteronism: sensitivity in 29 patients. AJR Am J Roentgenol 1993;160:321–4.

41. Patel SM, Lingam RK, Beaconsfield TI, et al. Role of radiology in the management of primary aldosteronism. Radiographics 2007;27:1145–57.

42. Young WF, Stanson AW, Thompson GB, et al. Role for adrenal venous sampling in primary aldosteronism. Surgery 2004;136:1227–35.

43. Miskulin J, Shulkin BL, Dohery GM, et al. Is preoperative iodine 123 meta-iodobenzylguanidine scintigraphy routinely necessary before initial adrenalectomy for pheochromocytoma? Surgery 2003;134:918–23.

44. Greenblatt DY, Shenker Y, Chen H. The utility of Metaiodobenzylguanidine (MIBG) scintigraphy in patients with pheochromocytom. Ann Surg Oncol 2008;15:900–5.

45. Berland LL, Silverman SG, Gore RM, et al. Managing incidental findings on abdominal CT: white paper of the American College of Radiology Incidental Findings Committee. J Am Coll Radiol 2010;7:754–77.

Recent Advances in Imaging Cancer of the Kidney and Urinary Tract

Susan Hilton, MD*, Lisa P. Jones, MD, PhD

KEYWORDS

- Kidney cancer • Bladder cancer • Urothelial cancer • Urinary tract cancer
- Radiologic imaging • Computed tomography • Magnetic resonance imaging
- Ultrasonography

KEY POINTS

- Cancer of the kidney and urinary tract continue to affect significant numbers of patients, and the incidence of renal cancer is increasing.
- New and evolving techniques in radiologic imaging have improved the detection, characterization, staging, and treatment planning of cancer of the kidney and urinary tract.
- For reassessment of advanced stage or recurrent kidney and urinary tract cancer after treatment, new, more functional radiologic imaging techniques such as diffusion-weighted magnetic resonance imaging have been shown to be useful.

CANCER OF THE KIDNEY
Epidemiology of Renal Cancer

More than 80% of renal cancers are adenocarcinomas arising from the renal parenchyma, that is, renal cell carcinoma (RCC).[1] It is difficult to obtain population-based data on the incidence and mortality of RCC, because published population data from different geographic regions combine RCC and cancer of the renal pelvis as 1 group. Thus, in this article, epidemiologic data regarding renal cancer refers to cancers of the renal parenchyma and renal pelvis. It was estimated that 65,150 new cases of cancer of the kidney and renal pelvis would be diagnosed in the United States in 2013.[2] Incidence rates for renal cancer in the United States have been increasing steadily for more than 3 decades, more rapidly for African Americans than whites. In the United States, the annual incidence of renal cancer increased by 2.6% per year between 1997 and 2007.[3] The increased incidence of renal cancer occurred across

Dr Jones is a consultant for Bioclinica.
Department of Radiology, Hospital of the University of Pennsylvania, 3400 Spruce Street, Philadelphia, PA 19104, USA
* Corresponding author.
E-mail address: hiltons@uphs.upenn.edu

Surg Oncol Clin N Am 23 (2014) 863–910
http://dx.doi.org/10.1016/j.soc.2014.06.001
1055-3207/14/$ – see front matter © 2014 Elsevier Inc. All rights reserved.
surgonc.theclinics.com

all age groups, with the greatest increase in patients with localized tumors.[1] The increase in incidence of localized tumors can be attributed to the introduction and widespread use of cross-sectional abdominal imaging, including diagnostic ultrasonography (US), computed tomography (CT), and magnetic resonance imaging (MRI), which allow detection of asymptomatic localized renal tumors. Up to 50% to 60% of renal cancers may be found incidentally in asymptomatic patients on abdominal imaging studies performed for unrelated indications.[4] However, the incidence of more advanced renal cancers in the United States, including those with regional extension or distant metastasis, also increased in all race and sex categories.[1] The global incidence of renal cancer increased from the 1970s until the mid-1990s, then leveled off or decreased in many countries.

New and Expanded Roles for Radiologic Imaging of Renal Cancer

The large number of renal tumors detected on routine survey-type abdominal imaging studies has stimulated further expansion of the role of imaging, because more focused imaging studies are often required to characterize these lesions as benign or malignant. Although as many as 85% of renal lesions believed to warrant surgery for presumed renal cancer are malignant,[5,6] the number of benign lesions with features on imaging that are indistinguishable from malignancy is not insignificant. In a series of 292 partial nephrectomies for presumed renal neoplasms, 22% of the lesions were benign.[7] Benign histology is more common in small lesions. In a series of 2675 patients treated surgically for renal lesions, the percentage of benign histology for lesions for those with diameter less than 1 cm was 38%.[8]

The task of modern imaging of renal lesions is not only to detect and stage lesions suspicious for cancer but also to provide definitive characterization of these lesions in as many cases as possible, to minimize unnecessary invasive procedures. For lesions believed likely to represent cancer, imaging is used for planning and execution of percutaneous and intraoperative biopsies and ablative procedures as well as for surgical planning. For patients undergoing nonsurgical treatment of unresectable, metastatic, residual, or recurrent renal cancer, radiologic imaging is used for staging to determine extent of disease and subsequently to assess treatment response. In recent years, novel methods have been introduced to determine treatment response beyond simple tumor bidirectional size measurements, using functional parameters.

Radiologic Imaging for Detection, Characterization, and Staging of RCC

Most renal masses are incidentally discovered on medical imaging studies obtained to investigate a large variety of abdominal conditions. Once it has been shown that the morphology of a renal mass is not in keeping with an uncomplicated simple cyst, the presence of vascularity in a renal mass is the most reliable finding to characterize the lesion as a neoplasm.[9]

When a renal mass has been defined as a probable cancer, radiologic imaging is used to stage the tumor. In the 1960s, the Robson classification was developed to stage renal cell cancers. In this system, stage I tumors were confined to the renal capsule; stage II tumors extended to the perirenal fat or ipsilateral adrenal gland; stage III tumors had vascular (A) or nodal (B) extension, or both (C); and stage IV indicated distant disease.[10] This system has been widely replaced with the TNM (tumor, node, metastasis) classification of the International Union Against Cancer (Union International Contre le Cancer [UICC]), which is being used worldwide (**Table 1**).[11] US, CT, and MRI are the standard imaging modalities used to evaluate renal masses.

Table 1 TNM staging of renal cancer			
Definition of TNM			
Primary Tumor (T)			
TX	Primary tumor cannot be assessed		
T0	No evidence of primary tumor		
T1	Tumor ≤7 cm, limited to kidney		
T1a	Tumor ≤4 cm, limited to kidney		
T1b	Tumor 4–7 cm, limited to kidney		
T2	Tumor >7 cm, limited to the kidney		
T2a	Tumor >7 cm but ≤10 cm in greatest dimension		
T2b	Tumor >10 cm, limited to the kidney		
T3	Tumor extends into major veins or perinephric tissues but not into the ipsilateral adrenal gland and not beyond Gerota's fascia		
T3a	Tumor grossly extends into the renal vein or its segmental (muscle containing) branches, or tumor invades perirenal and/or renal sinus fat but not beyond Gerota's fascia		
T3b	Tumor grossly extends into the vena cava below the diaphragm		
T3c	Tumor grossly extends into the vena cava above the diaphragm or invades the wall of the vena cava		
T4	Tumor invades beyond Gerota's fascia (Including contiguous extension into the ipsilateral adrenal gland)		
Regional Lymph Nodes (N)			
NX	Regional lymph nodes cannot be assessed		
N0	No regional lymph node metastasis		
N1	Metastasis in regional lymph node(s)		
Distant Metastasis (M)			
M0	No distant metastasis		
M1	Distant metastasis		
Anatomic Stage/Prognostic Groups			
Stage I	T1	N0	M0
Stage II	T2	N0	M0
Stage III	T1 or T2	N1	M0
Stage IV	T4	Any N	M0
	Any T	Any N	M1

Used with the permission of the American Joint Committee on Cancer (AJCC), Chicago, Illinois. The original source for this material is the AJCC Cancer Staging Manual, Seventh Edition (2010) published by Springer Science and Business Media LLC, www.springer.com.

US

The advantage of renal US is its low cost, wide availability, and lack of ionizing radiation or intravenous (IV) contrast material. In many cases, use of US to define a renal lesion can obviate more costly imaging tests.

For detection of small renal cancers, US lacks the sensitivity of CT. In a study by Jamis-Dow and colleagues,[12] CT and US detection rates for renal lesions measuring 15 to 20 mm at surgical pathology, were, respectively, 100% and 58%; for lesions measuring 20 to 25 mm, 100% and 79%.

For characterization of renal lesions, US is useful and definitive in many cases, because most space-occupying renal lesions are cysts that are easily characterized with US. US is also useful to detect characteristics in cystic renal lesions that raise suspicion that the lesion represents a neoplasm, including nodularity, thickened septations, and vascularity (**Fig. 1**). US can distinguish cystic from solid renal lesions. Although contrast-enhanced US would be potentially useful for determining vascularity of renal lesions, it is not approved by the US Food and Drug Administration (FDA) for use in the United States. Echogenicity of solid renal lesions as seen on US is not specific for differentiating benign from malignant lesions, because the echogenicity of RCC is variable. Both RCC and angiomyolipoma (AML), a benign macroscopic fat-containing lesion, can appear hyperechoic (**Figs. 2** and **3**).

CT

CT is the modality of choice for both detection and characterization of RCC. CT excels in its high spatial resolution and its ability to detect enhancement of a lesion. Newer, multidetector CT (MDCT) scanners, which use ever-increasing numbers of rows of detectors, allow high-quality multiplanar reconstructions of image datasets, with spatial resolution nearly equivalent in all planes (**Fig. 4**).

For detection of renal masses measuring 15 mm or larger, CT has excellent sensitivity (**Fig. 5**). For detection of smaller renal lesions measuring 0 to 5 mm, CT and US

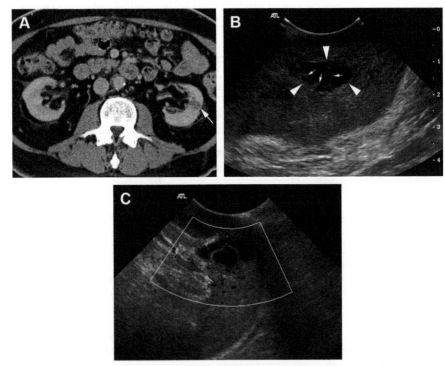

Fig. 1. Small left renal mass characterized by US in a 62-year-old man. (*A*) Axial contrast-enhanced CT image shows a low-density mass (*arrow*). (*B, C*) Sagittal intraoperative grayscale (*B*) color Doppler (*C*) images of the left kidney show a cystic mass (*arrowheads*) with multiple internal septations (*arrows*), which show internal color signal on Doppler, reflecting vascularity. Surgical pathology showed a multicystic Fuhrman grade I/IV RCC.

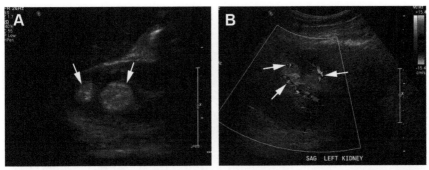

Fig. 2. Typical US appearance of an AML. A 42-year-old woman with incidentally detected renal masses on US. Sagittal grayscale (*A*) and color Doppler (*B*) images of the upper pole of the right kidney show 2 echogenic masses (*A, arrows*), which show internal areas of color signal, representing internal vascularity (*B, arrows*).

detection rates in the study by Jamis-Dow and colleagues[12] were respectively 47% and 0%, and for lesions measuring 5 to 10 mm, 60% and 21%.

Contrast enhancement of a mass lesion suspected to represent cancer is the most important feature used in radiologic imaging to confirm that the lesion is a neoplasm, because enhancement shows that the lesion has vascularity. Enhancement on CT is defined as an increase in density measured by Hounsfield unit (HU) of at least 15 to 20 HU after IV contrast is given. Before the introduction of helical scanners, thresholds for enhancement were as low as 10 HU, but the phenomenon of pseudoenhancement, which creates an artifactual increase in measured HU density of a lesion after IV contrast is given, has been problematic with helical scanners (**Fig. 6**).[13] Pseudoenhancement is related to hardening of the radiograph beam (loss of low-energy

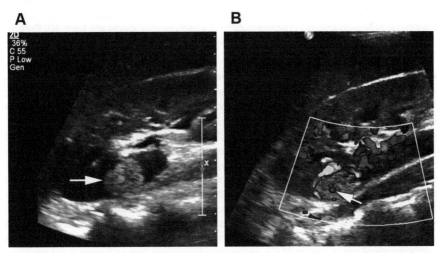

Fig. 3. Small echogenic RCC mimicking an AML on US. Sagittal grayscale (*A*) and color Doppler (*B*) US images of the right kidney show the presence of an echogenic mass (*arrow, A*) in the upper pole of the kidney with areas of internal color signal on the Doppler image (*arrow, B*), reflecting areas of vascularity. The mass is indistinguishable from an AML by US (see **Fig. 2**). Surgical pathology showed a Fuhrman Grade II clear cell RCC.

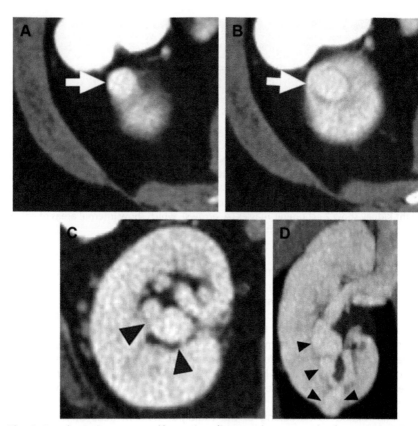

Fig. 4. Renal arteriovenous malformation diagnosed on coronal reformatted CT images. A 53-year-old woman with incidentally discovered right renal lesion. (*A, B*) Axial images of an IV contrast-enhanced abdominal CT scan show a focus of bright enhancement in the right lower renal pole (*arrows*). (*C*) Prominent central vessels (*arrowheads*) are seen. (*D*) Coronal reformat best shows the entirety of an arteriovenous malformation (*arrowheads*).

photons) as it passes through enhancing renal tissue surrounding a small lesion. Increase in HU attenuation number as a result of pseudoenhancement is usually mild; higher HU thresholds for defining enhancement should be used to avoid false-positive interpretation for enhancement.

Although in some instances, a single-phase survey-type IV contrast-enhanced abdominal CT scan shows that a renal mass is obviously enhancing and morphologically in keeping with a renal cancer, in many cases, a dedicated, multiphase CT study obtained before and after IV contrast administration is necessary to determine that there is a significant increase in density after IV contrast, thereby confirming tumor enhancement, and to best define the lesion. Several investigators[14,15] have presented evidence that the degree of vascularity of a renal tumor as assessed on a multiphase examination has predictive value in differentiating subtypes of renal carcinoma. A dedicated renal mass protocol CT study should include thin ($\leq$3 mm) axial sections before and after IV contrast. Although a multiphase CT study, with more than 1 post-contrast phase (**Table 2**), provides the most information, a renal mass protocol may be streamlined to minimize radiation dose, by restricting the number of scanning phases to include only those phases necessary to determine that the lesion enhances. For

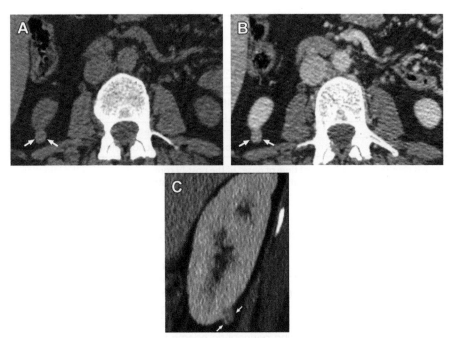

Fig. 5. Tiny enhancing renal mass. (*A*) Axial CT image without IV contrast shows a 7-mm right lower pole renal mass. (*B*) After IV contrast, the mass enhances from 53 HU before IV contrast to 120 HU after contrast. (*C*) Sagittal CT image shows the mass projecting inferoposteriorly (*arrows*).

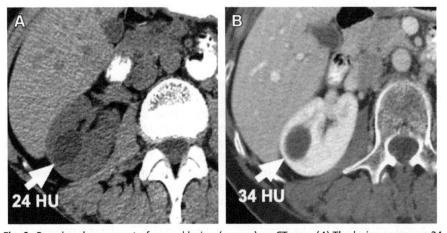

Fig. 6. Pseudoenhancement of a renal lesion (*arrows*) on CT scan. (*A*) The lesion measures 24 HU in density on an axial section before administration of IV contrast. (*B*) The lesion measures 34 HU after IV contrast administration, which is less than the threshold for true enhancement. This lesion had been unchanged for more than 5 years and likely represents a hemorrhagic or proteinaceous cyst.

Table 2		
Phases of renal contrast enhancement on CT		
Phase	**Time After Start of Contrast Injection**	**Use for Detection of**
Non-enhanced	Before injection	Renal calcifications, baseline density of mass
Corticomedullary	25–80 s	Differentiate bulges of normal variant renal parenchyma from true renal mass
Nephrographic	60–136 s	Parenchymal mass lesions, enhancement of mass
Excretory	3–5 min	Collecting system abnormalities

There is considerable variation of time of onset of the post-IV contrast phases after the initiation of contrast injection, which may be influenced by patient age, contrast injection rate, and volume of contrast administered.[98,99]

surgical planning studies, additional phases may be added, depending on the information needed.

CT is the mainstay modality for staging RCC, with a reported overall staging accuracy of up to at least 90%,[16–19] similar to MRI. Although historically, MRI had the advantage over CT for delineating extent of tumor thrombus, newer multidetector helical CT scanners allow high-quality multiplanar imaging, which may achieve this purpose in more cases than was possible in the past.[20] Limitations in staging accuracy include difficulty in distinguishing perinephric edema from perinephric tumor extension[18] and difficulty in distinguishing enlarged lymph nodes because of reactive inflammation from lymph nodes involved with tumor, because the diagnosis of lymph node involvement with tumor using CT depends only on size criteria. False-positive rates for retroperitoneal nodal involvement have been reported as high as 40% to 50%.[21,22] False-negative results, reported as approximately 4%,[18] may occur as a result of microscopic involvement of normal-sized nodes.

Limitations of CT Although CT is of tremendous value for detecting and characterizing renal cancer, disadvantages of CT include its limited ability to characterize small lesions less than 1 cm in diameter, the potentially adverse effects of iodinated IV contrast (including nephrotoxicity and allergic reactions), and the exposure of patients undergoing CT to ionizing radiation.

MRI

MRI is a robust modality to characterize renal mass lesions, because of its superior tissue contrast. MRI can detect IV gadolinium contrast enhancement with high sensitivity. The ability of MRI to depict morphologic detail of cystic lesions, including nodular enhancing elements, is superior to CT (**Fig. 7**). MRI is performed on a 1.5-T or 3-T magnet using a phased-array body coil.[23] The standard MRI protocol for renal mass imaging should include T2-weighted sequences, T1-weighted opposed-phase imaging (with in-phase and out-of-phase sequences) for detection of intratumoral fat, and fat-suppressed T1-weighted gradient-echo acquisition before and after administration of IV gadolinium contrast in corticomedullary, nephrographic, and urographic phases of renal enhancement.[24]

Overall accuracy of MRI for staging RCC is similar to MDCT, although because of its higher cost and lower availability, it is often reserved as a problem-solving tool rather than a first-line imaging modality for RCC characterization and staging. In a prospective study by Hallscheidt and colleagues[17] of 82 RCCs in 47 patients staged with both MDCT and MRI and correlated with histopathologic results, CT staged 68 and

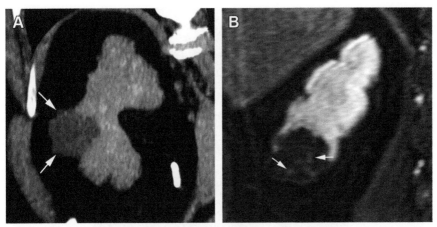

Fig. 7. Morphologic detail of cystic RCC better shown on MRI than CT in a 70-year-old man. (*A*) Coronal contrast-enhanced CT image shows a partially exophytic renal mass (*arrows*), which measured fluid density in attenuation, reflecting cystic nature. Little if any internal complexity was appreciable on the CT. (*B*) Postgadolinium fat-saturated T1-weighted coronal MRI shows the presence of enhancing nodular septations (*arrows*), a feature concerning for malignancy. Surgical pathology showed cystic RCC.

66 tumors correctly (independent readers 1 and 2, with overall accuracy of 0.83 and 0.80, respectively), and MRI staged 71 and 64 tumors staged correctly by readers 1 and 2 (overall accuracy of 0.87 and 0.78, respectively). Regarding tumor extension into the renal veins, the 2 readers correctly diagnosed venous infiltration by means of MRI in 15 and 16 cases. Compared with MRI, even MDCT with three-dimensional (3D) and multiplanar reconstruction had limited certainty in depicting the superior extension of a caval thrombus into the inferior vena cava, although the number of cases with caval thrombus was few in the study group. Differentiating reactive from tumor-involved lymph nodes is problematic for both modalities (**Fig. 8**); in a study by Beer[20] comparing 16 MDCT and MRI for characterization of renal lesions, overstaging with both modalities was always the result of false classification of enlarged lymph nodes (>15 mm) as malignant lymph nodes.

Limitations of MRI Although MRI offers many advantages for evaluating renal mass lesions, especially small lesions, several factors limit its widespread use for this purpose. Gadolinium contrast agents are considered nonnephrotoxic at the dose used for MRI; however, an association of administration of gadolinium-based contrast agents (GDBCAs) with development of nephrogenic systemic fibrosis (NSF) in patients with severely impaired renal function (<30 mL/min/1.73 m^2), has prompted the FDA to issue a black box warning for use of GDBCAs in patients with severe renal insufficiency.[25] The American College of Radiology (ACR) Committee on Drugs and Contrast Media advises that patients with any of the following conditions are at risk of developing NSF after administration of GDBCA: patients on dialysis, patients with severe or end-stage chronic kidney disease (CKD) (CKD 4 or 5, estimated glomerular filtration rate [eGFR] <30 mL/min/1.73 m^2) without dialysis, patients with eGFR 30 to 40 mL/min/1.73 m^2 without dialysis, and patients with acute kidney injury. Identification of 1 or more of these risk factors should prompt consideration to withhold use of GDBCA and use alternative diagnostic examinations, unless there are compelling potential benefits, which require review with both patient and referring physician.[26]

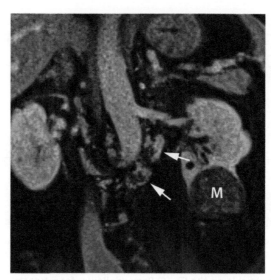

Fig. 8. Reactive lymph nodes indeterminate for metastatic RCC on MRI. A 55-year-old man with left renal mass incidentally detected on CT obtained for unrelated symptoms. Coronal postgadolinium fat-saturated T1-weighted image shows an enhancing partially exophytic renal mass (M) as well as enlarged left para-aortic lymph nodes (*arrows*). Partial nephrectomy showed papillary type II RCC, Fuhrman grade III/IV. The lymph nodes were stable at 5-year imaging follow-up, in keeping with reactive lymph nodes.

The presence of a pacemaker or implantable cardioverter-defibrillator (ICD) is considered a relative contraindication to MRI. Published studies examining the safety of MRI in patients with cardiac devices have reported varying effects of MRI on pacemakers, including impedance changes, battery depletion, and an increase in pacing thresholds. Although some reports included no deaths or device/lead failures, others reported some serious adverse events in patients undergoing inadvertent MRI, especially in patients with older devices.[27] In 2011, the FDA approved an MRI-conditional pacemaker for marketing in the United States (Revo MRI SureScan pacing system; Medtronic, Minneapolis, MN). However, significant risks preclude routine elective replacement of conventional pacemaker systems solely for the purpose of undergoing MRI. Despite recent studies suggesting that MRI can be performed with minimal risk in non–pacemaker-dependent patients with pacemakers or ICDs, controversy remains, and ongoing multicenter studies[27] should better define the risks of performing MRI for patients with implanted cardiac devices.

MRI is more costly than other imaging modalities and less widely available than CT.

Positron emission tomography

Although positron emission tomography (PET) with [18F]-labeled fluoro-2-deoxy-2-glucose (FDG) is helpful for diagnosis and surveillance for many types of cancer, for initial diagnosis of RCC, its role is limited, because uptake is often mild and similar in intensity to adjacent renal parenchyma. Also, excreted radiotracer in the renal collecting system may obscure renal masses.[10]

Imaging of Histologic Subtypes of RCC

The World Health Organization (WHO), in collaboration with the UICC and the American Joint Committee on Cancer (AJCC), adopted the Heidelberg classification of renal cancer[28] in 1997 (**Table 3**). Because biological behavior and prognosis are different for

Table 3
Renal carcinoma: histologic subtypes and prognosis[14]

Type	Frequency (%)	Prognosis (%)
Conventional (clear cell) carcinoma	70 of renal cancers	Second worst prognosis; 5-y survival of 55–60
Papillary carcinoma	15–20 of renal cancers	High 5-year survival: 80–90
Chromophobe renal carcinoma	6–11 of renal cancers	Best prognosis: 5-y survival approximately 90
Unclassified	3–5 of renal cancers	Uncertain
Collecting duct carcinoma	<1 of renal cancers	Worst prognosis: 5-y survival rate <5

the various subtypes of RCC, knowledge of the particular histopathology of a newly diagnosed RCC is important for treatment planning and optimal patient management.

The major differentiating features on CT and MRI include degree of tumor enhancement and lesion morphology, and on MRI, presence of intracellular lipid and, as suggested by recent literature, apparent diffusion coefficient (ADC) values on diffusion-weighted imaging (DWI).

Clear cell renal carcinoma, the most common RCC subtype responsible for 70% of renal cancers, has a poorer prognosis than the other histologic subtypes (with the exception of the rare collecting duct carcinoma). Clear cell RCC is characterized by glycogen and lipid-rich clear cells and a regular network of small, thin-walled blood vessels.[4] Thus, the tumor typically shows brisk hyperenhancement and heterogeneity at imaging (**Fig. 9**),[14,15] because of its vascularity and central necrosis. On MRI on opposed-phase images, up to 60% of clear cell RCCs show relative focal and diffuse loss of signal intensity (SI) as a result of intracytoplasmic lipid content (**Fig. 10**).[29] This lipid is distinguished from the focal macroscopic fat seen in fat-predominant AMLs, which is isointense relative to fat on all MRI sequences (**Fig. 11**). On MRI, the presence of tumor necrosis, retroperitoneal vascular collaterals and renal vein thrombosis is

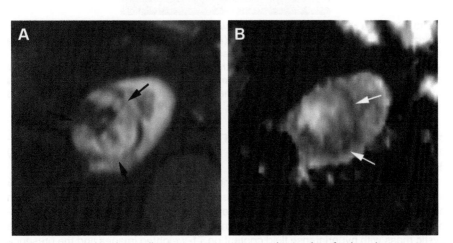

Fig. 9. Hypervascular clear cell RCC on MRI. MRI was obtained to further characterize an incidentally detected renal mass on staging CT in a 67-year-old woman. (*A*) Axial postgadolinium fat-saturated T1-weighted image shows an avidly enhancing mass (*arrows*) with a central area of necrosis (*central dark area*). (*B*) Axial ADC image shows low signal in the periphery of the mass (*arrows*) caused by restricted diffusion in areas of viable tumor. The central necrotic area does not restrict diffusion and appears bright.

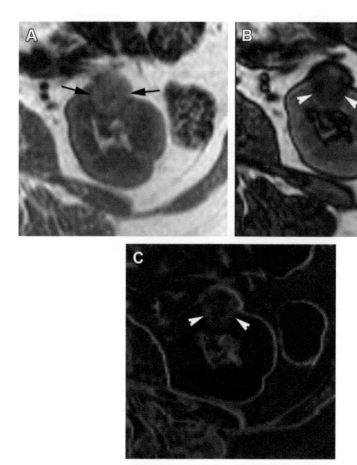

Fig. 10. Lipid in a clear cell RCC on MRI. MRI was obtained in a 60-year-old woman to characterize an incidentally detected renal mass. (*A*) In-phase T1-weighted axial image shows a mass (*black arrows*) that is brighter than adjacent renal parenchyma. (*B*) Out-of-phase T1-weighted axial image shows dark areas within the mass (*arrowheads*), reflecting signal loss in areas where both lipid and water are present. (*C*) Image produced from subtracting the out-of-phase image from the in-phase images shows the areas of intralesional lipid as bright areas (*arrowheads*). Surgical pathology showed Fuhrman II/IV clear cell RCC.

correlated with high-grade clear cell RCC (**Fig. 12**).[30] Cystic lesions with minimal or little solid enhancing component correlate with low-grade clear cell histopathology (**Fig. 13**).[30]

Papillary RCC is the second most common histology subtype, accounting for 15% to 20% of renal cancers. Papillary RCCs are typically hypoenhancing[31] compared with adjacent renal parenchyma and often homogeneous (**Fig. 14**). Papillary RCC often undergoes internal hemorrhage, which accounts for its common appearance on MRI as a cystic mass with hyperintense fluid content on T1-weighted images and the presence of enhancing papillary projections from the wall of the mass (**Fig. 15**).[23] Calcifications may occur in papillary carcinomas (see **Fig. 14**). Papillary carcinomas may be multifocal in 20% to 40% of patients.[23]

Chromophobe RCCs account for 6% to 11% of renal cancers. Chromophobe tumors tend to show homogeneous enhancement, with an intermediate degree of

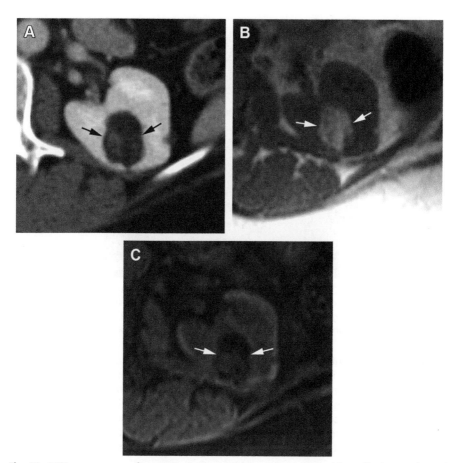

Fig. 11. MRI appearance of an AML. A 53-year-old woman with incidentally detected renal mass. (*A*) Axial enhanced CT image shows that most of the mass is dark (*arrows*), similar to perirenal fat. (*B, C*) Axial non–fat-saturated T1-weighted (*B*) and axial fat-saturated T1-weighted (*C*) images show that the most of the mass (*arrows*) is the same SI as perirenal fat (*bright in B, dark in C*), indicating macroscopic fat, a feature typical of AML.

enhancement compared with clear cell RCC and papillary subtypes (**Fig. 16**). They can often grow to a large size without undergoing central necrosis. On imaging, chromophobe RCCs can be heterogeneous, mimicking clear cell RCC (**Fig. 17**).[29] Patients with chromophobe RCC have the best prognosis, with a 5-year survival of approximately 90%.[14] Collecting duct tumors are infiltrative and involve the medulla (**Fig. 18**),[32] and are associated with a poor prognosis.

Unclassified RCC, representing 3% to 5% of renal cancers, tends to carry a poor prognosis. Specific imaging features of these tumors have not been reported.

New Techniques of Radiologic Imaging for Detection, Characterization, and Staging of RCC

CT
Dual-energy CT If a CT imaging technique could reliably identify the presence of iodinated contrast molecules within a renal mass lesion on images obtained only with IV

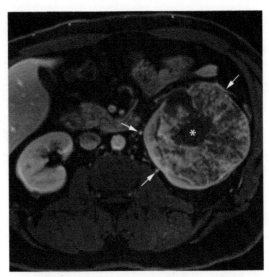

Fig. 12. High-grade RCC with retroperitoneal collaterals on MRI. A 55-year-old man with suspected RCC based on mediastinal lymph node biopsy. Axial post-gadolinium fat-saturated T1-weighted image shows multiple collateral vessels (*arrows*) in the perinephric fat surrounding a large enhancing renal mass with areas of central necrosis (*asterisk*).

contrast, thereby confirming enhancement, there would be no need to perform 2 separate scanning series both before and after administration of IV contrast to determine whether a lesion enhances. Dual-energy CT (DECT) is a technique that can potentially accomplish this goal, thereby omitting the need for the noncontrast scanning sequence and decreasing radiation dose for the examination.[33–36]

DECT refers to CT that uses 2 photon spectra; therefore, DECT is sometimes also referred to as spectral CT. The 2 different spectra are generated either by switching

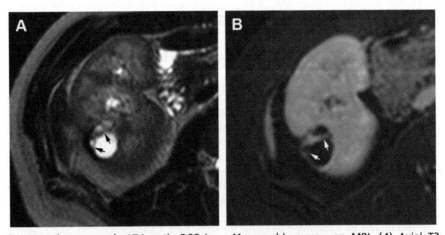

Fig. 13. Fuhrman grade I/IV cystic RCC in a 41-year-old woman on MRI. (*A*) Axial T2-weighted image shows a mass, which is primarily bright (reflecting cystic areas), with a few thickened septations (*arrows*). (*B*) Postgadolinium fat-saturated axial T1-weighted image shows that the septations (*arrows*) appear as bright as renal parenchyma, reflecting enhancement, whereas the fluid areas remain dark.

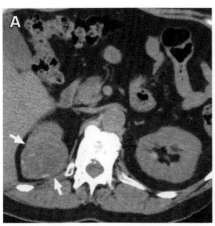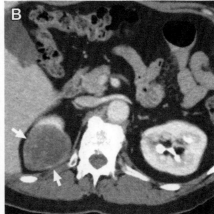

Fig. 14. Mildly enhancing papillary RCC, on CT scan. (*A*) The right upper pole renal mass (*arrows*), which measures 50 HU, contains some faint calcifications on the axial section before IV contrast. (*B*) After IV contrast, the density of the mass (*arrows*) increased to 70 HU.

the voltage of 1 radiograph tube or by running 2 tubes at different voltages, and spectral information is typically gained from 2 sets of absorption measurements obtained with CT detectors.[37] Based on a principle called 3-material decomposition, DECT can differentiate materials in the scan field using different postprocessing algorithms that enable identification of iodine (as well as calcium, or uric acid) in the image. So-called virtual nonenhanced images with near-equivalent image quality and CT number stability of true nonenhanced images can be created. In addition, color-coded display of the iodine distribution in the scan field can potentially allow the radiologist to determine the presence of enhancement within a renal mass without the need for CT number measurements.[34]

CT scanning with lower radiation dose There has been a significant[38] increase in per capita effective radiation dose from diagnostic medical procedures over the past several decades. Widely publicized serious errors in diagnostic and therapeutic radiation dose delivery have heightened general concern.[39] Although the degree of cancer risk caused by medical radiation remains controversial, contemporary heightened popular concern has had a beneficial effect by accelerating development of CT technology that allows scanning at considerably lower radiation doses than was possible only a few years ago. Automated dose-minimizing scanning techniques such as mA modulation and automated kVp selection allow lower dose scanning.[40,41] CT images obtained with lower radiation dose protocols can be created using newer commercially available iterative reconstruction computer algorithms, to reduce image noise and maintain acceptable image quality.[42] Standards for CT radiation dose limits for each type of CT examination, enforced by ACR accreditation of equipment, have become more stringent.[43]

MRI

DWI DWI allows measurement of random water motion (Brownian motion) in biological tissue. Restriction of the random motion of water by the local microenvironment can be assessed qualitatively or quantitatively. A simple method of obtaining DWI is to apply pairs of opposing and balanced magnetic field gradients (but of differing durations and amplitudes) around a spin-echo refocusing pulse of a T2-weighted sequence.[44]

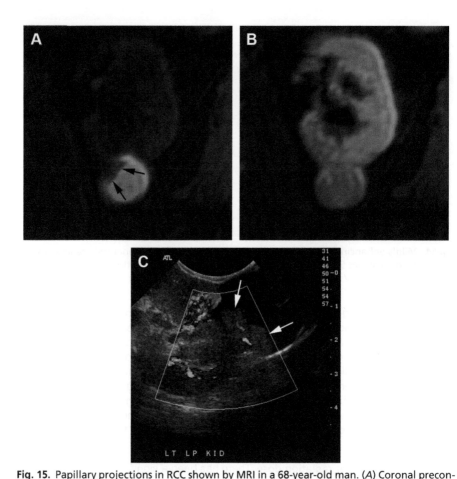

Fig. 15. Papillary projections in RCC shown by MRI in a 68-year-old man. (*A*) Coronal precontrast fat-saturated T1-weighted image shows an exophytic mass consisting of hemorrhagic fluid (which appears bright) surrounding a papillary projection (*arrows*). (*B*) Coronal postcontrast fat-saturated T1-weighted image shows that the papillary projection becomes similar in signal to the remainder of the mass as a result of enhancement, and therefore is no longer visible. (*C*) Intraoperative color Doppler sagittal US image shows the papillary projection (*arrows*) as a soft tissue area with internal flow. Surgical pathology showed type II papillary RCC with macroscopic papillary excrescences.

The degree of diffusion weighting applied is indicated by the b value (measured in s/mm^2). The decay of SI as a function of increasing diffusion-weighting factor (b value) is approximated by a monoexponential function to quantitatively assess restriction to the diffusion. The rate of decay is called the ADC and can be mapped on a voxel by voxel basis as an ADC map.[45] In biological tissues that are highly cellular (such as neoplasms), the higher density of cell membranes restricts the diffusion of water protons. This restriction to diffusion results in less signal loss and therefore higher signal on high b value DWI sequences, with corresponding lower signal on ADC. Conversely, benign less cellular structures have higher mobility of water molecules, and manifest as lower SI on DWI acquisition with corresponding high ADC.[46]

Accumulating evidence over the past decade has suggested that DWI can be used to diagnose malignant renal tumors, and that it may also be possible to use DWI to

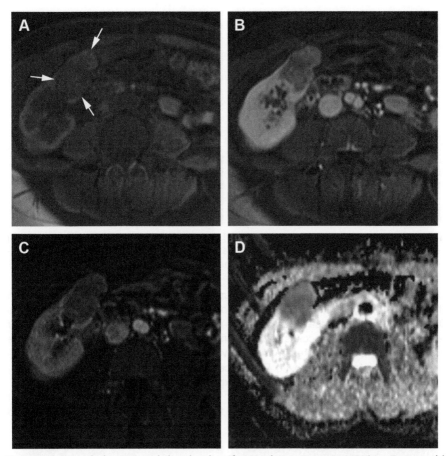

Fig. 16. Chromophobe RCC with low-level uniform enhancement on MRI in a 51-year-old woman. (*A–C*) Axial fat-saturated precontrast (*A*) and postcontrast (*B*) T1-weighted images show the presence of an exophytic renal mass (*arrows, A*), which becomes brighter after IV gadolinium, indicating enhancement, best depicted as homogeneous internal signal on a subtraction image (*C*, generated by subtracting unenhanced images from enhanced images). (*D*) Axial ADC image shows dark signal throughout the mass reflecting diffusion restriction. Surgical pathology showed 4.3 cm chromophobe type RCC.

assess renal cancer subtype and grade. Given the large number of incidentally discovered small renal masses and the availability of a wide array of treatment options for renal neoplasms, the capability of preoperative radiological imaging to predict the histopathology of the tumor and its potential biological behavior with reasonable certainty should prove useful as an aid to therapeutic decision making. For patients with renal dysfunction who are at risk for NSF, DWI could also serve as a reasonable alternative to contrast-enhanced MRI (see **Figs. 9** and **16; Fig. 19**) and contrast-enhanced CT for the diagnosis of malignant renal neoplasms. Results of several studies have suggested that change in ADC on DWI may be useful for assessing treatment response in at least several cancers in the body, with many of the published studies focusing on hepatic cancer.[47] Use of DWI to assess ADC change as an indicator of treatment response is especially useful in tumors for which change in measured size using

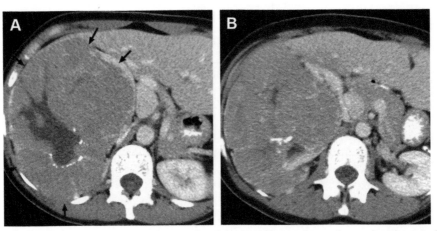

Fig. 17. Large chromophobe RCC on CT. (*A, B*) Large right renal mass (*arrows*) with central necrosis is seen on CT after IV contrast. The patient was a 29-year-old woman with an incidentally shown renal mass on imaging obtained to investigate gastrointestinal symptoms.

criteria such as RECIST (Response Evaluation Criteria in Solid Tumors) has been shown to be inadequate as an indicator of treatment response (**Fig. 20**). Because DWI can assess response to systemic or regional treatment of cancer at a cellular level, it should detect successful treatment earlier than anatomic measures.[47] The possibility that DWI ADC change may prove similarly useful as an indicator of treatment response for patients with RCC receiving targeted therapy for unresectable, advanced, or recurrent disease is being explored.[46]

Studies of Cova and colleagues[48] and Squillaci and colleagues[49] reported that ADCs of RCC were significantly lower than ADCs of renal cysts. Zhang and

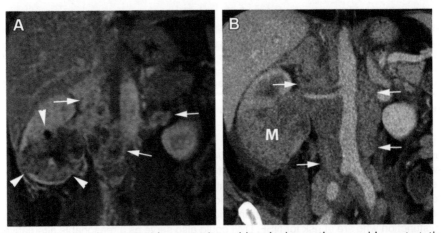

Fig. 18. Collecting duct RCC with retroperitoneal lymphadenopathy caused by metastatic disease, in a 36-year-old man, on both CT and MRI. (*A*) Coronal postgadolinium fat-saturated T1-weighted MRI shows an infiltrative mass in the lower pole of the right kidney (*arrowheads*) with adjacent retroperitoneal lymphadenopathy (*arrows*). (*B*) Coronal contrast-enhanced CT image obtained 1 month later shows the mass (M) again and progression of the retroperitoneal lymphadenopathy (*arrows*). Surgical pathology showed collecting duct RCC.

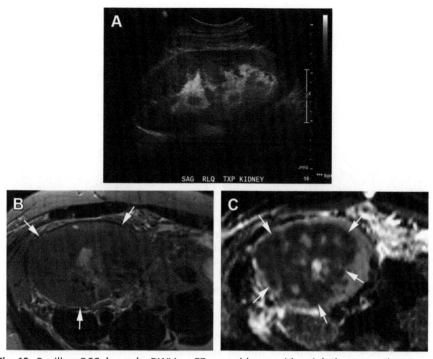

Fig. 19. Papillary RCC shown by DWI in a 57-year-old man with a right lower quadrant renal transplant. (*A*) Sagittal grayscale US image of the right lower quadrant transplant obtained before biopsy shows an enlarged but otherwise grossly normal kidney. The renal biopsy showed carcinoma and therefore, MRI was obtained for further evaluation. (*B*) Axial T2-weighted MRI image shows a transplant kidney (*arrows*) with mild nonspecific parenchymal heterogeneity. (*C*) Axial ADC MRI image showed marked restricted diffusion (*dark areas, arrows*) throughout much of the kidney, reflecting extensive tumor. Explanted kidney surgical pathology showed a 10.9 cm Fuhrman grade III/IV RCC.

colleagues[50] reported use of DWI to evaluate 25 renal masses and found lower ADCs in cystic/necrotic portions of renal neoplasms compared with ADCs of simple cysts. Results of a study by Taouli and colleagues[51] suggest that DWI can be used to characterize renal lesions, although compared with contrast-enhanced MRI, these investigators found it to be less accurate. These investigators suggest that DWI can be used to differentiate solid RCCs from oncocytomas and characterize the histologic subtypes of RCC. The mean ADCs for RCCs were significantly lower than those for benign renal lesions, and oncocytomas had significantly higher ADCs compared with solid RCCs, but the mean ADC for papillary RCCs was significantly lower than that for non-papillary RCCs (**Fig. 21**). However, AMLs had the lowest mean ADC values (**Fig. 22**). The area under the receiver operating characteristic curve (AUC), sensitivity, and specificity of DWI for the diagnosis of RCC (excluding AMLs, which could be diagnosed at unenhanced imaging) were 0.856, 86%, and 80%, respectively, with use of a cutoff ADC of equal to or less than 1.92×10^{-3} mm^2/s. The AUC, sensitivity, and specificity of contrast-enhanced MRI in the diagnosis of RCC, with AMLs excluded, were 0.944, 100%, and 89%, respectively. Results of Sandrasegaran and colleagues[52] were in agreement that benign and malignant renal lesions could be differentiated.

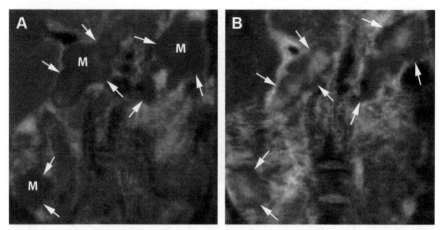

Fig. 20. Decreased ADC in metastases, indicating a treatment response, in a 56-year-old woman with clear cell RCC. (*A*) Coronal ADC image from abdominal MRI before treatment shows multiple metastatic lesions (M, *arrows*), which appear dark, reflecting restricted diffusion. (*B*) Coronal ADC image after 6 weeks of therapy with sunitinib shows little change in the size of the lesions (*arrows*), but the lesions appear brighter, indicating reduction in the degree of restricted diffusion.

The DWI scanning technique typically used for abdominal imaging is a single-shot spin-echo echo-planar protocol with fat suppression.[46] DWI is routinely performed without gadolinium IV contrast administration, and can be obtained within a breath hold or with free breathing. The strength of diffusion weighting is set at the MRI scanner by changing the b value. There is no agreement regarding the optimal b values to be used in renal imaging, and therefore, it should be kept in mind when evaluating

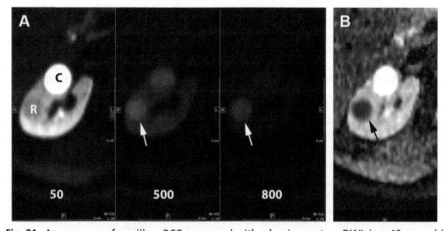

Fig. 21. Appearance of papillary RCC compared with a benign cyst on DWI, in a 46-year-old man. (*A*) Diffusion-weighted axial images with b values of 50, 500, and 800, respectively (*left to right*), show a cyst (C) and a papillary RCC (R). Note that the RCC loses less signal on high b value images compared with the cyst, reflecting restricted diffusion of the cancer (RCC stays bright on the high b value images, *arrow*). (*B*) Axial ADC image shows that the RCC (*arrow*) appears dark because of restricted diffusion, whereas the cyst appears bright, reflecting relatively free diffusion in the cyst.

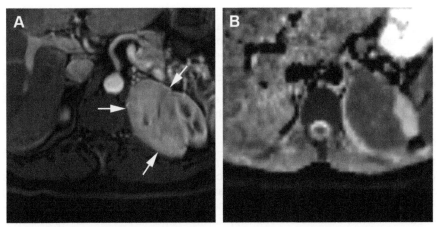

Fig. 22. Minimal fat AML with restricted diffusion on MRI in a 52-year-old woman. (A) Axial postgadolinium fat-saturated T1-weighted image shows an enhancing mass (*arrows*), which on other sequences (not shown) did not contain macroscopic fat. (B) Axial ADC image shows dark signal throughout the mass, reflecting restricted diffusion. Core biopsy histopathology showed AML, and the patient subsequently underwent therapeutic embolization.

studies from different investigators that quantitative ADC values depend on the b value used for the imaging study. For interpretation, visual inspection is routinely used in clinical practice to detect and assess renal lesions by noting different signal attenuation between renal parenchyma and lesions. Cellular lesions such as renal neoplasms show less signal loss on high b value (>400 s/mm^2) images and lower ADC values. Quantitative ADC value determination may be obtained by placing a region of interest (ROI) cursor on the ADC map. ADC is usually expressed in ($\times 10^{-3}$) mm^2/s.

Limitations of DWI include low signal-to-noise ratio, limited spatial resolution, and multiple artifacts, such as distortion, ghosting, and blurring.[46] Standardized methods for quantitative ADC analysis should be developed and deployed by commercial vendors.

Perfusion-weighted imaging Given that contrast enhancement as an indicator of tumor vascularity is the key factor in evaluating renal masses, it follows that assessment of dynamics of tumor perfusion should provide meaningful information about the nature of a variety of renal neoplasms and potentially quantify perfusion and angiogenic activity in tumors as a monitor of antiangiogenic treatment response. Perfusion-weighted imaging (PWI) uses high-temporal resolution imaging for measurement of perfusion dynamics of parenchymal organs and tumors arising from them.[24] Although this method has been used in neuroimaging, use of PWI in the abdomen is especially technically challenging. Recent technical advances in MRI have allowed initiation of its use in the abdomen, and early studies have focused on PWI of the hepatic parenchyma and hepatic neoplasms.[53] For PWI analysis, an SI versus time curve is generated by placing ROIs over the tissue of interest. The analysis can be performed by semiquantitative or quantitative techniques.

Immuno-PET

Research is under way to develop monoclonal antibodies labeled with PET radiotracers (immuno-PET) to target RCC antigens for imaging (radioimmunoscintigraphy) and therapy (radioimmunotherapy). Because of its high resolution and sensitivity and its unique ability to measure tissue concentrations of radioactivity in 3 dimensions,

PET is an excellent method for in vivo imaging of therapeutic and diagnostic antibodies. The radioiodinated antibody G250 and its chimeric form cG250 bind to the antigen carbonic anhydrase IX, a transmembrane glycoprotein expressed in clear cell RCC. In a study performed to assess whether iodine[124]-labeled antibody chimeric G250 ([124]I-cG250) PET could predict clear cell RCC, 15 of 16 clear cell carcinomas were identified accurately by antibody PET, and all 9 non–clear cell renal masses were negative for the tracer (**Fig. 23**). The sensitivity of [124]I-cG250 PET for clear cell kidney carcinoma in this trial was 94 and the negative predictive value was 90%.[54]

Follow-Up After Treatment of RCC

Monitoring after local ablative or surgical treatment

For follow-up of patients with treated renal carcinoma, radiologic imaging is a valuable tool and the cornerstone of surveillance management of these patients. The widening array of treatment options for locally confined RCC, which include observation, ablation, and minimally invasive and open approaches to partial and radical nephrectomy, points to the need for evidence-based directives for imaging follow-up. Although updated guidelines for follow-up of renal cancer have been published,[55] much of the available source material for compilation of guidelines is based on observational and case studies.[56] Additional prospective scientific studies are needed to further define the most accurate and cost-effective posttreatment imaging strategies.

Patients who have undergone ablative treatment of renal tumors are subsequently followed with radiologic imaging, using CT or MRI. Radiologic imaging to rule out early treatment failure should be obtained initially at 3 and 6 months after the ablative

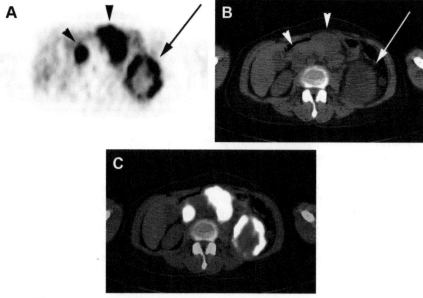

Fig. 23. [124]I-cG250 PET identifies clear cell renal carcinoma in a patient with advanced left renal carcinoma and extensive retroperitoneal nodal metastases. (*A*) [124]I-cG250 PET axial image. The centrally necrotic primary tumor (*arrow*) has intense antibody binding (*black*), as does the upper abdominal lymphadenopathy (*arrowheads*). (*B*) Low-dose axial CT scan image. Tumor (*arrow*) and lymphadenopathy (*arrowheads*) are seen. (*C*) Fused CT-PET axial image. (*Courtesy of* C.R. Divgi, MD, New York, NY; and D.A. Pryma, MD, Philadelphia, PA.)

procedure. Radiologic evolution of cryoablated tumors is characterized by significant shrinkage and loss of contrast enhancement on CT (**Fig. 24**). Tumors successfully treated with radiofrequency ablation (RFA) show no IV contrast enhancement, but with minimal shrinkage on CT. On MRI, the imaging hallmark of successful renal tumor ablation is lack of tumor enhancement at gadolinium-enhanced imaging (**Fig. 25**). Cryoablated or RFA renal tumors generally appear relatively hypointense on T2-weighted images compared with the intermediate or high SI tumor seen on preablation images (see **Fig. 24**).

The overall incidence of metastatic disease after RCC surgery is approximately 20% to 50%. Most disease relapses occur within the first 3 years,[55] but late recurrences can occur (**Fig. 26**).[57] Although the prognosis for patients with untreated metastatic disease is poor, with 5-year survival of 2.7% to 9%, response rates of 5% to 20%

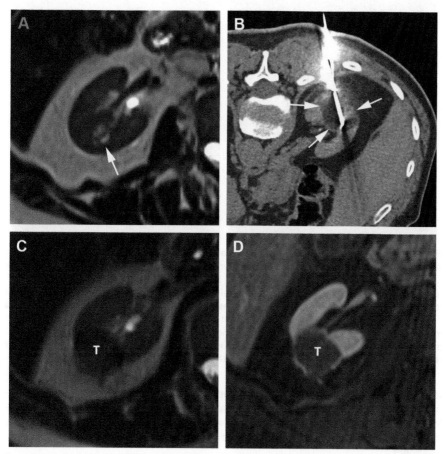

Fig. 24. Small papillary RCC in a 67-year-old man on MRI, treated with cryoablation. (*A*) Axial T2-weighted image shows a heterogeneous mass (*arrow*), which enhanced after IV gadolinium (not shown) and was found to represent papillary RCC on biopsy. (*B*) Prone unenhanced axial CT image during cryoablation shows an ice ball (*arrows*) encompassing the expected location of the mass. (*C, D*) Axial T2-weighted (*C*) and axial postgadolinium fat-saturated T1-weighted (*D*) images show replacement of the RCC by a nonenhancing treatment zone (T), which appears dark in both the T2-weighted and postgadolinium images.

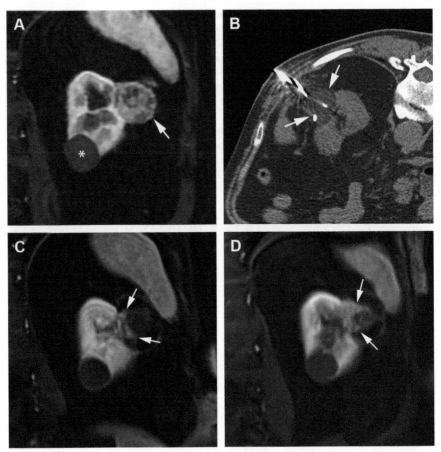

Fig. 25. Enlarging residual tumor after cryoablation on MRI in an 81-year-old man with an RCC. (*A*) Coronal postgadolinium fat-saturated T1-weighted image shows a heterogeneously enhancing mass (*arrow*), representing RCC. Note also a nonenhancing cyst (*asterisk*). (*B*) Prone unenhanced axial CT image obtained during cryoablation shows an ice ball (*arrows*) in the expected location of the mass. (*C*) Coronal postgadolinium fat-saturated T1-weighted image 2 months later shows that most of the mass now appears dark (reflecting necrosis), with a residual bright, enhancing area medially (*arrows*). (*D*) Coronal postgadolinium fat-saturated T1-weighted image 6 months after ablation shows enlargement of the enhancing area (*arrows*) caused by growth of viable tumor.

to systemic immunotherapy or chemotherapy have been reported.[56] There are also reports of survival improvement with surgical treatment of solitary metastases. Therefore, the rationale for surveillance of patients after partial or radical nephrectomy is to detect recurrent or distant metastatic disease and improve outcome through treatment.

After partial or radical nephrectomy, disease relapse and cancer-specific survival are highly related to pathologic tumor stage. Published guidelines for radiologic imaging follow-up of patients who have been surgically treated for RCC are based on stage-specific risk of recurrence, although the specific recommended types of imaging studies and time intervals between studies vary among the guidelines. Patients with familial RCC syndromes require close serial monitoring.

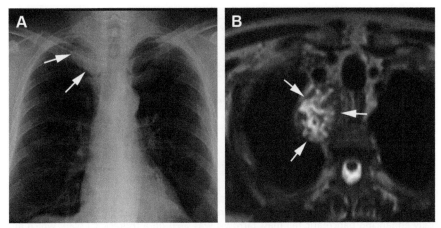

Fig. 26. Late recurrence of clear cell RCC in a 71-year-old man. (*A*) Frontal radiograph of the chest obtained 17 years after nephrectomy for RCC shows a right apical mass (*arrows*). MRI was obtained for further evaluation. (*B*) Axial T2-weighted image shows a right superior mediastinal mass (*arrows*), with internal bright areas, reflecting areas of necrosis. The mass showed avid enhancement and intralesional lipid (not shown), raising suspicion for metastatic clear cell RCC, which was confirmed on excision.

Determining response after treatment of metastatic disease

Approximately 20% to 30% of patients with RCC have metastatic disease at presentation, and nearly 50% of patients with advanced disease die within 5 years of diagnosis.[4] The most common sites of metastatic disease, in decreasing order of frequency, include lung, bone, lymph nodes, liver, adrenal gland, and brain (**Fig. 27**).[58] Atypical sites of metastatic disease that are uncommon but not rare include the peritoneum and the pancreas (**Fig. 28**). In general, the hypervascular metastatic foci of clear cell RCC are most conspicuous during the arterial phase of imaging.

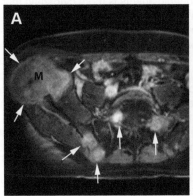
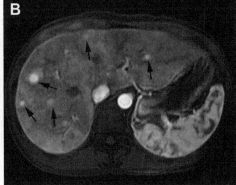

Fig. 27. Examples of metastatic RCC on MRI. (*A*) Axial postgadolinium fat-saturated T1-weighted image through the pelvis shows the presence of multiple enhancing osseous metastases (*bright-appearing lesions, arrows*). The dominant lesion (M) has a large extraosseous soft tissue component extending into adjacent musculature. (*B*) Axial enhanced arterial-phase fat-saturated T1-weighted image in a different patient shows the presence of multiple early-enhancing hepatic lesions (*arrows*), representing RCC metastases, which are often hypervascular, as in this case.

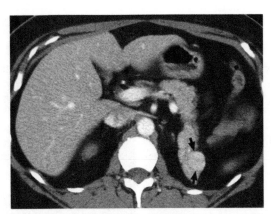

Fig. 28. Metastatic clear cell RCC to the pancreatic tail, IV contrast-enhanced CT scan. This briskly enhancing pancreatic tail mass (*arrows*) was seen on a thoracic CT scan, which also showed pulmonary metastases. The patient had undergone a nephrectomy for RCC 4 years before the scan.

For many years, the mainstay of treatment of metastatic RCC was immunotherapy with interferon α or interleukin 2. Response rates for these therapies were low, in the range of 10% to 20%. With better understanding of the molecular biology of RCC, newer, antiangiogenic drugs have been developed, which induce stabilization of disease rather than regression.[58,59]

Clear cell RCC is characterized by the loss of the Von Hippel-Lindau gene. The tumor secretes growth factors and proteolytic enzymes, which stimulate tumor neoangiogenesis. These hypoxia-inducible factors (HIFs) induce the release of proangiogenic growth factors, including the vascular endothelial growth factor and the platelet-derived growth factor. In addition, increased expression of HIF is caused by constitutive activation of the mammalian target of rapamycin. Antiangiogenic therapies disrupt the signaling pathways of key angiogenic growth factors.

Because the mechanism of action of antiangiogenic agents is more cytostatic than cytotoxic,[60] classification systems to assess tumor response based on change in size such as RECIST 1.1 (Response Evaluation Criteria in Solid Tumors) have proved inadequate to differentiate patients with early tumor progression from those with stable disease and prolonged survival. As a result of early necrosis, tumors responding to treatment may increase in size on posttreatment imaging studies (**Fig. 29**), rendering size measurements misleading.[58] Subsequent criteria schemes, which are based on tumor attenuation, include the Choi criteria,[61] and the modified Choi criteria.[62] The SACT (size and attenuation CT) criteria[63] and the MASS (morphology, attenuation, size, and structure) criteria[64] have been shown to be better predictors of clinical response. The initial degree of vascularity of the tumor correlates with likelihood of response to treatment,[65] and loss of vascularity as assessed by attenuation decrease in the tumor indicates response to treatment. Newer, more functional imaging schemes that have been introduced to monitor patients receiving antiangiogenic therapy include dynamic contrast-enhanced MRI and CT.

CANCER OF THE URINARY BLADDER
Epidemiology and Pathology of Bladder Cancer

Cancer of the urinary bladder is the sixth most common cancer in the United States, with an estimated 72,570 cases to be diagnosed in the United States in 2013.[2] Bladder

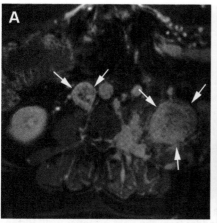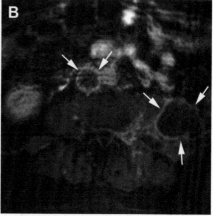

Fig. 29. Decreased enhancement in metastases, reflecting treatment response to a cytostatic agent. (A) Axial postgadolinium fat-saturated T1-weighted image before therapy shows metastatic lesions (*arrows*), which appear bright because of enhancement of viable tumor. (B) Axial postgadolinium fat-saturated T1-weighted image after 6 weeks of pazopanib therapy shows similar size lesions (*arrows*), which no longer appear bright, reflecting interval necrosis.

cancer is the most common cancer of the urinary tract, and occurs 3 to 4 times as frequently in men as in women. Cancer of the urinary bladder has a significant recurrence rate and therefore requires long-term surveillance after surgical treatment. It is estimated that the 5-year cost of treating Medicare patients with this condition is about $1 billion, seventh highest among all cancers.[66] Cigarette smoking is the most common risk factor for development of bladder cancer,[67] with other risk factors including chemical carcinogens such as aniline dyes. Risk factors for squamous cell cancer include long-term catheterization, nonfunctioning bladder, urinary tract calculi, and chronic infection by *Schistosoma haematobium*.[68]

More than 95% of bladder tumors arise from the uroepithelium (epithelial tumors), including urothelial tumors (>90%), squamous cell carcinomas (6%–8%), and adenocarcinomas (2%). The WHO/International Society Of Urological Pathology consensus classification system of urothelial (transitional cell) neoplasms of the urinary bladder covers neoplastic conditions as well as preneoplastic lesions.[68] Rarer epithelial tumors include small cell/neuroendocrine carcinoma, carcinoid tumors, and melanoma.[69]

Radiologic Imaging for Detection of Bladder Cancer

Hematuria usually prompts the diagnostic workup for bladder cancer, because 85% of patients with bladder cancer present with painless microscopic or macroscopic hematuria.[68] However, the rate of bladder cancer in patients with microscopic hematuria is only in the range of 0.5% to 10.5%.[70] The recommended workup of patients with hematuria includes cystoscopy and at least 1 imaging study to evaluate both the upper and lower urinary tracts. Multiphase CT urography (CTU), performed without and with IV contrast is recommended by the American Urological Association (AUA) guideline as the imaging procedure of choice for evaluation of the patient with asymptomatic microhematuria, because it has the highest sensitivity and specificity for evaluation of the upper urinary tract (**Fig. 30**). The ACR Appropriateness Criteria rank CTU as the best initial imaging examination for the evaluation of patients with hematuria.[71] For patients with relative or absolute contraindications that preclude use of multiphasic CT (such as iodinated contrast allergy, pregnancy), magnetic resonance urography

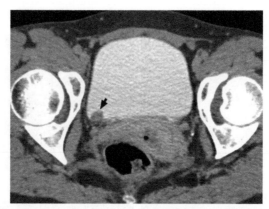

Fig. 30. Tiny bladder carcinoma on CTU in a 40-year-old woman with hematuria. A tiny polypoid lesion (*arrow*) protrudes into the bladder from the right posterior wall. Histopathology after transurethral resection showed a papillary urothelial carcinoma, with no bladder wall invasion.

(MRU) (without/with IV contrast) is advocated by the AUA as an acceptable alternative imaging approach. US alone, or in combination with conventional IV urography (IVU), although in previous widespread use and recommended in other clinical guideline papers as recently as 2009,[72] has been shown in numerous studies to be less sensitive for detection of both solid mass lesions and urothelial malignancy. For patients with significantly compromised function who cannot receive IV contrast for CT (because of risk of contrast-induced renal failure) or MRI (because of risk of NSF), retrograde pyelography (RUP) provides an alternative for visualization of the upper urinary tracts (**Fig. 31**).

Despite the present capabilities of CTU and MRI to detect bladder lesions, cystoscopic evaluation is still considered essential in the workup of most patients with

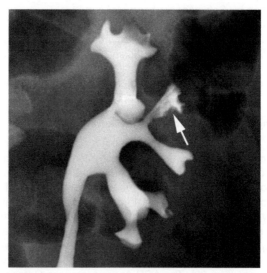

Fig. 31. Small urothelial carcinoma on retrograde pyelogram in a 71-year-old man. Image from a left retrograde pyelogram shows an irregular filling defect in the superior interpolar calyx (*arrow*), found to represent a 1-cm papillary urothelial carcinoma on nephroureterectomy.

suspected bladder cancer, because flat lesions and lesions at the base of the bladder near the prostate gland cannot be visualized confidently, and thickening of the bladder wall caused by inflammatory cause may be indistinguishable from thickening caused by tumor. CT has limited ability to detect small bladder lesions.[73]

Evolving techniques for detection of bladder cancer

MRI Recent improvements in MRI include multiplanar image acquisition and reconstruction, using 3D sequences. These sequences offer the advantages of shorter acquisition time, volumetric coverage without intersection gaps, and an improved signal-to-noise ratio.[74,75] Rapid acquisition minimizes artifacts produced by bowel peristalsis and respiration. Although MRI has good sensitivity and positive predictive value (PPV) for detecting bladder cancer, its role for this purpose remains to be defined (**Fig. 32**). In 1 prospective study of 36 patients with a history of bladder cancer comparing CT and MRI, the sensitivity and PPVs for tumor detection were 93% and 96%, respectively, for CT; 94% and 94%, respectively, for MRI on T2-weighted imaging; and 100% and 93%, respectively, for dynamic gadolinium-enhanced MRI.[76]

Radiologic Imaging for Staging of Bladder Cancer

Clinical and pathologic staging of bladder cancer is according to the TNM system (**Table 4**). Although staging for local tumor extent is aided by radiologic imaging, and new imaging techniques are showing promise in improving staging accuracy, staging for depth of bladder wall involvement before treatment is performed using endoscopic transurethral resection.[70] For assessment of lymph node involvement and distant metastases, cross-sectional imaging using CT or MRI are important imaging tools.

CT

The same imaging study used for detection of bladder cancer, CTU, is often used for staging of a detected cancer, or, once a bladder cancer is detected with cystoscopy, CT or CTU is frequently performed to stage the tumor (**Fig. 33**). For local staging of the

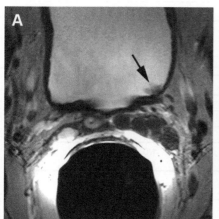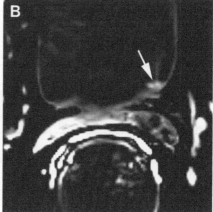

Fig. 32. Incidentally detected papillary urothelial carcinoma on MRI obtained for local staging of newly diagnosed prostate cancer in a 72-year-old man. (*A*) Axial T2-weighted image shows a papillary lesion along the posterior left urinary bladder wall (*arrow*). (*B*) Axial subtraction image obtained by subtracting precontrast images from postcontrast images shows that the lesion (*arrow*) appears bright, indicating internal vascularity. Histopathology after transurethral resection showed a urothelial carcinoma, with no bladder wall invasion.

Table 4
TNM staging of cancer of the urinary bladder

Primary Tumor (T)

TX	Primary tumor cannot be assessed
T0	No evidence of primary tumor
Ta	Noninvasive papillary carcinoma
Tis	Carcinoma in situ: "flat tumor"
T1	Tumor invades subepithelial connective tissue
T2	Tumor invades muscularis propria
pT2a	Tumor invades superficial muscularis propria (inner half)
pT2b	Timor invades deep muscularis propria (outer half)
T3	Tumor invades perivesical tissue
pT3a	Microscopically
pT3b	Macroscopically (extravesical mass)
T4	Tumor invades any of the following: prostatic stroma, seminal vesicles, uterus, vagina, pelvic wall, abdominal wall
T4a	Tumor invades prostatic stroma, uterus, vagina
T4b	Tumor invades pelvic wall, abdominal wall

Regional Lymph Nodes (N)

NX	Lymph nodes cannot be assessed
N0	No lymph node metastasis
N1	Single regional lymph node metastasis in the true pelvis (hypogastric, obturator, external iliac, or presacral lymph node metastasis)
N2	Multiple regional lymph node metastasis in the true pelvis (hypogastric, obturator, external iliac, or presacral lymph node metastasis)
N3	Lymph node metastasis to the common iliac lymph nodes

Distant Metastasis (M)

M0	No distant metastasis
M1	Distant metastasis

Distant Metastasis (M)

M0	No distant metastasis
M1	Distant metastasis

Anatomic Stage/Prognostic Groups

Stage 0a	Ta	N0	M0
Stage 0is	Tis	N0	M0
Stage I	T1	N0	M0
Stage II	T2a	N0	M0
	T2b	N0	M0
Stage III	T3a	N0	M0
	T3b	N0	M0
Stage IV	T4a	N0	M0
	T4b	N0	M0
	Any T	N1–3	M0
	Any T	Any N	M1

Used with the permission of the American Joint Committee on Cancer (AJCC), Chicago, Illinois. The original source for this material is the AJCC Cancer Staging Manual, Seventh Edition (2010) published by Springer Science and Business Media LLC, www.springer.com.

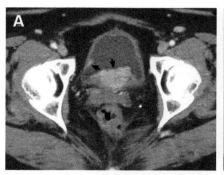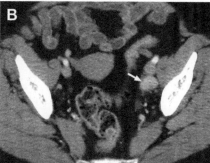

Fig. 33. Multifocal bladder carcinoma, with metastasis to a left obturator lymph node on CTU. These IV contrast-enhanced scans were obtained during the nephrographic phase, before excretion of contrast. (*A*) Two sites of bladder carcinoma are seen (*arrows*), with brisk enhancement of the lesions. (*B*) An enlarged left obturator lymph node is present (*arrow*), with enhancement similar to the bladder lesions. Transurethral biopsy of the bladder lesions showed high-grade papillary urothelial carcinoma. The patient was a 74-year-old woman with gross hematuria.

bladder cancer, the disadvantage of CT is that it cannot depict the individual layers of the bladder wall, and therefore, it cannot accurately assess depth of bladder wall invasion except in cases in which there is obvious extravesical tumor extension. In addition, inflammatory changes after transurethral resection of a bladder tumor (ie, infiltrative changes of the perivesical fat) are not distinguishable from tumor extension on CT (**Figs. 34** and **35**). In a study by Kim and colleagues,[77] sensitivity and specificity for diagnosis of perivesical invasion were 89% and 95%, respectively, in 67 patients with bladder cancer who underwent diagnosis and staging with CT, and increased to 92% and 98%, respectively, for the 44 patients within this group who had a time interval of 7 or more days between transurethral resection of the bladder and CT examination. The accuracy of contrast-enhanced CT in the local staging of bladder cancer is reported to be in the range of 60%.[78]

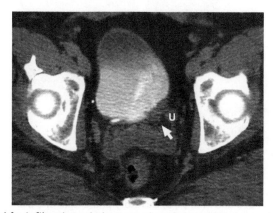

Fig. 34. Perivesical fat infiltration mimics tumor invasion on CTU. A mass lesion arising from the left posterolateral wall of the bladder obstructs the ureter (U) and produces some infiltration of the left perivesical fat (*arrow*). Histopathology at transurethral resection showed high-grade urothelial carcinoma without involvement of the detrusor muscle in the specimen. The patient was a 52-year-old man with hematuria.

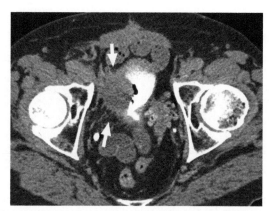

Fig. 35. Locally advanced bladder cancer on CTU. This right-sided bladder wall mass (*arrows*) transgresses the bladder wall and penetrates the perivesical fat, with a spiculated outer margin (a little gas along the inner aspect of the mass is caused by instrumentation.) At cystoprostatectomy, surgical histopathology showed invasion of the perivesical fat, and 2 of 5 resected right obturator lymph nodes were involved with tumor. The patient was a 78-year-old man who had undergone previous partial cystectomy for bladder cancer.

For staging of lymph node involvement, accuracy of CT is in the range of 70% to 90%, with false-negative rates of 25% to 40%.[79,80] Staging of lymph nodes on CT is mainly limited because lymph nodes are evaluated on CT only with respect to size; therefore, enlarged lymph nodes with an inflammatory cause cannot be differentiated from tumor-involved nodes, and small lymph nodes harboring microscopic tumor spread cannot be diagnosed (**Fig. 36**).

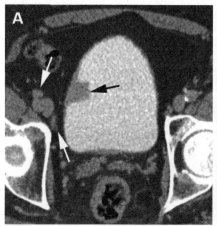
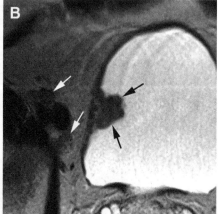

Fig. 36. Presumed reactive lymph nodes in a 75-year-old man with low-grade papillary urothelial carcinoma, on CTU and MRI. (*A*, *B*) Excretory-phase axial CT (*A*) and axial T2-weighted MRI (*B*) images show a mass (*black arrows*) in the urinary bladder, representing the bladder carcinoma, as well as enlarged right external iliac lymph nodes (*white arrows*). Histopathology from transurethral resection of the bladder carcinoma showed invasion into the lamina propria only. Two-year clinical follow-up showed no signs of tumor recurrence, favoring reactive cause for the lymph nodes.

MRI

MRI has been shown to be more accurate than CT for local staging of bladder cancer, because of its superior tissue contrast and ability to visualize the layers of the bladder wall (**Figs. 37–40**). MRI scanning protocols for imaging bladder cancer typically include both conventional and functional sequences. Axial spin-echo (SE) T1-weighted images with a large field of view (FOV) are useful for evaluating the perivesical fat planes for extravesical tumor infiltration, pelvic lymphadenopathy, and bone metastases. High-resolution fast SE T2-weighted images of the bladder obtained in the 3 orthogonal planes with a small FOV and a large matrix are used to evaluate the detrusor muscle for tumor depth and invasion of the surrounding organs.[75] The detrusor muscle appears as a hypointense line on T2-weighted images (**Fig. 41**).

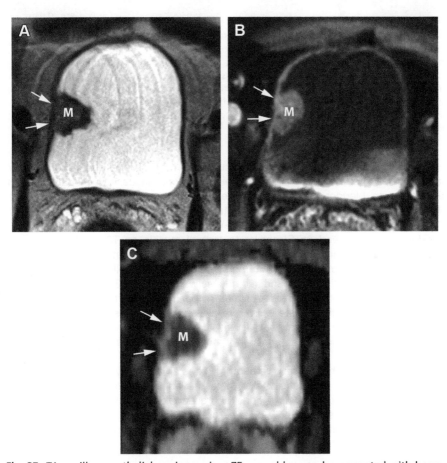

Fig. 37. T1 papillary urothelial carcinoma in a 75-year-old man who presented with hematuria (same patient as in **Fig. 36**). (*A*) Axial T2-weighted image shows an intraluminal bladder mass (M), with apparent irregularity of the detrusor muscle (*arrows*), concerning for muscle invasion. (*B, C*) Axial T1-weighted fat-saturated postgadolinium (*B*) and axial ADC (*C*) images show an intact detrusor muscle (*arrows*), which appears brighter than the tumor on both images. Histopathology from transurethral resection showed a low-grade urothelial carcinoma, with invasion of the lamina propria only.

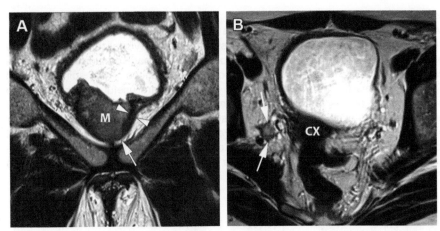

Fig. 38. Bladder neck/urethral T2 urothelial carcinoma with a metastatic lymph node in a 58-year-old woman with hematuria. (*A*) Coronal T2-weighted image shows a mass (M), involving the bladder neck and upper urethra. There is marked focal thinning of the detrusor muscle inferiorly (*large arrow*), suspicious for muscle invasion, compared with other areas, where the detrusor muscle is of normal thickness (*arrowheads*). At cystourethrectomy, histopathology showed muscle invasion without perivesical extension. (*B*) Axial T2-weighted image shows an abnormal obturator lymph node (*arrow*), proved to represent a metastasis. CX, cervix.

Despite superiority over CT, overall accuracy of MRI for local staging of bladder cancer is only moderate. In a study by Tekes and colleagues,[81] of 71 patients with biopsy-proven bladder cancer who underwent MRI on a 1.5-T scanner with a phased-array pelvic coil, on a stage by stage basis, MRI accuracy was 62%, with overstaging the most common error (32%). The investigators reported that 81% of bladder tumors showed an SI similar to that of muscle on T2-weighted images, creating difficulty in distinguishing tumor from intact detrusor muscle (see **Figs. 37 and 39**). In a study of 52 bladder tumors evaluated with MRI, Takeuchi and colleagues[82] found that the tumor and submucosa were of similar SI in 60% (31 of 52) of the dynamic contrast-enhanced examinations, rendering it difficult to distinguish an intact submucosa and thus differentiate T1 from T2 disease. Nevertheless, staging accuracies of 85% and 82% were achieved for differentiating superficial from invasive tumors and organ-confined from non–organ-confined tumors, respectively, in the study by Tekes and colleagues.

For staging of lymph node involvement, MRI has an accuracy of 64% to 92% (see **Figs. 38** and **39**).[75,79] MRI suffers from the same limitations as CT in that only size criteria are used to evaluate lymph nodes for presence of tumor involvement; enlarged reactive (benign) nodes, and small nodes harboring microscopic tumor are missed unless additional functional MRI such as DWI can be proved of additional value and can be incorporated into the imaging protocol.

New Imaging Techniques for Staging of Bladder Cancer

Diffusion-weighted MRI

Recent studies have shown DWI to be of potential value for both the diagnosis and staging of bladder cancer (see **Fig. 36**). Matsuki and colleagues[83] reported that the ADCs of urinary bladder cancers were lower than those of surrounding structures and that the tumors were clearly depicted as lesions with high SI on diffudion-weighted

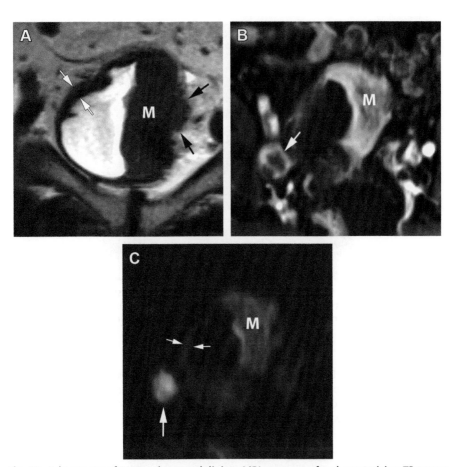

Fig. 39. Advantages of DWI and postgadolinium MRI sequences for characterizing T3 tumor, in a 65-year-old man. (*A*) Coronal T2-weighted image shows the tumor as an area of irregular thickening of the left urinary bladder wall (M), which is nearly isointense to detrusor muscle (*white arrows*). There is extension of tumor into the perivesical fat (*black arrows*). (*B*) Axial postgadolinium fat-saturated T1-weighted image shows that the SI of the mass is conspicuously brighter than the bladder wall, because of contrast enhancement of the tumor. (*C*) Axial diffusion-weighted (C, b value of 800) image. Here, the increase in signal within the tumor because of restricted diffusion improves differentiation of the tumor from the muscle (*small arrows*). A centrally necrotic right external iliac lymph node (*large arrow, B, C*) caused by a metastasis is also seen.

images (see **Fig. 39; Fig. 42**). In a study by Watanabe and colleagues,[84] 16% of tumors were overstaged with sequences that included gadolinium-enhanced images versus 5% with the addition of diffusion-weighted images. Although a statistically significant difference between the methods without and with DWI was not found, results suggested that addition of DWI might be helpful for preoperative staging of bladder cancer. In a study of 52 bladder tumors in 40 patients, Takeuchi and colleagues[82] reported overall accuracy of T stage diagnosis was 67% for T2-weighted images alone, 88% for T2-weighted plus diffusion-weighted images, 79% for T2-weighted plus contrast-enhanced images, and 92% for all 3 image types together, suggesting incremental value for DWI.

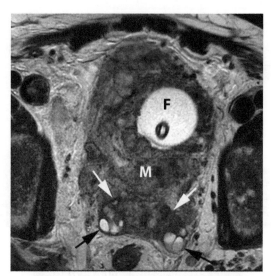

Fig. 40. T4 tumor in a 58-year-old man. Axial T2-weighted image shows diffuse irregular thickening of the urinary bladder wall caused by extensive tumor (M), which extends contiguously (*white arrows*) into the seminal vesicles (*black arrows*). F, Foley catheter balloon.

PET

The use of PET with FDG for local staging of bladder cancer is limited by obscuration caused by urinary excretion of the radiotracer. Radiotracers such as carbon 11 [^{11}C] methionine or [^{11}C]choline are not excreted in urine and may be of more use as PET agents, but they have not yet been approved by the FDA.[75]

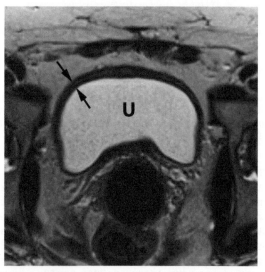

Fig. 41. Normal detrusor muscle on MRI. Axial T2-weighted image shows the detrusor muscle as a dark structure (*arrows*), separating the bright urine (U) in the bladder from adjacent bright perivesical fat.

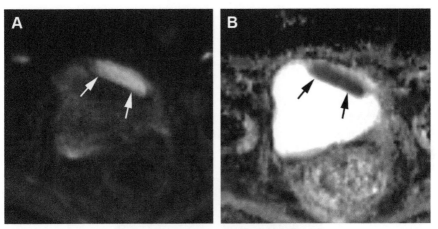

Fig. 42. T3 urothelial carcinoma of the urinary bladder showing restricted diffusion in a 50-year-old woman. Axial diffusion-weighted (*A*, b value 800) and axial ADC image (*B*) show a urothelial carcinoma (*arrows*), which appears bright on the diffusion-weighted image and dark on the ADC image.

Imaging Surveillance After Treatment of Bladder Cancer

The necessity and frequency of follow-up radiologic imaging for surveillance of patients treated for bladder cancer is based on the pathologic stage and grade of the tumor.

For patients diagnosed with superficial bladder cancer, doubts exist as to the necessity of upper tract (UT) imaging after treatment in patients without positive urine cytology or concerning symptoms, because subsequent development of UT tumors is rare in this group.

After radical cystectomy for invasive bladder cancer, overall recurrence rates are in the range of 25% to 46%, with most recurrences occurring within the first 2 to 3 years.[85] The most common sites for recurrence include bone, lung, pelvis, and liver. Although there is lack of agreement on surveillance imaging protocols for patients with stage T2 disease, most investigators agree on the necessity of close surveillance for patients treated for T3 disease, warranting abdominopelvic CT scans and chest radiographs at least every 3 to 6 months in the first several years. Metachronous UT tumors are reported to occur in 2.4% to 6.6% of patients at a mean interval of 30 to 80 months after cystectomy (**Fig. 43**).[85] Periodic evaluation of the upper urinary tract with CTU carries the advantage over conventional IVU of simultaneous evaluation of the abdominal and pelvic contents.

UPPER URINARY TRACT UROTHELIAL CANCER
Epidemiology and Patterns of Involvement of UT Urothelial Cancer

The risk factors for the development of UT urothelial cancers are similar to those for bladder cancer. In addition, in Eastern Europe, an endemic degenerative interstitial nephropathy called Balkan nephropathy is associated with 100 to 200 times greater risk of UT transitional cell carcinoma (TCC).[86] UT tumors develop in 2.4% to 6.6% of patients with bladder cancer,[85] and approximately 40% (range, 20%–70%) of patients with UT TCC develop TCC of the lower urinary tract. The renal pelvis is the second most common site of urothelial cancer after the bladder. In the ureter, the distal ureter is the most common site of TCC, accounting for 73% of all ureteral TCCs;

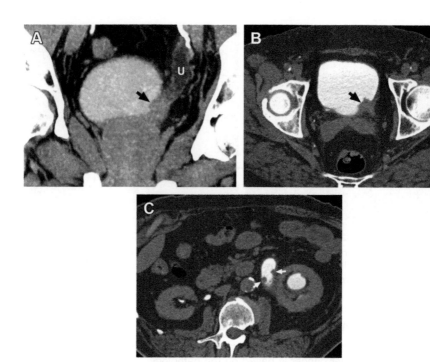

Fig. 43. Recurrent bladder cancer and new upper urinary tract urothelial carcinoma, on CTU. The patient was a 68-year-old man with previous history of bladder cancer. (*A*) A left-sided bladder mass (*arrow*) obstructs the ureter (U). (*B*) More of the left-sided mass lesion (*arrow*) is shown on a lower section. (*C*) A 2-hour delayed scan (enabling contrast opacification of the obstructed left urinary tract) shows 2 additional sites of carcinoma (*arrows*) in the left renal pelvis.

24% occur in the midureter and only 3% in the proximal ureter. In 2% to 5% of UT TCCs, the disease is bilateral. 85% of UT TCCs are low stage and superficial, and approximately 15% are infiltrating.[86]

Radiologic Imaging for Detection and Staging of UT Urothelial Cancer

Unlike bladder cancer, which is most often detected using cystoscopy, detection of UT urothelial cancer depends mainly on radiologic imaging.

MDCT urography

Traditionally, IVU has been the radiologic imaging examination of choice for detection of urothelial cancer. However, the introduction of thin collimation MDCT in the past decade has enabled detailed imaging of the urinary tract using MDCT urography (MDCTU).[87–89] In addition to assessing the urinary tract for calculi and renal mass lesions, CTU allows assessment of the urinary tract for urothelial lesions (**Figs. 44–46**), including small lesions not normally visible on CT without opacification and distension of the urinary tract with contrast (see **Fig. 46**). The CTU examination is usually performed with a combination of unenhanced and timed nephrographic and excretory-phase imaging after administration of iodinated IV contrast. The sensitivity of IVU for detection of upper urinary tract lesions has been reported in the range of 50% to 75%.[90] Reported sensitivity, specificity, and overall accuracy for MDCTU for detection of UT urothelial tumors is superior to IVU. In a meta-analysis of the published literature

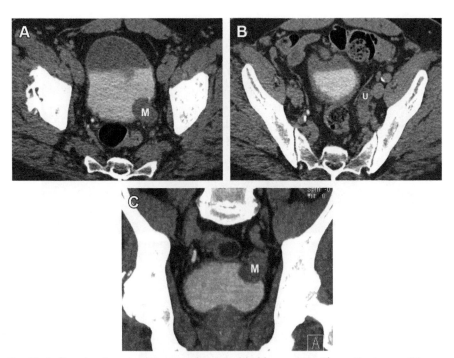

Fig. 44. Left ureteral carcinoma protruding into bladder, on CTU. The patient was a 57-year-old man with a sensation of incomplete bladder emptying. (*A*) Axial CTU image shows an obstructing left ureteral mass (M) protruding into the bladder. (*B*) Axial section at a higher level shows the dilated left ureter (U) and the upper aspect of the soft tissue mass. (*C*) Coronal image shows the mass (M). At left nephroureterectomy, histopathology showed papillary urothelial carcinoma with no invasion.

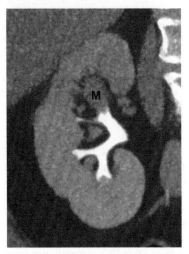

Fig. 45. Invasive urothelial carcinoma of the right renal collecting system in a 55-year-old man. Coronal CTU image shows a mass (M) in the right upper pole collecting system. Surgical histopathology at right nephroureterectomy showed papillary carcinoma invading the renal parenchyma and renal sinus fat. The invasion was difficult to predict from the CT image.

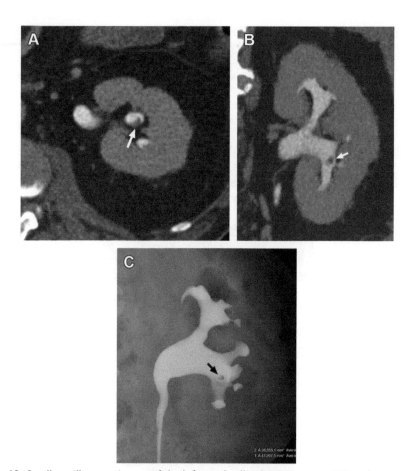

Fig. 46. Small papillary carcinoma of the left renal collecting system, on CTU and retrograde pyelogram, in a 61-year-old man with a history of low-grade bladder cancer and a positive urine fluorescence in situ hybridization test. (*A*) CTU axial section shows a tiny filling defect (*arrow*) in the left lower pole collecting system. (*B*) The lesion (*arrow*) is shown more conspicuously on a coronal reconstruction from the CTU. (*C*) Retrograde pyelogram shows the lesion (*arrow*) again. On endoscopic biopsy, the lesion was a low-grade papillary urothelial carcinoma, which was treated with endoscopic laser ablation.

reported by Chlapoutakis and colleagues,[91] sensitivity of MDCTU for detection of UT urothelial tumors ranged between 88% and 100%, and specificity between 93% and 100%. Pooled sensitivity was 96% (95% confidence interval [CI], 88%–100%) and pooled specificity was 99% (95% CI, 98%–100%), and direct comparison of the method with IVU confirmed the superiority of CTU over IVU in terms of sensitivity and specificity. In a study by Jinzaki and colleagues[90] of 104 patients at high risk for urothelial carcinoma, in which upper urinary tract urothelial carcinoma was diagnosed in 77 (14%) segments of 46 (44%) patients, per patient sensitivity, specificity, overall accuracy, and AUCs for detecting carcinomas with CTU (93.5%, 94.8%, 94.2%, and 0.963, respectively) were significantly greater than those for excretory urography (80.4%, 81.0%, 80.8%, and 0.831, respectively) ($P = .041$, $P = .027$, $P = .001$, and $P<.001$, respectively).

A disadvantage of MDCTU is that the radiation dose of the study is higher than for conventional abdominopelvic CT examinations, largely because of the use of multi-phase imaging protocols, which require repeat scanning sequences through the abdomen and pelvis. Since the introduction of CTU in the late 1990s, several important measures have been taken to decrease the radiation dose for this examination, including reduction of the number of scanning sequences, tailoring of dose settings for individual scan phases, and introduction by scanner manufacturers of dose-optimizing automated tube current modulation. These measures have succeeded in decreasing overall dose for MDCTU,[92] and further initiatives are ongoing.

RUP and retrograde ureteropyeloscopy

The diagnostic workup for patients who are undergoing urinary tract surveillance for urothelial cancer or who present with hematuria includes urinary cytology, MDCTU, and cystoscopy. For patients with contraindications to iodinated contrast medium used for MDCTU such as renal insufficiency or contrast allergy, RUP or retrograde ureteropyeloscopy may be performed (see **Fig. 31**). For RUP, sensitivity and specificity reported by Cowan and colleagues[87] was 0.96 and 0.97, respectively. Chen and colleagues[93] reported a sensitivity of 71.7% and specificity of 84.7% for RUP read in the endoscopy room. The superior sensitivity of RUP is caused by the higher spatial resolution of the radiographs used for the study. Ureteroscopic biopsy/cytology, which allows direct vision and sampling of visualized lesions, has a reported sensitivity as high as 93.4%.[93] Although these examinations are accurate diagnostic tools, they are relatively invasive, requiring cannulation of the ureters under general anesthesia.

MRU

MRU is a less invasive alternative to RUP for patients with contraindications to MDCTU, if the level of abnormal renal function, if present, does not preclude use of IV gadolinium contrast material because of risk of NSF (see discussion of NSF in the cancer of the kidney section, in the section on MRI under radiologic imaging for detection, characterization, and staging of RCC). MRU involves performing multiple MRI sequences through the kidneys, urinary tract, and bladder, with image acquisition in multiple planes, both before and after IV injection of a diuretic, typically furosemide, and gadolinium contrast. Because TCC is isointense to the renal parenchyma in both T1-weighted and T2-weighted sequences, MRU is best performed with the use of IV gadolinium.[94] The post-IV contrast scans are generally obtained in at least 2 phases, including nephrographic and excretory phases. Takahashi and colleagues,[95] in a study to assess the ability of MRU to detect UT small urothelial lesions smaller than 2 cm, reported a sensitivity of 74%. Lee and colleagues[96] reported a sensitivity of MRU for detection of upper urinary tract neoplasms of 63%. Previous reports have indicated sensitivities approaching 88%, but in these reports, the tumors were larger, as indicated by the presence of secondary urinary obstruction.[96] MRU should be reserved for patients for whom MDCTU is contraindicated, because spatial resolution of CT is better than MRI.[95]

Staging of UT urothelial cancer with radiologic imaging

The TNM system (**Table 5**) is most frequently used for staging upper urinary tract tumors. CTU permits staging and assessment of the upper urinary tract in a single examination. When a fat plane or a layer of contrast medium separates the mass from the renal parenchyma, the tumor can be classified as T1 or T2. Loss of renal sinus fat and abnormal enhancement of the adjacent parenchyma are signs of a T3 tumor.[86] In addition to assessing depth of local tumor involvement, CT can determine the

Table 5	
TNM staging of cancer of the renal pelvis and ureter	
Primary Tumor (T)	
Tx	Primary tumor cannot be assessed
T0	No evidence of primary tumor
Ta	Papillary noninvasive carcinoma
Tis	Carcinoma in situ
T1	Tumor invades subepithelial connective tissue
T2	Tumor invades the muscularis
T3	(For renal pelvis only): tumor invades beyond muscularis into peripelvic fat or the renal parenchyma T3; (for ureter only): tumor invades beyond muscularis into periureteric fat
T4	Tumor invades adjacent organs, or through the kidney into the perinephric fat
Regional Lymph Nodes (N)[a]	
NX	Regional lymph nodes cannot be assessed
N0	No regional lymph node metastasis
N1	Metastasis in a single lymph node, $\leq$2 cm in greatest dimension
N2	Metastasis in a single lymph node, >2 cm but not >5 cm in greatest dimension; or multiple lymph nodes, none >5 cm in greatest dimension
N3	Metastasis in a lymph node, >5 cm in greatest dimension
Distant Metastasis (M)	
M0	No distant metastasis
M1	Distant metastasis

Anatomic Stage/Prognostic Groups			
Stage 0a	Ta	N0	M0
Stage 0is	Tis	N0	M0
Stage I	T1	N0	M0
Stage II	T2	N0	M0
Stage III	T3	N0	M0
Stage IV	T4	N0	M0
	Any T	N1	N0
	Any T	N2	M0
	Any T	N3	M0
	Any T	Any N	M1

[a] Laterality does not affect the N classification.

Used with the permission of the American Joint Committee on Cancer (AJCC), Chicago, Illinois. The original source for this material is the AJCC Cancer Staging Manual, Seventh Edition (2010) published by Springer Science and Business Media LLC, www.springer.com.

presence of lymph nodal and distant metastases (**Fig. 47**). MRI also has the ability to identify nodal metastases with similar accuracy to CT. However, as noted in previous sections on nodal staging of RCC and carcinoma of the urinary bladder, staging of lymph nodes with both CT and MRI is limited, because only size criteria are applied to distinguish normal from abnormal lymph nodes.

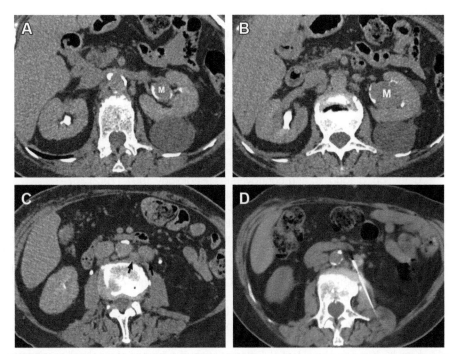

Fig. 47. Urothelial carcinoma of the left renal pelvis with metastatic involvement of left para-aortic lymph nodes shown on CTU, in a 76-year-old woman with hematuria. (*A, B*) A soft tissue mass (M) expands the contrast-opacified left renal pelvis. There are incidental left renal cysts. (*C*) A more caudal axial section shows enlarged retroperitoneal lymph nodes (*arrows*). (*D*) Image from a subsequent percutaneous CT-guided biopsy of an enlarged left para-aortic lymph node, which yielded metastatic TCC.

Surveillance of Patients Diagnosed with UT Urothelial Cancer with Radiologic Imaging

The multicentric synchronous and metachronous patterns of occurrence of urinary tract TCC emphasize the need for continuous surveillance of the urinary tract at risk in patients diagnosed with UT urothelial cancer. Periodic follow-up with upper urinary tract imaging, using the methods described herein, is essential.

For patients who have undergone nephroureterectomy for invasive disease, evidence-based guidelines for specific posttreatment imaging regimens are lacking, but most investigators agree that close follow-up with cross-sectional imaging is indicated. The European Association of Urology 2011 guideline recommends MDCTU every 6 months for 2 years and then yearly for at least 5 years.[97]

REFERENCES

1. Pantuck AJ, Zisman A, Belldegrun AS. The changing natural history of renal cell carcinoma. J Urol 2001;166(5):1611–23.
2. Siegel R, Naishadham D, Jemal A. Cancer statistics, 2013. CA Cancer J Clin 2013;63(1):11–30.
3. Cho E, Adami HO, Lindblad P. Epidemiology of renal cell cancer. Hematol Oncol Clin North Am 2011;25(4):651–65.
4. Choudhary S, Sudarshan S, Choyke PL, et al. Renal cell carcinoma: recent advances in genetics and imaging. Semin Ultrasound CT MR 2009;30(4):315–25.

5. Frank I, Blute ML, Cheville JC, et al. Solid renal tumors: an analysis of pathological features related to tumor size. J Urol 2003;170(6 Pt 1):2217–20.

6. Snyder ME, Bach A, Kattan MW, et al. Incidence of benign lesions for clinically localized renal masses smaller than 7 cm in radiological diameter: influence of sex. J Urol 2006;176(6 Pt 1):2391–5 [discussion: 5–6].

7. McKiernan J, Yossepowitch O, Kattan MW, et al. Partial nephrectomy for renal cortical tumors: pathologic findings and impact on outcome. Urology 2002; 60(6):1003–9.

8. Thompson RH, Kurta JM, Kaag M, et al. Tumor size is associated with malignant potential in renal cell carcinoma cases. J Urol 2009;181(5):2033–6.

9. Bosniak MA. The small (less than or equal to 3.0 cm) renal parenchymal tumor: detection, diagnosis, and controversies. Radiology 1991;179(2):307–17.

10. Krajewski KM, Giardino AA, Zukotynski K, et al. Imaging in renal cell carcinoma. Hematol Oncol Clin North Am 2011;25(4):687–715.

11. Compton CC, Byrd DR, Garcia-Aguilar J, et al, editors. AJCC Cancer Staging Atlas. 2nd edition. A Companion to the Seventh Editions of the AJCC Cancer Staging Manual and Handbook. New York: Springer; 2012. p. 637.

12. Jamis-Dow CA, Choyke PL, Jennings SB, et al. Small (< or = 3-cm) renal masses: detection with CT versus US and pathologic correlation. Radiology 1996;198(3):785–8.

13. Birnbaum BA, Maki DD, Chakraborty DP, et al. Renal cyst pseudoenhancement: evaluation with an anthropomorphic body CT phantom. Radiology 2002;225(1): 83–90.

14. Kim JK, Kim TK, Ahn HJ, et al. Differentiation of subtypes of renal cell carcinoma on helical CT scans. AJR Am J Roentgenol 2002;178(6):1499–506.

15. Sun MR, Ngo L, Genega EM, et al. Renal cell carcinoma: dynamic contrast-enhanced MR imaging for differentiation of tumor subtypes–correlation with pathologic findings. Radiology 2009;250(3):793–802.

16. Reznek RH. CT/MRI in staging renal cell carcinoma. Cancer Imaging 2004; 4(Spec No A):S25–32.

17. Hallscheidt PJ, Bock M, Riedasch G, et al. Diagnostic accuracy of staging renal cell carcinomas using multidetector-row computed tomography and magnetic resonance imaging: a prospective study with histopathologic correlation. J Comput Assist Tomogr 2004;28(3):333–9.

18. Catalano C, Fraioli F, Laghi A, et al. High-resolution multidetector CT in the preoperative evaluation of patients with renal cell carcinoma. AJR Am J Roentgenol 2003;180(5):1271–7.

19. Kopka L, Fischer U, Zoeller G, et al. Dual-phase helical CT of the kidney: value of the corticomedullary and nephrographic phase for evaluation of renal lesions and preoperative staging of renal cell carcinoma. AJR Am J Roentgenol 1997; 169(6):1573–8.

20. Beer AJ, Dobritz M, Zantl N, et al. Comparison of 16-MDCT and MRI for characterization of kidney lesions. AJR Am J Roentgenol 2006;186(6):1639–50.

21. Studer UE, Scherz S, Scheidegger J, et al. Enlargement of regional lymph nodes in renal cell carcinoma is often not due to metastases. J Urol 1990; 144(2 Pt 1):243–5.

22. Johnson CD, Dunnick NR, Cohan RH, et al. Renal adenocarcinoma: CT staging of 100 tumors. AJR Am J Roentgenol 1987;148(1):59–63.

23. Sun MR, Pedrosa I. Magnetic resonance imaging of renal masses. Semin Ultrasound CT MR 2009;30(4):326–51.

24. Kang SK, Chandarana H. Contemporary imaging of the renal mass. Urol Clin North Am 2012;39(2):161–70, vi.
25. Prince MR, Zhang HL, Prowda JC, et al. Nephrogenic systemic fibrosis and its impact on abdominal imaging. Radiographics 2009;29(6):1565–74.
26. ACR Committee on Drugs and Contrast Media. ACR manual on contrast media version 9. 2013. p. 123. Available at: http://www.acr.org/quality-safety/resources/contrast-manual. Accessed July 29, 2014.
27. Russo RJ. Determining the risks of clinically indicated nonthoracic magnetic resonance imaging at 1.5 T for patients with pacemakers and implantable cardioverter-defibrillators: rationale and design of the MagnaSafe Registry. Am Heart J 2013;165(3):266–72.
28. Kovacs G, Akhtar M, Beckwith BJ, et al. The Heidelberg classification of renal cell tumours. J Pathol 1997;183(2):131–3.
29. Pedrosa I, Sun MR, Spencer M, et al. MR imaging of renal masses: correlation with findings at surgery and pathologic analysis. Radiographics 2008;28(4):985–1003.
30. Pedrosa I, Chou MT, Ngo L, et al. MR classification of renal masses with pathologic correlation. Eur Radiol 2008;18(2):365–75.
31. Ruppert-Kohlmayr AJ, Uggowitzer M, Meissnitzer T, et al. Differentiation of renal clear cell carcinoma and renal papillary carcinoma using quantitative CT enhancement parameters. AJR Am J Roentgenol 2004;183(5):1387–91.
32. Pickhardt PJ, Siegel CL, McLarney JK. Collecting duct carcinoma of the kidney: are imaging findings suggestive of the diagnosis? AJR Am J Roentgenol 2001;176(3):627–33.
33. Graser A, Johnson TR, Hecht EM, et al. Dual-energy CT in patients suspected of having renal masses: can virtual nonenhanced images replace true nonenhanced images? Radiology 2009;252(2):433–40.
34. Graser A, Becker CR, Staehler M, et al. Single-phase dual-energy CT allows for characterization of renal masses as benign or malignant. Invest Radiol 2010;45(7):399–405.
35. Chandarana H, Megibow AJ, Cohen BA, et al. Iodine quantification with dual-energy CT: phantom study and preliminary experience with renal masses. AJR Am J Roentgenol 2011;196(6):W693–700.
36. Kaza RK, Caoili EM, Cohan RH, et al. Distinguishing enhancing from nonenhancing renal lesions with fast kilovoltage-switching dual-energy CT. AJR Am J Roentgenol 2011;197(6):1375–81.
37. Johnson TR. Dual-energy CT: general principles. AJR Am J Roentgenol 2012;199(Suppl 5):S3–8.
38. Hricak H, Brenner DJ, Adelstein SJ, et al. Managing radiation use in medical imaging: a multifaceted challenge. Radiology 2011;258(3):889–905.
39. Coakley FV, Gould R, Yeh BM, et al. CT radiation dose: what can you do right now in your practice? AJR Am J Roentgenol 2011;196(3):619–25.
40. McCollough CH, Bruesewitz MR, Kofler JM Jr. CT dose reduction and dose management tools: overview of available options. Radiographics 2006;26(2):503–12.
41. Yu L, Li H, Fletcher JG, et al. Automatic selection of tube potential for radiation dose reduction in CT: a general strategy. Med Phys 2010;37(1):234–43.
42. Singh S, Kalra MK, Hsieh J, et al. Abdominal CT: comparison of adaptive statistical iterative and filtered back projection reconstruction techniques. Radiology 2010;257(2):373–83.

43. American College of Radiology CT Accreditation Requirements. 2013. Available at: http://www.acr.org/Quality-Safety/Accreditation/CT. Accessed July 30, 2014.
44. Koh DM, Padhani AR. Diffusion-weighted MRI: a new functional clinical technique for tumour imaging. Br J Radiol 2006;79(944):633–5.
45. Chandarana H, Kang SK, Wong S, et al. Diffusion-weighted intravoxel incoherent motion imaging of renal tumors with histopathologic correlation. Invest Radiol 2012;47(12):688–96.
46. Gilet AG, Kang SK, Kim D, et al. Advanced renal mass imaging: diffusion and perfusion MRI. Curr Urol Rep 2012;13(1):93–8.
47. Bonekamp S, Corona-Villalobos CP, Kamel IR. Oncologic applications of diffusion-weighted MRI in the body. J Magn Reson Imaging 2012;35(2):257–79.
48. Cova M, Squillaci E, Stacul F, et al. Diffusion-weighted MRI in the evaluation of renal lesions: preliminary results. Br J Radiol 2004;77(922):851–7.
49. Squillaci E, Manenti G, Di Stefano F, et al. Diffusion-weighted MR imaging in the evaluation of renal tumours. J Exp Clin Cancer Res 2004;23(1):39–45.
50. Zhang J, Tehrani YM, Wang L, et al. Renal masses: characterization with diffusion-weighted MR imaging–a preliminary experience [Erratum appears in Radiology 2010;255(3):1011]. Radiology 2008;247(2):458–64.
51. Taouli B, Thakur RK, Mannelli L, et al. Renal lesions: characterization with diffusion-weighted imaging versus contrast-enhanced MR imaging. Radiology 2009;251(2):398–407.
52. Sandrasegaran K, Sundaram CP, Ramaswamy R, et al. Usefulness of diffusion-weighted imaging in the evaluation of renal masses. AJR Am J Roentgenol 2010;194(2):438–45.
53. Chandarana H, Taouli B. Diffusion and perfusion imaging of the liver. Eur J Radiol 2010;76(3):348–58.
54. Divgi CR, Pandit-Taskar N, Jungbluth AA, et al. Preoperative characterisation of clear-cell renal carcinoma using iodine-124-labelled antibody chimeric G250 (124I-cG250) and PET in patients with renal masses: a phase I trial. Lancet Oncol 2007;8(4):304–10.
55. Donat SM, Diaz M, Bishoff JT, et al. Follow-up for clinically localized renal neoplasms: AUA Guideline. J Urol 2013;190(2):407–16.
56. Skolarikos A, Alivizatos G, Laguna P, et al. A review on follow-up strategies for renal cell carcinoma after nephrectomy. Eur Urol 2007;51(6):1490–500 [discussion: 501].
57. Newmark JR, Newmark GM, Epstein JI, et al. Solitary late recurrence of renal cell carcinoma. Urology 1994;43(5):725–8.
58. Brufau BP, Cerqueda CS, Villalba LB, et al. Metastatic renal cell carcinoma: radiologic findings and assessment of response to targeted antiangiogenic therapy by using multidetector CT. Radiographics 2013;33:1691–716.
59. Larkin J, Gore M. Is advanced renal cell carcinoma becoming a chronic disease? Lancet 2010;376(9741):574–5.
60. Cuenod CA, Fournier L, Balvay D, et al. Tumor angiogenesis: pathophysiology and implications for contrast-enhanced MRI and CT assessment. Abdom Imaging 2006;31(2):188–93.
61. Choi H. Response evaluation of gastrointestinal stromal tumors. Oncologist 2008;13(Suppl 2):4–7.
62. Nathan PD, Vinayan A, Stott D, et al. CT response assessment combining reduction in both size and arterial phase density correlates with time to progression in metastatic renal cancer patients treated with targeted therapies. Cancer Biol Ther 2010;9(1):15–9.

63. Smith AD, Lieber ML, Shah SN. Assessing tumor response and detecting recurrence in metastatic renal cell carcinoma on targeted therapy: importance of size and attenuation on contrast-enhanced CT. AJR Am J Roentgenol 2010;194(1): 157–65.

64. Smith AD, Shah SN, Rini BI, et al. Morphology, attenuation, size, and structure (MASS) criteria: assessing response and predicting clinical outcome in metastatic renal cell carcinoma on antiangiogenic targeted therapy. AJR Am J Roentgenol 2010;194(6):1470–8.

65. Han KS, Jung DC, Choi HJ, et al. Pretreatment assessment of tumor enhancement on contrast-enhanced computed tomography as a potential predictor of treatment outcome in metastatic renal cell carcinoma patients receiving antiangiogenic therapy. Cancer 2010;116(10):2332–42.

66. Yabroff KR, Lamont EB, Mariotto A, et al. Cost of care for elderly cancer patients in the United States. J Natl Cancer Inst 2008;100(9):630–41.

67. Zeegers MP, Tan FE, Dorant E, et al. The impact of characteristics of cigarette smoking on urinary tract cancer risk: a meta-analysis of epidemiologic studies. Cancer 2000;89(3):630–9.

68. Kirkali Z, Chan T, Manoharan M, et al. Bladder cancer: epidemiology, staging and grading, and diagnosis. Urology 2005;66(6 Suppl 1):4–34.

69. Wong-You-Cheong JJ, Woodward PJ, Manning MA, et al. From the archives of the AFIP: neoplasms of the urinary bladder: radiologic-pathologic correlation. Radiographics 2006;26(2):553–80.

70. Carmack AJ, Soloway MS. The diagnosis and staging of bladder cancer: from RBCs to TURs. Urology 2006;67(3 Suppl 1):3–8 [discussion: 8–10].

71. ACR appropriateness criteria. 2013. Available at: http://www.acr.org/Quality-Safety/Appropriateness-Criteria. Accessed July 30, 2014.

72. Wollin T, Laroche B, Psooy K. Canadian guidelines for the management of asymptomatic microscopic hematuria in adults. Can Urol Assoc J 2009;3:77.

73. Jinzaki M, Tanimoto A, Shinmoto H, et al. Detection of bladder tumors with dynamic contrast-enhanced MDCT. AJR Am J Roentgenol 2007;188(4): 913–8.

74. Purysko AS, Leao Filho HM, Herts BR. Radiologic imaging of patients with bladder cancer. Semin Oncol 2012;39(5):543–58.

75. Verma S, Rajesh A, Prasad SR, et al. Urinary bladder cancer: role of MR imaging. Radiographics 2012;32(2):371–87.

76. Kim B, Semelka RC, Ascher SM, et al. Bladder tumor staging: comparison of contrast-enhanced CT, T1- and T2-weighted MR imaging, dynamic gadolinium-enhanced imaging, and late gadolinium-enhanced imaging. Radiology 1994; 193(1):239–45.

77. Kim JK, Park SY, Ahn HJ, et al. Bladder cancer: analysis of multi-detector row helical CT enhancement pattern and accuracy in tumor detection and perivesical staging. Radiology 2004;231(3):725–31.

78. Zhang J, Gerst S, Lefkowitz RA, et al. Imaging of bladder cancer. Radiol Clin North Am 2007;45(1):183–205.

79. Drieskens O, Oyen R, Van Poppel H, et al. FDG-PET for preoperative staging of bladder cancer. Eur J Nucl Med Mol Imaging 2005;32(12):1412–7.

80. Paik ML, Scolieri MJ, Brown SL, et al. Limitations of computerized tomography in staging invasive bladder cancer before radical cystectomy. J Urol 2000;163(6): 1693–6.

81. Tekes A, Kamel I, Imam K, et al. Dynamic MRI of bladder cancer: evaluation of staging accuracy. AJR Am J Roentgenol 2005;184(1):121–7.

82. Takeuchi M, Sasaki S, Ito M, et al. Urinary bladder cancer: diffusion-weighted MR imaging–accuracy for diagnosing T stage and estimating histologic grade. Radiology 2009;251(1):112–21.

83. Matsuki M, Inada Y, Tatsugami F, et al. Diffusion-weighted MR imaging for urinary bladder carcinoma: initial results. Eur Radiol 2007;17(1):201–4.

84. Watanabe H, Kanematsu M, Kondo H, et al. Preoperative T staging of urinary bladder cancer: does diffusion-weighted MRI have supplementary value? AJR Am J Roentgenol 2009;192(5):1361–6.

85. Bradford TJ, Montie JE, Hafez KS. The role of imaging in the surveillance of urologic malignancies. Urol Clin North Am 2006;33(3):377–96.

86. Vikram R, Sandler CM, Ng CS. Imaging and staging of transitional cell carcinoma: part 2, upper urinary tract. AJR Am J Roentgenol 2009;192(6):1488–93.

87. Cowan NC, Turney BW, Taylor NJ, et al. Multidetector computed tomography urography for diagnosing upper urinary tract urothelial tumour. BJU Int 2007;99(6): 1363–70.

88. Vrtiska TJ, Hartman RP, Kofler JM, et al. Spatial resolution and radiation dose of a 64-MDCT scanner compared with published CT urography protocols. AJR Am J Roentgenol 2009;192(4):941–8.

89. Silverman SG, Leyendecker JR, Amis ES Jr. What is the current role of CT urography and MR urography in the evaluation of the urinary tract? Radiology 2009; 250(2):309–23.

90. Jinzaki M, Matsumoto K, Kikuchi E, et al. Comparison of CT urography and excretory urography in the detection and localization of urothelial carcinoma of the upper urinary tract. AJR Am J Roentgenol 2011;196(5):1102–9.

91. Chlapoutakis K, Theocharopoulos N, Yarmenitis S, et al. Performance of computed tomographic urography in diagnosis of upper urinary tract urothelial carcinoma, in patients presenting with hematuria: systematic review and meta-analysis. Eur J Radiol 2010;73(2):334–8.

92. Dahlman P, Jangland L, Segelsjo M, et al. Optimization of computed tomography urography protocol, 1997 to 2008: effects on radiation dose. Acta Radiol 2009;50(4):446–54.

93. Chen GL, El-Gabry EA, Bagley DH. Surveillance of upper urinary tract transitional cell carcinoma: the role of ureteroscopy, retrograde pyelography, cytology and urinalysis. J Urol 2000;164(6):1901–4.

94. Browne RF, Meehan CP, Colville J, et al. Transitional cell carcinoma of the upper urinary tract: spectrum of imaging findings. Radiographics 2005;25(6):1609–27.

95. Takahashi N, Kawashima A, Glockner JF, et al. Small (<2-cm) upper-tract urothelial carcinoma: evaluation with gadolinium-enhanced three-dimensional spoiled gradient-recalled echo MR urography. Radiology 2008;247(2):451–7.

96. Lee KS, Zeikus E, DeWolf WC, et al. MR urography versus retrograde pyelography/ureteroscopy for the exclusion of upper urinary tract malignancy. Clin Radiol 2010;65(3):185–92.

97. Roupret M, Zigeuner R, Palou J, et al. European guidelines for the diagnosis and management of upper urinary tract urothelial cell carcinomas: 2011 update. Eur Urol 2011;59(4):584–94.

98. Yuh BI, Cohan RH. Different phases of renal enhancement: role in detecting and characterizing renal masses during helical CT. AJR American Journal of Roentgenology 1999;173(3):747–55.

99. Birnbaum BA, Jacobs JE, Langlotz CP, Ramchandani P. Assessment of a bolus-tracking technique in helical renal CT to optimize nephrographic phase imaging. Radiology 1999;211(1):87–94.

Radiology of Soft Tissue Tumors

Paul I. Mallinson, MBChB*, Hong Chou, MBBS, Bruce B. Forster, MD,
Peter L. Munk, MD

KEYWORDS

- Soft tissue tumor • Sarcoma • Radiology • Biopsy

KEY POINTS

- Magnetic resonance imaging is the mainstay of diagnostic imaging for soft tissue masses, but plain film, ultrasonography, and computed tomography have roles. Nuclear medicine contributes to staging and detection of recurrence.
- A subset of lesions has specific imaging features that enable a confident radiological diagnosis with appropriate clinical correlation.
- Many soft tissue masses have nonspecific appearances and should be considered for biopsy in a specialist center.
- When a biopsy is required for definitive diagnosis, careful multidisciplinary planning is essential to avoid contamination of unaffected tissue, leading to recurrence and unnecessary amputations.

INTRODUCTION
Background

The soft tissue mass is a common complaint that raises concern and anxiety for malignancy in patients and physicians alike. However, incidence of benign tumors is estimated at 3000 per million population and a benign cause is found in 95% of patients presenting to primary care with a soft tissue mass.[1,2] It is important to establish a good clinical history and perform careful examination before imaging, as such masses may have a nonpathological explanation or nonsoft tissue etiology. These include the following:

- Normal anatomy
  - Ribs
  - The sternoclavicular joint, particularly after age-related degenerative hypertrophy

The authors have nothing to disclose.
Radiology Department, Vancouver General Hospital, Jim Pattison Pavilion, 899 West 12th Avenue, Vancouver, British Columbia V5Z 1M9, Canada
* Corresponding author.
E-mail address: dr_pmallinson@hotmail.com

Surg Oncol Clin N Am 23 (2014) 911–936
http://dx.doi.org/10.1016/j.soc.2014.06.006
1055-3207/14/$ – see front matter © 2014 Elsevier Inc. All rights reserved.

surgonc.theclinics.com

- Subcutaneous fat irregularity in larger patients
- The subcutaneous fat pad overlying the cervicothoracic junction
- Masses arising from a bone or abdominal organ
  - Old fractures
  - Bone tumors
  - Hepato/splenomegaly, gallbladder masses, and hernias
- Imaginary masses
  - Overanxious patient
  - Obesity
  - Family history of cancer

Important factors to note in the history are summarized in **Table 1**. In addition to these, the patient's age and the location of the lesion can further reduce the differential diagnosis.[3] For example, many mesenchymal tumor types occur in adults, angiomas occur in all ages, and dermatofibrosarcoma protuberans (DFSP) and epithelioid sarcoma peak in the 20 to 40 age range. DFSP often involves the skin, malignant fibrous histiocytoma is often deep, liposarcomas are usually found in the extremities and retroperitoneum, and epithelioid sarcoma is most common in the fingers, hands, and forearms.

These features help the referring physician decide on the necessity for imaging and the best initial modality to request (eg, a radiograph for a suspected bony mass or an ultrasound for soft tissue). This information allows the radiologist to appropriately protocol the requested studies to expedite patient care; for example, changing a modality or arranging the most appropriate sequences and orthogonal planes on magnetic resonance imaging (MRI). Furthermore, the information provides valuable clues as to the likely pathology, to correlate with the imaging. This can be particularly useful when faced with nonspecific imaging appearances.

All physicians should be wary of a history of trauma; although this is a common cause for a mass, sometimes the event has drawn the patient's attention to the affected area for the first time and can result in a misleading diagnosis.

Sarcomas

A rare, but perhaps the most feared, cause of a soft tissue mass is the soft tissue sarcoma. They are tumors of mesenchymal origin that histologically resemble, but do not necessarily arise from, the tissue they are named for. More than 50 histologically distinct subtypes exist. The major categories are summarized in **Table 2**.

Table 1	
A list of useful features in the clinical history that may guide diagnosis	
History Says...	**Could Be**
Previous or known primary malignancy	Metastasis or recurrence Radiation-induced sarcomas
Previous trauma or on anticoagulation	Hematoma or myositis ossificans
Painful lesion	Inflammatory or neural origin
Rapid increase in size	May be malignant
Stable size over long period	Likely benign
Variation in size	Hemangioma or ganglia
Multiple lesions	Lipomatosis or neurofibromatosis Metastases

Table 2	
Nomenclature of the major categories of soft tissue sarcoma	
Tumor Resembles	**Tumor Name**
Fat	Liposarcoma
Skeletal muscle	Rhabdomyosarcoma
Peripheral nerves	(Malignant) peripheral nerve sheath tumor (M)PNST
Blood vessels	Angiosarcoma
Fibrous tissue	Fibrosarcoma
Bone	Osteosarcoma
Cartilage	Chondrosarcoma

Sarcomas account for fewer than 1% of solid adult tumors. They were estimated to have caused 3490 deaths in the United States in 2005, with an international incidence of 1.8 to 5.0 per 100,000 people per year.[4–6] The vast majority are soft tissue tumors, with just more than 10% occurring in bone.[7] Two-thirds of soft tissue sarcomas occur within the limbs.[8]

The risk factors are not well understood and are dependent on subtype. They are often sporadic but associated with familial cancer syndromes and previous radiation exposure.[1,9] Sarcomas have traditionally been associated with poor survival because of vague, nonspecific, early symptoms, leading to delayed presentation, delayed diagnosis, and metastases. They occur more frequently in adolescents and young adults than do other cancers, leading to substantial loss of years of life and morbidity from limb loss.

Role of the Radiologist

The radiologist has several roles in the diagnosis and management of soft tissue masses:

- Detection of the mass and confirmation of the existence of the mass.
- Characterizing the mass: size, location, related structures, and likely composition and giving a differential diagnosis.
- Staging, in the case of malignancy.
- Image-guided biopsy to establish/confirm the histologic diagnosis.
- Follow-up to assess treatment response, recurrence, and posttreatment complications.

In this article, we discuss appearances of the soft tissue mass, both benign and malignant, from the common lipoma through to rare malignancies; the strengths and limitations of the various imaging modalities; and the basic principles of guided biopsy and subsequent surgical management.

PREIMAGING PLANNING

Following the discovery and clinical evaluation of a suspected soft tissue mass, a variety of imaging modalities are available to the referring clinician. Each has its advantages and limitations. MRI is widely acknowledged to be the gold standard for soft tissue imaging, but plain films, ultrasound, computed tomography (CT), and nucleotide imaging can all serve a purpose.[10] The attributes of each modality are summarized in **Table 3**.

Although MRI is usually the most informative imaging modality, ultrasound may be preferable as an initial screening test that is well tolerated by patients, can confirm the

Table 3
Summary of imaging modalities for soft tissue mass assessment

Modality	Advantages	Disadvantages
Plain film	• Quick to perform. • Cheap. • Readily available. • Allows evaluation of calcification within lesions and bone involvement. • A useful adjunct to MRI.	• Very limited soft tissue information.
Ultrasound	• Cheap and readily available. • Useful for initial evaluation. • Allows differentiation of cystic vs solid and assessment of vascularity. • Useful in the presence of metal prostheses. Optimal modality for guided biopsy. • Well tolerated.	• Limited at depth/in obese patients. • Operator dependent and has to be focused on an area. • Questionable accuracy.[14]
MRI	• Exquisite soft tissue detail. • Wide field of view.	• More costly and less readily available than US and plain film. • Contraindications such as pacemaker. • Movement artifact
CT	• Excellent bone and calcium detail. • Characterize osteoid/calcific matrix and level of bone destruction. • Useful where MRI contraindicated to provide cross-sectional imaging. • Contrast improves soft tissue detail. • Wide field of view useful for extensive tumors.	• Ionizing radiation. • Soft tissue detail inferior to MRI and US.
PET	• Most sensitive for the detection of early metastases, especially when combined with CT. • Excellent for staging and useful in assessing recurrence after significant postoperative interval. • Uptake can indicate grade of lesion. • More sensitive than CT and MRI for recurrence.[85]	• Ionizing radiation. • Very limited soft tissue detail. Limited availability.
Angiography	Evaluation of tumor blood supply and embolization can aid surgery.	Very limited information in tumor characterization.

Abbreviations: CT, computed tomography; MRI, magnetic resonance imaging; PET, positron emission tomography; US, ultrasound.

presence and size of a lesion, give an indication of benign or malignant nature, and evaluate the need for further investigation.[10–12] It provides dynamic evaluation of hernia and is diagnostic for simple lipoma. Accurate definitive diagnosis of many lesions is not possible however.[13,14]

Radiographs are often unrewarding in the context of soft tissue mass, but give added information on calcium and are therefore a useful adjunct to an MRI.[15] Disrupted tissue planes, lucent fatty lesions, and evidence of erosions suggesting the possibility of tophi also may be seen.

CT provides excellent calcium detail and is very useful where osteoid/chondroid matrix and/or bone involvement is suspected.[16] Positron emission tomography (PET) CT is reserved for staging malignancy and detecting recurrence. Angiography may provide useful images for preoperative planning and embolization of tumors before resection or for palliative pain management.[17]

DIAGNOSTIC IMAGING TECHNIQUE

A few simple principles will optimize image quality for soft tissue imaging.

- Plain films: Always obtain at least 2 orthogonal plains. They are recommended as a routine adjunct to MRI when evaluating limbs and pelvic or shoulder girdle lesions.
- Ultrasound: In general, start with the highest-frequency probe available and then reduce as required. Linear probes of approximately 17 MHz are ideal for superficial lesions, but curvilinear probes in the 5-MHz range may be necessary for deeper lesions and larger patients. Evaluate any internal vascular flow with color Doppler. Acoustic shadowing may represent calcification, whereas posterior acoustic enhancement suggests a cystic lesion. Check for peristalsis in suspected bowel herniae.
- MRI
  ○ Skin markers are strongly advised for subtle, doubtful, or diffuse lesions. These should be placed over small lesions, or at the outer limits of ill-defined ones.
  ○ At least 2 orthogonal planes should be used, with the choice tailored to the location and orientation of the lesion.
  ○ Field of view should be kept focused of the lesion. A wider field of view may be used for initial detection and where multiple lesions are suspected, but avoid trying to characterize 2 or more widely spaced lesions in a single broad field, or imaging both limbs together.[18] A full-length view of the bone on one sequence is advised to identify any skip lesions.
  ○ Sequences: We recommend our tumor protocol consisting of axial T1, axial T2, axial T2 Fat Saturated (FS), sagittal gradient echo (GRE), and a coronal short-tau inversion recovery (STIR) sequence.
    ■ T1 and T2 Turbo spin echo (SE) are performed to ascertain basic signal characteristics, define the location, and begin substance characterization.
    ■ T2 FS confirms the presence of fat and increases conspicuity of nonfat and fluid, such as edema.
    ■ STIR is similar to T2 FS in revealing lesions with a high water content and edema and confirming fat content.
    ■ T2* GRE sequence is useful for identification of hemosiderin as low signal with blooming artifact, therefore useful in diagnosing hemangiomas, pigmented villonodular synovitis (PVNS), and mature hematomas.

Routine use of Gadolinium is controversial. It is advocated in some centers, but in others it is reserved purely for follow-up and problem solving, for example identifying areas of recurrence postoperatively or targeting of solid components during biopsy.[10]

Pearls and Pitfalls

- When contrast is selected, it is vital to have a similar fat-saturated sequence, preferably T1 FS, for comparison.
- The previous protocol should be modified to take into account the orientation of the lesion. Review of the localizer images before formal sequence acquisition is

useful where the lesion topography is uncertain, before acquiring the formal sequences.

INTERPRETATION/ASSESSMENT OF CLINICAL IMAGES

Interpretation begins with a description of the lesion, which should attempt to answer the following questions:

- *What is it the composition?* Including fat, calcification, hemosiderin, and fluid.
- *What is the shape and structure?* Presence of lobulation, septation, cystic/solid, fluid levels, and lesion dimensions.
- *Where is it?* The report should include the location, adjacent structures, and any invasion. The relationship to neurovascular bundles, muscle compartments, bones, and joints must be included.
- *Where is the nodal/metastatic disease?*

The radiologist must then try to determine *what is it?* Some lesions have specific appearances. Recognition of these can spare the patient unnecessary biopsy, anxiety, and, in the worse cases, surgery due to misdiagnosis. **Box 1** lists the lesions that may be recognized by their imaging features alone.

In the event of nonspecific appearances, commentary should be made on the likelihood of *benign versus malignant nature.* There are many imaging features that are suggestive of malignancy; these are summarized in **Box 2**. However, there are no absolute rules or formulas and biopsy and/or follow-up imaging is required when there is doubt. The following example cases demonstrate how imaging appearances can be deceptive.

Synovial Sarcoma

These can be small, well-defined, slow-growing lesions with calcifications (**Fig. 1**). No pathognomonic features on MRI.

Fibromatosis

A benign lesion with locally aggressive features. The example in **Fig. 2** shows displacement of the adjacent muscles and surrounding edema. Low signal intensity fibrous bands, sometimes seen within, are characteristic.

Box 1
Lesions that may be recognized by their imaging features alone

Lipoma and lipomatous lesions

Hemangiomas

Ganglia

Peripheral nerve sheath tumors

Giant cell tumors of the tendon sheath

Pigmented villonodular synovitis

Myositis ossificans

Hematomas

Morton neuroma

Morel Lavallée lesion

| **Box 2** |
| **Imaging features that are suggestive of malignancy** |
| Large size |
| Deep lesions |
| Heterogeneous signal |
| Increased rate and amount of contrast enhancement |
| Presence of central necrosis |
| Irregular margins |
| Signal change in surrounding tissues |
| Invasion of adjacent structures |

Myxoma

A solid lesion with a cystic appearance. The example in **Fig. 3** shows a well-circumscribed, homogeneously T2 hyperintense mass, with mild perilesional edema. However, the heterogeneous enhancement indicates a solid lesion.

Nodular Fasciitis

A tumorlike inflammatory lesion, which is commonly a lobulated, T1 hypointense and T2 hyperintense, enhancing mass, closely associated with the fascia, which has nonspecific features and can mimic a sarcoma by its rapid growth.

Interpreting Soft Tissue Masses on Radiographs

Important radiographic features are summarized in **Table 4**. Radiographs may allow spot diagnoses of hemangiomas, synovial chondromatosis, and myositis ossificans and identify chronic bone remodeling versus more aggressive destruction patterns. They are a valuable adjunct to MRI.[18]

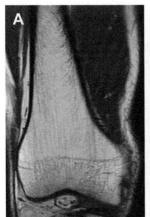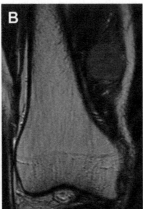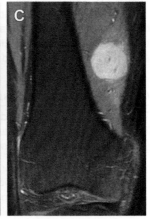

Fig. 1. Coronal T1 (*A*), T2 (*B*), and PD FS (*C*) MRI images showing a small well-defined lesion with little surrounding edema, later proven to be a synovia sarcoma.

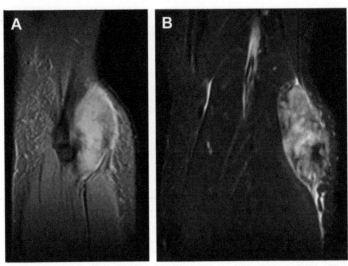

Fig. 2. Sagittal GRE (*A*) and coronal STIR (*B*) show a heterogeneous lesion with muscular displacement and surrounding edema. Appearances are aggressive but proved to be benign fibromatosis.

Interpreting Soft Tissue Masses on CT

CT has an increased sensitivity for subtle calcifications or mineralization compared with radiographs, which is useful to characterize chondroid versus osteoid matrix. Their density may further characterize the soft tissues, for example:

- Hypodense tissue like fat or fluid (approximately −100 and 0 HU, respectively)
- Hyperdense tissue can indicate acute blood (60–70 HU)
- Calcium, typically greater than 100 HU

Bony changes adjacent to lesions, such as lysis of bone and periosteal reaction, are best demonstrated on CT. CT also offers the potential for guided biopsy and may be advantageous over ultrasound for deep-seated lesions. The recent advent of dual-energy CT (DECT) allows detection of urate deposits in cases of suspected gout. This new technology exploits the photoelectric effect when scanning patients at 2 different energy levels, to gain additional tissue data. A decomposition algorithm is then used to separate calcium from urate, which can be color coded (eg, green) and fused onto the standard gray-scale CT images (**Fig. 4**).[19,20]

Interpreting Soft Tissue Masses on MRI

Tissues can be characterized by their signal intensities. The 2 more distinct characteristics are T1 hyperintensity and T2 hyperintensity.

A T1 *hyperintense* tissue/substance may represent fat:

- Correlate with fat-suppression sequences and the T2 sequence. Presence most commonly indicates lipomatous lesions. Consider mature myositis ossificans or hemangiomas if calcium is present.
- If not fat, consider melanin (melanoma), proteinaceous fluid in a cystic lesion such as ganglion or abscess, or methemoglobin relating to a hematoma or hemorrhagic tumor.

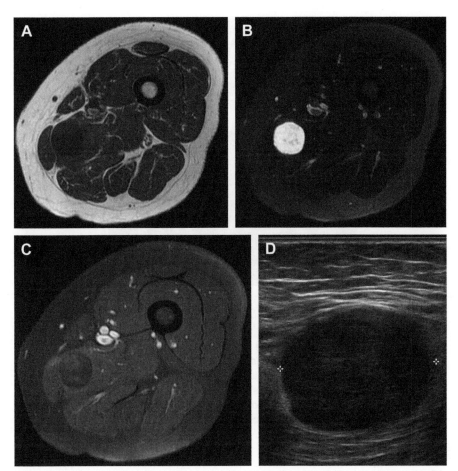

Fig. 3. Axial T1 (*A*), T2 FS (*B*), and T1 FS post gadolinium (*C*) MRI images show a well-circumscribed mass, homogeneously T2 hyperintense and T1 hypointense. However, the heterogeneous enhancement and ultrasound (*D*) indicate a solid lesion.

Table 4
Summary of important radiographic features

Radiographic Finding	Possible Diagnosis
Phleboliths	Hemangioma
Juxta-articular osteo-cartilaginous masses	Synovial chondromatosis
Mature ossification (history of trauma)	Myositis ossificans
Dystrophic calcification (associated with slowly growing lower extremity soft tissue mass)	Synovial sarcoma
Destructive bone lesion	Underlying primary osseous malignancy
Peripheral calcification	Chronic unresolved hematoma
Hazy calcification (with para-articular erosions)	Gouty tophus

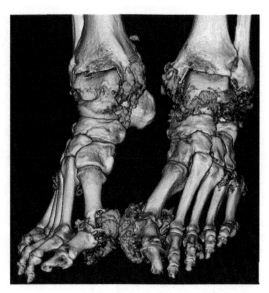

Fig. 4. DECT gout.

A T2 *hypointense* tissue/substance may represent:

- Mineralization: correlate with the radiographs; dystrophic calcification, phlebo-liths, and uric acid deposits (consider DECT to confirm).
- Fibrous lesions: correlate with history, morphology, and location. Can indicate scar, fibromas and fibrosarcomas, elastofibromas, leiomyoma, desmoid tumors.
- Hemosiderin: consider PVNS and its tendon sheath equivalent, giant cell tumor of the tendon sheath (GCT-TS), chronic hematoma, and hemorrhagic mass.

EXAMPLES OF SPECIFIC LESIONS
Lipomas and Lipomatous Lesions

A typical lipoma

- Is encapsulated, contains only fat, no nodularity or thick septations, is isointense to fat on all sequences, with complete fat saturation.[21,22]
- However, they may contain fat necrosis and associated calcifications, myxoid change, inflammation, fibrosis, and hemorrhage.[23,24]
- Lipomas and well-differentiated liposarcomas can have similar imaging appearances (**Fig. 5**).

Features suspicious of liposarcoma include[21–23,25]:

- Size greater than 5 cm
- Lesion composition of less than 75% fat
- Thick septations (>2 mm)
- Nonfat nodules
- Deep intramuscular location (**Fig. 6**)

Hemangiomas and Vascular Malformations

These terms cover a wide range of lesions that can be broadly classified into true neoplastic lesions with proliferation of the vascular endothelium (hemangiomas) and malformed vessels (vascular malformations).[26–31] Another important distinction is

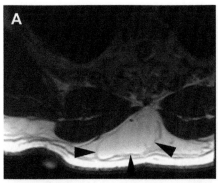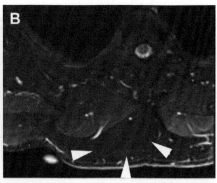

Fig. 5. Axial T1 (*A*) and T2 FS (*B*) images demonstrate a simple encapsulated lesion (*arrowheads*) with no internal nodules or thick septations that follow fat on all sequences. Appearances are typical of a lipoma.

high flow (commonly treated by embolization) versus low flow (commonly treated by sclerotherapy).[32–35] Low-flow lesions account for 90% of those outside the central nervous system.[36] Clinical characteristics, such as presence at birth, growth patterns, involution, and appearance, further aid diagnosis.

Ultrasound is often first used, but MRI is now considered superior (**Fig. 7**).[37] Typical imaging appearances include serpentine vessels, fat (in hemangiomas), calcification (phleboliths), and hemosiderin.[23] On MRI, typical appearances are of lobulated septated masses with intermediate to low T1 and increased T2 or STIR signal corresponding to stagnant blood in venous lakes.[34,38,39] Hemangiomas may show T1 hyperintensity in area of fat and hemorrhage and GRE blooming in areas of hemosiderin (**Fig. 8**). Vascular malformations are often infiltrating, non-masslike, nondisplacing, and do not respect tissue planes (**Fig. 9**).[32] They should not demonstrate a soft tissue component. Flow voids are indicative of high-flow lesions. Additional CT or radiograph is useful to identify any phleboliths present (see **Fig. 9**C).

Ganglion

The term is a misnomer; these lesions are not related to nerves. They may represent synovial herniation, or be the consequence of cystic degenerative change in the tendon sheath or joint capsule.[40] Typical imaging characteristics are the following[11,24,25]:

- MRI: T1 hypointense, T2 hyperintense, cystic lesions with thin septations and faint rim enhancement post-gadolinium (**Fig. 10**).
- Ultrasound: Anechoic lesion with posterior acoustic enhancement, unilocular or multilocular, which can be septated and noncompressible.
- Typically near a joint or tendon sheath.
- They can also
  - Show pericystic edema.
  - Be T1 hyperintense, if the fluid within is highly proteinaceous.
  - Occur away from joints.

Peripheral Nerve Sheath Tumors

Peripheral nerve sheath tumors (PNSTs) include neurofibromas, schwannoma and their malignant equivalents, neurofibrosarcoma and malignant schwannoma (MPNSTs). Appearances can often be nonspecific; however, typically they show the following:

- T1 isointense and T2 hyperintense characteristics on MRI.[25]
- Fusiform morphology with a dural tail, but a schwannoma may be eccentric.[25,41]

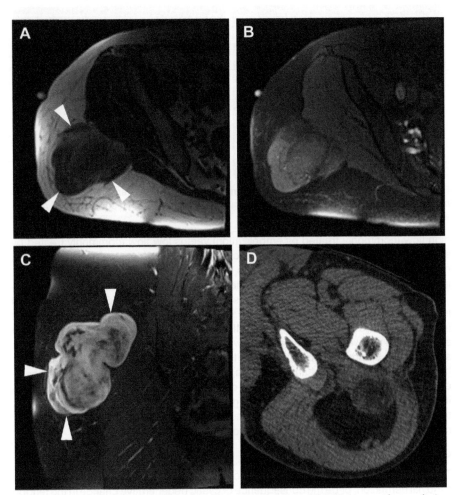

Fig. 6. Axial T1 (*A*), T2 FS (*B*), and cor T1 FS post gadolinium (*C*) MRI images show a lesion (*arrowheads*) that is only partially fat with a soft tissue component and avid gadolinium enhancement. There is extension into the gluteal muscle. Another lesion shows fat and smoky soft tissue density of CT (*D*). Appearances are those of a liposarcoma.

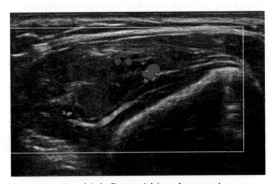

Fig. 7. Ultrasound demonstrating high flow within a hemangioma.

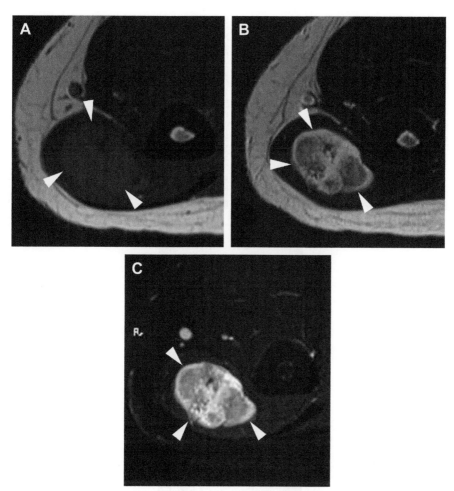

Fig. 8. Axial T1 (*A*), T2 (*B*), and T2 FS (*C*) demonstrating a hemangioma (*arrows*) with lower T1 signal than muscle due to fat content, with internal vessels and low signal calcification.

- Sometimes the near pathognomonic "Target" sign on transverse T2 images, with a low-density center composed of fibrocollagenous tissue and a bright outer rim of myxomatous tissue.[42,43] The entering and exiting nerve may also be seen.
- Sometimes the "split fat sign"; displaced fat from the neurovascular bundle seen surrounding the tumor in a thin rind.
- Enhancing solid and cystic components.

Malignant forms: may have ill-defined margins, central necrosis, and exhibit rapid growth (**Fig. 11**).

GCT-TS

A GCT-TS is part of the spectrum of benign proliferative synovial disease, which includes PVNS. When disease is focal and extra-articular, it is described as GCT-TS. Clinically, it may present with triggering of the fingers. MRI appearances are of a generally T1 and T2 intermediate/hypointense nodular/tubular lesion surrounding or adjacent to the tendon (**Fig. 12**). Blooming may be seen on GRE sequence due to

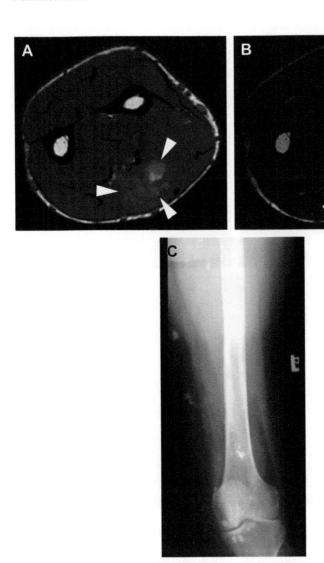

Fig. 9. Axial T1 (*A*) and T2 FS (*B*) images demonstrate a serpentine lesion (*arrowheads*) with venous lakes, no soft tissue component, and no flow voids. Appearances are typical of a venous malformation. A plain film (*C*) demonstrates multiple phleboliths in a venous malformation.

hemosiderin deposition, which may also cause high signal areas on T2. Gadolinium enhancement is homogeneous.[25,44,45]

Myositis Ossificans

Myositis ossificans is a benign, ossifying, self-limiting soft tissue mass, typically arising in the skeletal muscle of young adults. Although it may be associated with trauma, this history is often absent. There is an association with burns, paraplegia, and neuromuscular disorders.[46] No primary inflammation of muscle is found and there is no evidence that this lesion is premalignant.[47] Appearances include the following:

- A usually well-circumscribed mass with a compressed fibrous connective tissue rim.

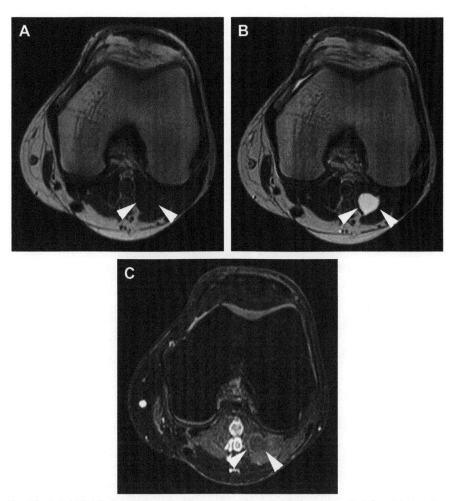

Fig. 10. Axial T1 (*A*), T2 (*B*), and T1 FS post gadolinium (*C*) show a well-defined lesion (*arrowheads*) with fluid characteristics and a mildly enhancing periphery. These are typical appearances of a ganglion cyst.

- Faint calcifications on radiograph at 2 to 6 weeks, progressing to a bony mass at 6 to 8 weeks.[48–50] CT usually shows a peripheral calcified rim at 4 to 6 weeks, sometimes with decreased attenuation in the center (**Fig. 13**).[51–53]
- Peripheral calcification pattern, which matures and fills centripetally. An important distinction from osteosarcomas, which progress in a centrifugal pattern.
- T1 hypointense/isointense to skeletal muscle and T2 hyperintensity, with mild adjacent edema.[47] Calcifications appear as hypointensities on T2* GRE (**Fig. 14**).
- Chronic lesions mature to dense bone.
- Intense uptake on bone scan, including blood flow and blood pool images.

Hematoma

A history of trauma or anticoagulation is supportive of the diagnosis, but hematoma can be a difficult diagnosis to make with confidence. The physician should be wary

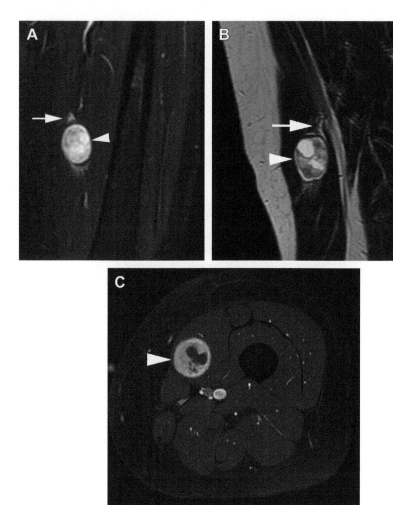

Fig. 11. Coronal T2 FS (*A*), sagittal T2 (*B*), and axial T1 FS post gadolinium (*C*) show a mixed cystic and solid lesion (*arrowhead*) with dural tail (*arrow*) and avid enhancement in keeping with a peripheral nerve tumor.

of the underlying tumor that has spontaneously hemorrhaged. Lack of, or minimal, surrounding edema, nodularity of the lesion wall, and lack of, or limited, hemosiderin in chronic cases, are all concerning for underlying tumor.[18] A density of 60 to 70 HU on CT is compatible with acute blood.

MRI appearances have a typically evolving pattern.[54] Acute hematomas from 0 to 2 days show T1 isointensity and T2 hypointensity due to intracellular deoxyhemoglobin. At 2 to 7 days this becomes intracellular methemoglobin at the periphery with a rim of high T1 and low T2 signal. At 1 to 4 weeks, the methemoglobin leaves the cells and becomes high signal on both T1 and T2. Finally, chronic hematomas demonstrate an even rim of low signal on all sequences and blooming on GRE, due to hemosiderin (**Fig. 15**). Chronic hematomas may organize to produce septations and fluid levels.[46] Peripheral calcification suggests early myositis ossificans. Where doubt exists, the lesion can be biopsied, or followed to resolution.[23]

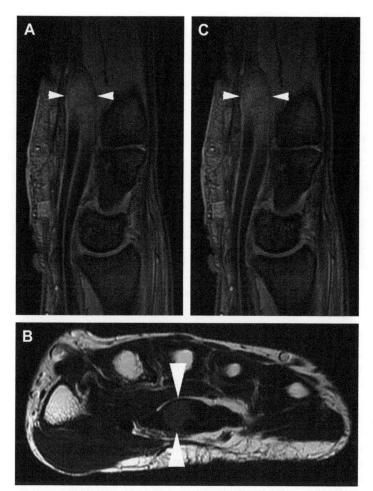

Fig. 12. Axial T1 (*A*) and T2 (*B*) and sagittal GRE (*C*) MRI images demonstrate a GCT-TS (*arrowheads*) as an intermediate signal lesion wrapping around the tendons of the flexor compartment of the wrist.

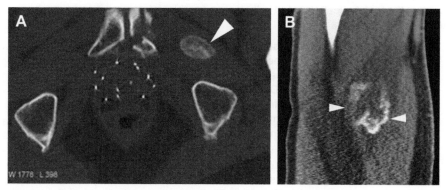

Fig. 13. CT shows 2 examples (*A, B*) of well-defined calcified lesions (*arrowheads*) with lower density centers typical of myositis ossificans.

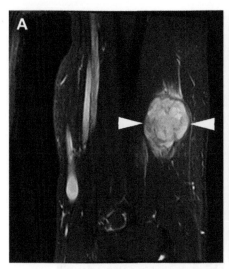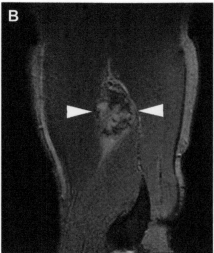

Fig. 14. Coronal STIR (*A*) and sagittal T2*GRE (*B*) MRI images demonstrate a lesion (*arrowheads*) with mild peripheral edema and low peripheral signal on GRE, corresponding to calcium in myositis ossificans.

Morel Lavallée Lesion

These lesions are effusions resulting from a de-gloving injury in which the skin and subcutaneous fat separate from the underlying fascia (**Fig. 16**). Damaged capillaries drain into the cavity, filling it with blood and debris.[55]

- May be present for years and grow slowly.
- Typically has oval/fusiform morphology.
- Can become peripherally encapsulated with hemosiderin/fibrous tissue, which is of low signal intensity and enhances with gadolinium.
- Can contain debris, blood, lobules of fat/fat signal, separated by fluid.
- Heterogeneous or homogeneous appearance
- Typical location in the trochanteric region and proximal thigh adjacent to fascia.

Morton Neuroma

Another misnomer, Morton neuroma is actually perineural fibrosis around a digital nerve in the foot, typically located in the second or third interspace.[56] Imaging characteristics are as follows (**Fig. 17**):

- Well-demarcated typical teardrop/spindle-shaped mass.
- Located in the vicinity of the neurovascular bundle, on the plantar side of the transverse metatarsal ligament.
- Hypoechoic on ultrasound. Dynamic imaging while squeezing the forefoot allows the motion of the neuroma from between the metatarsal heads to be tracked.
- MRI signal is isointense to muscle on T1 and hypointense to fat on T2.
- May or may not show enhancement with gadolinium.

Elastofibroma

Elastofibroma is a benign fibroelastic pseudotumor that is most easily recognizable by its typical subscapular location (**Fig. 18**).[46] Etiology is unclear, but may relate to repetitive trauma between scapula and chest wall. Intermediate signal on T1 and T2 fibrous

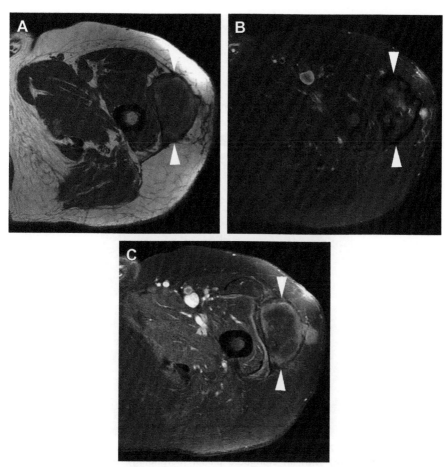

Fig. 15. Axial T1 (*A*), T2 FS (*B*), and T1 FS post gadolinium (*C*) show a well-defined lesion (*arrowheads*) with a low signal hemosiderin rim and mild peripheral enhancement typical of a hematoma.

components mixed with high-signal T1 fat components. They can be mildly enhancing and are often bilateral. Biopsy is to be avoided because of the extremely tough nature of the lesion, which is resistant to sample collection.

BIOPSY

Although some lesions have image-specific appearances, many lesions do not, and biopsy is required either to confirm diagnosis, or separate the benign from the malignant variants. However, biopsy is the most frequently mismanaged aspect of the soft tissue mass workup. Biopsy technique can dramatically alter both patient management and outcome and is therefore best carried out in specialist centers.

The key issue is the potential for seeding sarcoma cells into the tissues along the track of the biopsy. Sarcoma surgeons often choose to resect the biopsy track to reduce the risk of local recurrence. If performed incorrectly, unaffected compartments can be contaminated, resulting in unnecessary amputations or more extensive debilitating resections.[57,58] In addition, unidentifiable tracks may be incompletely resected,

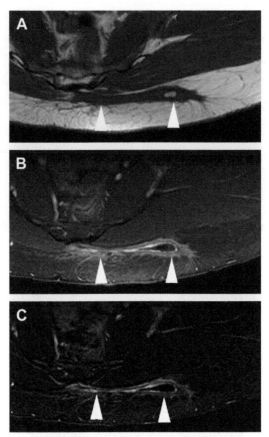

Fig. 16. Axial T1 (*A*), T2 FS (*B*), and T1 FS post gadolinium (*C*) show an encapsulated fluid collection (*arrowheads*) with an elongated planar morphology, subcutaneous location, and peripheral enhancement typical of a shearing injury and Morel Lavallée lesion.

resulting in local recurrence with the associated morbidity and mortality. Good communication with the surgeons and pathologists is essential. Many surgeons will specify the path to take, sometimes marking the site personally. A study of 25 surgeons, 21 institutions, and 597 patients demonstrated the capacity for harm from mismanaged biopsy of primary musculoskeletal tumors.[59]

A different or more complex procedure was performed after poorly planned biopsy in 19.3% and an unnecessary amputation had to be performed in almost 5%. Errors, complications, and changes in course and outcome were 2 to 12 times greater (*P*<.001) when biopsy was done in a referring institution instead of treatment center.

Preplanning of the soft tissue biopsy should include review of the relevant cross-sectional imaging, preferably an MRI.[60] Prior cross-sectional imaging is vital, not just for planning, but also because the post biopsy imaging appearance will often have been dramatically altered by the procedure. The biopsy route must be planned with the surgeon so that the track can be excised. Neurovascular bundles, unaffected compartments, and any infected sites must be avoided. Necrotic/cystic lesions are prone to nondiagnostic biopsies. Contrast-enhanced imaging may assist planning in these cases, by revealing the solid/enhancing components, which have a better diagnostic yield.

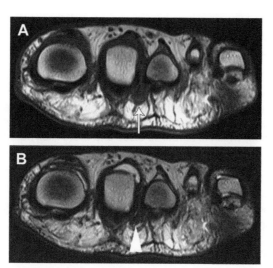

Fig. 17. Axial T1 (*A*) and T2 (*B*) MRI images show the typical low to intermediate signal "tear-drop"–shaped morphology and intermetatarsal location of a Morton neuroma (*arrowheads*).

Technique

The usual modality of choice is ultrasound, which offers real-time imaging in any chosen plane and superior soft tissue detail to CT, particularly in the absence of contrast. Doppler facilitates the avoidance of vascular bundles. CT may be necessary for deeper lesions, or those that are not seen on ultrasound, in which case they may be revealed by a contrast CT performed before needle placement.

- Aseptic technique: gloves, drapes, skin preparation, and probe cover.
- Local anesthetic (Lidocaine 1%).
- Fine-needle aspiration is generally inadequate for sarcomas and lymphomas. An 18-G core biopsy needle with 1 cm throw is our standard choice.
- A minimum of 3 biopsy cores is recommended to avoid insufficient sampling.
- The skin incision should be 5 to 10 mm and leave a suitable identifiable scar for the surgeon at time of resection.
- Always biopsy longitudinal to limb (this facilitates a desirable longitudinal surgical incision).

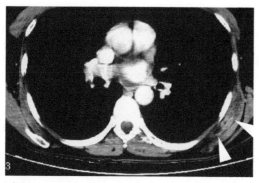

Fig. 18. Contrast axial CT images through the thorax show the typical location and striated appearance of the elastofibroma (*arrowheads*).

- Within the surgeon's specified marked area if present.
- Biopsy in-line with/over the lesion.
- Apply a dressing for 48 hours.

Pitfalls

- The biopsy result is not always definitive and a repeat sample may be necessary.
- Review of imaging with the pathologist can help where uncertainty exists.
- Do not biopsy transversely across a limb, as this necessitates a transverse surgical incision, which is harder to close and more likely to dehisce.

Tips

- If the needle tip cannot be identified, an ultrasound, then a gentle bouncing motion may reveal the location.
- PNSTs can be excruciating when biopsied, regardless of local anesthetic. Warn the patient preprocedure and only take one core if painful.

OPTIONS/PATHWAYS FOR SURGICAL INTERVENTION

Surgery is the cornerstone of sarcoma management, and typically the sole treatment modality in small lesions.[61–64] In some limb-salvage cases, radiotherapy is used preoperatively or postoperatively to reduce local recurrence rates, but does not appear to improve long-term survival rates in large high-grade tumors.[65–67] The decision to use preoperative or postoperative radiation balances the advantages of smaller treatment areas and radiation doses against increased rates of postoperative wound complications.[66,68–70] The role of chemotherapy for soft tissue sarcomas is limited by their relative chemo-resistance and modest survival benefits.[61] Studies have yielded mixed results, causing controversy; however, consideration should be given for chemotherapy for all patients with or at high risk of metastases or local recurrence.[71–77] A better understanding of biology, better preoperative imaging, and improved surgical techniques from orthopedics and plastics have widened the possibilities for limb salvage. Amputation rates have fallen significantly over the past few decades from reports of 38% to 47% in the 1970s[8,78–81] to 6% to 21% in the 1990s and have continued to decrease since 2001.[82] Limb salvage and reconstruction are now the mainstay of treatment, but should be considered only if

- The cure rate is at least the same as an equivalent amputation.
- The function is at least the same as an equivalent amputation.
- The long-term results are satisfactory.
- It is acceptable to the patient.

Although several studies have demonstrated no difference in long-term survival for amputation versus limb salvage, it should be remembered that, even in modern practice, amputation can still be the best treatment available.[74,83,84] With modern prosthetics, surprisingly good function can be attained.

SUMMARY

- Background clinical information is important but should be interpreted with caution.
- MRI is the mainstay of imaging, but plain film, ultrasound, and CT have roles.
- A subset of lesions have specific imaging features that enable a confident diagnosis with appropriate clinical correlation.
- A large proportion of soft tissue masses have nonspecific appearances.

- Where biopsy is required for definitive diagnosis, careful multidisciplinary planning is essential.

REFERENCES

1. Williams KJ, Hayes AJ. A guide to oncological management of soft tissue tumours of the abdominal wall. Hernia 2014;18:91–7.
2. Rydholm A. Management of patients with soft-tissue tumors. Strategy developed at a regional oncology center. Acta Orthop Scand Suppl 1983;203:13–77.
3. Beaman FD, Kransdorf MJ, Andrews TR, et al. Superficial soft-tissue masses: analysis, diagnosis, and differential considerations. Radiographics 2007;27(2): 509–23.
4. Nystrom LM, Reimer NB, Reith JD, et al. Multidisciplinary management of soft tissue sarcoma. ScientificWorldJournal 2013;2013:852462.
5. Jemal A, Murray T, Ward E, et al. Cancer statistics. CA Cancer J Clin 2005;55(1): 10–30.
6. Wibmer C, Leithner A, Zielonke N, et al. Increasing incidence rates of soft tissue sarcomas? A population-based epidemiologic study and literature review. Ann Oncol 2010;21(5):1106–11.
7. Burningham Z, Hashibe M, Spector L. The epidemiology of sarcoma. Clin Sarcoma Res 2012;2(1):14.
8. Popov P. Soft tissue sarcomas of the lower extremity: surgical treatment and outcome. Eur J Surg Oncol 2000;26(7):679–85.
9. Karlsson P, Holmberg E, Samuelsson A. Soft tissue sarcoma after treatment for breast cancer—a Swedish population-based study. Eur J Cancer 1998;34(13): 2068–75.
10. James SLJ, Davies AM. Post-operative imaging of soft tissue sarcomas. Cancer Imaging 2008;8:8–18.
11. Smith S, Salanitri J, Lisle D. Ultrasound evaluation of soft tissue masses and fluid collections. Semin Musculoskelet Radiol 2007;11(2):174–91.
12. Lakkaraju A, Sinha R, Garikipati R, et al. Ultrasound for initial evaluation and triage of clinically suspicious soft-tissue masses. Clin Radiol 2009;64(6):615–21.
13. Wu S, Tu R, Liu G, et al. Role of ultrasound in the diagnosis of common soft tissue lesions of the limbs. Ultrasound Q 2013;29(1):67–71.
14. Kwok HC, Pinto CH, Doyle AJ. The pitfalls of ultrasonography in the evaluation of soft tissue masses. J Med Imaging Radiat Oncol 2012;56(5):519–24.
15. Gartner L, Pearce CJ, Saifuddin A. The role of the plain radiograph in the characterisation of soft tissue tumours. Skeletal Radiol 2008;38(6):549–58.
16. Subhawong TK, Fishman EK, Swart JE, et al. Soft-tissue masses and masslike conditions: what does CT add to diagnosis and management? Am J Roentgenol 2010;194(6):1559–67.
17. Mavrogenis AF, Rossi G, Altimari G, et al. Palliative embolisation for advanced bone sarcomas. Radiol Med 2013;118(8):1344–59.
18. Manaster BJ. Soft-tissue masses: optimal imaging protocol and reporting. Am J Roentgenol 2013;201(3):505–14.
19. Nicolaou S, Yong-Hing CJ, Galea-Soler S, et al. Dual-energy CT as a potential new diagnostic tool in the management of gout in the acute setting. AJR Am J Roentgenol 2010;194(4):1072–8.
20. Glazebrook KN, Guimaraes LS, Murthy NS, et al. Identification of intraarticular and periarticular uric acid crystals with dual-energy CT: initial evaluation. Radiology 2011;261(2):516–24.

21. Kransdorf MJ, Bancroft LW, Peterson JJ, et al. Imaging of fatty tumors: distinction of lipoma and well-differentiated liposarcoma. Radiology 2002;224(1):99–104.

22. Munk PL, Lee MJ, Janzen DL, et al. Lipoma and liposarcoma: evaluation using CT and MR imaging. AJR Am J Roentgenol 1997;169(2):589–94.

23. Wu JS, Hochman MG. Soft-tissue tumors and tumorlike lesions: a systematic imaging approach. Radiology 2009;253(2):297–316.

24. Woertler K. Soft tissue masses in the foot and ankle: characteristics on MR imaging. Semin Musculoskelet Radiol 2005;09(03):227–42.

25. Teh J, Whiteley G. MRI of soft tissue masses of the hand and wrist. Br J Radiol 2007;80(949):47–63.

26. Behr GG, Johnson C. Vascular anomalies: hemangiomas and beyond—part 1, fast-flow lesions. AJR Am J Roentgenol 2013;200(2):414–22.

27. Behr GG, Johnson CM. Vascular anomalies: hemangiomas and beyond—part 2, slow-flow lesions. AJR Am J Roentgenol 2013;200(2):423–36.

28. Mulliken JB, Glowacki J. Classification of pediatric vascular lesions. Plast Reconstr Surg 1982;70(1):120–1.

29. Enjolras O. Classification and management of the various superficial vascular anomalies: hemangiomas and vascular malformations. J Dermatol 1997; 24(11):701–10.

30. Garzon MC, Huang JT, Enjolras O, et al. Vascular malformations: part I. J Am Acad Dermatol 2007;56(3):353–70.

31. Enjolras O, Mulliken JB. Vascular tumors and vascular malformations (new issues). Adv Dermatol 1997;13:375–423.

32. Moukaddam H, Pollak J, Haims AH. MRI characteristics and classification of peripheral vascular malformations and tumors. Skeletal Radiol 2008;38(6):535–47.

33. Yakes WF, Rossi P, Odink H. How I do it. Arteriovenous malformation management. Cardiovasc Intervent Radiol 1996;19(2):65–71.

34. Donnelly LF, Adams DM. Vascular malformations and hemangiomas: a practical approach in a multidisciplinary clinic. AJR Am J Roentgenol 2000;174(3):597–608.

35. Yakes WF, Haas DK, Parker SH, et al. Symptomatic vascular malformations: ethanol embolotherapy. Radiology 1989;170(3 Pt 2):1059–66.

36. Lee BB, Choe YH, Ahn JM, et al. The new role of magnetic resonance imaging in the contemporary diagnosis of venous malformation: can it replace angiography? J Am Coll Surg 2004;198(4):549–58.

37. Abernethy LJ. Classification and imaging of vascular malformations in children. Eur Radiol 2003;13(11):2483–97.

38. Rak KM, Yakes WF, Ray RL, et al. MR imaging of symptomatic peripheral vascular malformations. AJR Am J Roentgenol 1992;159(1):107–12.

39. Dobson MJ, Hartley RW, Ashleigh R, et al. MR angiography and MR imaging of symptomatic vascular malformations. Clin Radiol 1997;52(8):595–602.

40. El-Noueam KI, Schweitzer ME, Blasbalg R, et al. Is a subset of wrist ganglia the sequela of internal derangements of the wrist joint? MR imaging findings. Radiology 1999;212(2):537–40.

41. Murphey MD, Smith WS, Smith SE, et al. From the archives of the AFIP. Imaging of musculoskeletal neurogenic tumors: radiologic-pathologic correlation. Radiographics 1999;19(5):1253–80.

42. Banks KP. The target sign: extremity. Radiology 2005;234(3):899–900.

43. Lin J, Martel W. Cross-sectional imaging of peripheral nerve sheath tumors: characteristic signs on CT, MR imaging, and sonography. AJR Am J Roentgenol 2001;176(1):75–82.

44. De Beuckeleer L, De Schepper A, De Belder F, et al. Magnetic resonance imaging of localized giant cell tumour of the tendon sheath (MRI of localized GCTTS). Eur Radiol 1997;7(2):198–201.
45. Walker EA, Song AJ, Murphey MD. Magnetic resonance imaging of soft-tissue masses. Semin Roentgenol 2010;45(4):277–97.
46. McKenzie G, Raby N, Ritchie D. Non-neoplastic soft-tissue masses. Br J Radiol 2009;82(981):775–85.
47. Kransdorf MJ, Meis JM. From the archives of the AFIP. Extraskeletal osseous and cartilaginous tumors of the extremities. Radiographics 1993;13(4): 853–84.
48. Ackerman LV. Extra-osseous localized non-neoplastic bone and cartilage formation (so-called myositis ossificans) clinical and pathological confusion with malignant neoplasms. J Bone Joint Surg Am 1958;40(2):279–98.
49. Norman A, Dorfman HD. Juxtacortical circumscribed myositis ossificans: evolution and radiographic features. Radiology 1970;96(2):301–6.
50. Goldman AB. Myositis ossificans circumscripta: a benign lesion with a malignant differential diagnosis. AJR Am J Roentgenol 1976;126(1):32–40.
51. Amendola MA, Glazer GM, Agha FP, et al. Myositis ossificans circumscripta: computed tomographic diagnosis. Radiology 1983;149(3):775–9.
52. Heiken JP, Lee JK, Smathers RL, et al. CT of benign soft-tissue masses of the extremities. AJR Am J Roentgenol 1984;142(3):575–80.
53. Zeanah WR, Hudson TM. Myositis ossificans. Clin Orthop Relat Res 1982;(168): 187–91.
54. Bush CH. The magnetic resonance imaging of musculoskeletal hemorrhage. Skeletal Radiol 2000;29(1):1–9.
55. Mellado JM, del Palomar LP, Diaz L. Long-standing Morel-Lavallée lesions of the trochanteric region and proximal thigh: MRI features in five patients. AJR Am J Roentgenol 2004;182(5):1289–94.
56. Zanetti M, Weishaupt D. MR imaging of the forefoot: Morton neuroma and differential diagnoses. Semin Musculoskelet Radiol 2005;9(3):175–86.
57. Gogna A, Peh WCG, Munk PL. Image-guided musculoskeletal biopsy. Radiol Clin North Am 2008;46(3):455–73.
58. Errani C, Traina F, Perna F, et al. Current concepts in the biopsy of musculoskeletal tumors. ScientificWorldJournal 2013;2013(368):1–7.
59. Mankin HJ, Mankin CJ, Simon MA. The hazards of the biopsy, revisited. J Bone Joint Surg Am 1996;78(5):656–63.
60. Khoo MM, Saifuddin A. The role of MRI in image-guided needle biopsy of focal bone and soft tissue neoplasms. Skeletal Radiol 2013;42(7):905–15.
61. Balach T, Stacey GS, Hydon RC. The clinical evaluation of soft tissue tumors. Radiol Clin North Am 2011;49(6):1185–96.
62. Gibbs CP, Peabody TD, Mundt AJ, et al. Oncological outcomes of operative treatment of subcutaneous soft-tissue sarcomas of the extremities. J Bone Joint Surg Am 1997;79(6):888–97.
63. Pisters PWT, Pollock RE, Lewis VO, et al. Long-term results of prospective trial of surgery alone with selective use of radiation for patients with T1 extremity and trunk soft tissue sarcomas. Ann Surg 2007;246(4):675–82.
64. Rydholm A, Gustafson P, Rööser B, et al. Subcutaneous sarcoma. A population-based study of 129 patients. J Bone Joint Surg Br 1991;73(4):662–7.
65. Mendenhall WM, Indelicato DJ, Scarborough MT, et al. The management of adult soft tissue sarcomas. Am J Clin Oncol 2009;32(4):436–42.

66. O'Sullivan B, Davis AM, Turcotte R, et al. Preoperative versus postoperative radiotherapy in soft-tissue sarcoma of the limbs: a randomised trial. Lancet 2002;359(9325):2235–41.

67. O'Sullivan B, Wylie J, Catton C, et al. The local management of soft tissue sarcoma. Semin Radiat Oncol 1999;9(4):328–48.

68. Davis A, O'Sullivan B, Turcotte R, et al. Late radiation morbidity following randomization to preoperative versus postoperative radiotherapy in extremity soft tissue sarcoma. Radiother Oncol 2005;75(1):48–53.

69. Davis AM. Function and health status outcomes in a randomized trial comparing preoperative and postoperative radiotherapy in extremity soft tissue sarcoma. J Clin Oncol 2002;20(22):4472–7.

70. Pollack A, Zagars GK, Goswitz MS, et al. Preoperative vs. postoperative radiotherapy in the treatment of soft tissue sarcomas: a matter of presentation. Int J Radiat Oncol Biol Phys 1998;42(3):563–72.

71. Cormier JN. Cohort analysis of patients with localized, high-risk, extremity soft tissue sarcoma treated at two cancer centers: chemotherapy-associated outcomes. J Clin Oncol 2004;22(22):4567–74.

72. Fernberg JO, Hall KS. Chemotherapy in soft tissue sarcoma The Scandinavian Sarcoma Group experience. Acta Orthop Scand Suppl 2004;75(311):77–86.

73. Frustaci S, Gherlinzoni F, De Paoli A, et al. Adjuvant chemotherapy for adult soft tissue sarcomas of the extremities and girdles: results of the Italian Randomized Cooperative Trial. J Clin Oncol 2001;19(5):1238–47.

74. Rosenberg SA, Tepper J, Glatstein E, et al. Prospective randomized evaluation of adjuvant chemotherapy in adults with soft tissue sarcomas of the extremities. Cancer 1983;52(3):424–34.

75. Blay JY, Le Cesne A. Adjuvant chemotherapy in localized soft tissue sarcomas: still not proven. Oncologist 2009;14(10):1013–20.

76. Benjamin RS. Evidence for using adjuvant chemotherapy as standard treatment of soft tissue sarcoma. Semin Radiat Oncol 1999;9(4):349–51.

77. King JJ, Fayssoux RS, Lackman RD, et al. Early outcomes of soft tissue sarcomas presenting with metastases and treated with chemotherapy. Am J Clin Oncol 2009;32(3):308–13.

78. Shiu MH, Castro EB, Hajdu SI, et al. Surgical treatment of 297 soft tissue sarcomas of the lower extremity. Ann Surg 1975;182(5):597–602.

79. Abbas JS, Holyoke ED, Moore R, et al. The surgical treatment and outcome of soft-tissue sarcoma. Arch Surg 1981;116(6):765–9.

80. Karakousis CP, Proimakis C, Walsh DL. Primary soft tissue sarcoma of the extremities in adults. Br J Surg 1995;82(9):1208–12.

81. Vraa S, Keller J, Nielsen OS, et al. Prognostic factors in soft tissue sarcomas: the Aarhus experience. Eur J Cancer 1998;34(12):1876–82.

82. Downing S, Ahuja N, Oyetunji TA, et al. Disparity in limb-salvage surgery among sarcoma patients. Am J Surg 2010;199(4):549–53.

83. Potter DA, Kinsella T, Glatstein E, et al. High-grade soft tissue sarcomas of the extremities. Cancer 1986;58(1):190–205.

84. Williard WC, Hajdu SI, Casper ES, et al. Comparison of amputation with limb-sparing operations for adult soft tissue sarcoma of the extremity. Ann Surg 1992;215(3):269–75.

85. Johnson GR, Zhuang H, Khan J, et al. Roles of positron emission tomography with fluorine-18-deoxyglucose in the detection of local recurrent and distant metastatic sarcoma. Clin Nucl Med 2003;28(10):815–20.

Image-Guided Interventions in Oncology

Bruno C. Odisio, MD*, Michael J. Wallace, MD

KEYWORDS

- Interventional oncology • Interventional radiology • Percutaneous therapies
- Image-guided procedures • Transarterial therapies

KEY POINTS

- Interventional radiology provides a wide range of minimally invasive procedures that play a critical role on the diagnosis, treatment, and palliation of patients with cancer.
- Percutaneous image-guided biopsy is an established method for obtaining tissue specimens with high diagnostic accuracy, few complications, and lower costs when compared with more invasive procedures.
- Percutaneous ablation can be used as an alternative to surgical resection in patients with primary and secondary malignancies with similar outcomes in selected cases.
- Image-guided procedures can be used in the management of the complications of malignancy, improving a patient's quality of life.

INTRODUCTION

In 1964, Dr Charles Dotter, using a combination of basic guidewires and catheters, successfully dilated a focal stenosis of the superficial femoral artery in a patient with painful leg ischemia and gangrene who had refused surgery, thereby reestablishing flow and saving her limb.[1] The success, and symbolism, of this procedure opened the way for a shift in a long-last paradigm in medicine: the use of medical imaging solely as a diagnostic tool. Over the subsequent 3 decades, the investigational mind and talent of many interventional radiologists and the unparalleled technological advances in medical imaging and material development were pivotal for the establishment of interventional radiology as a distinct medical specialty.

Interventional oncology, a term commonly used to refer to minimally invasive procedures performed by interventional radiologists for diagnosing and treating cancer,[2–5] accounts for a broad spectrum of procedures unique to interventional radiology that

Conflict of Interest: The authors have no conflict of interest to disclose.

Division of Diagnostic Imaging, Department of Interventional Radiology, The University of Texas MD Anderson Cancer Center, 1515 Holcombe, Unit 1471, Houston, TX 77030, USA

* Corresponding author.

E-mail address: BCOdisio@mdanderson.org

have demonstrated unequivocal clinical benefits and established their roles as an integral part of the multidisciplinary oncologic cancer care team.[2] This article provides an updated overview of the role of image-guided interventions in oncology.

CLINICAL USE OF IMAGE-GUIDED INTERVENTIONS
Cancer Diagnosis

The advances in morphologic and functional imaging of the past decade, along with an expanding accessibility and use of this technology, have led to dramatic improvements in diagnosing and monitoring cancer.[6-9] Nevertheless, accurate diagnosis invariably relies on obtaining adequate pathologic specimens. More recent understanding of molecular biology and the use of molecularly targeted agents in the cancer armamentarium have directed cancer treatment to targeted therapy. In this new horizon, the requirements for obtaining tumor tissue for diagnosis not only play a role in the diagnosis of the malignancy but also could potentially provide useful information that could tailor patient therapy, ultimately providing objective clinical response in selected patients.[10] Among the modalities for obtaining tumor tissue for histologic diagnosis, percutaneous image-guided biopsy (PIB) is a safe, well-established, and widely used method for obtaining tissue specimens with high diagnostic yield and few complications, making it the alternative for the vast majority of biopsies. PIB also reduces hospital length of stay, costs associated with biopsy, and patients' anxiety associated with a major surgical intervention.[11-13]

Various imaging modalities are used to guide percutaneous biopsies. These include fluoroscopy, ultrasonography, computed tomography (CT), CT fluoroscopy, magnetic resonance imaging, positron emission tomography-CT, and combinations of these modalities. The choice of imaging modality is based on the biopsy site, operation preference, potential access routes, ability to visualize the lesion, and the availability and cost of the equipment. Most interventional radiologists prefer the coaxial technique for PIB. This technique involves the initial placement of a thin-walled needle in or close to the target lesion and the advancement of fine-needle aspiration and cutting needles through the thin-walled needle to obtain tissue samples, which allows multiple tissue samples to be obtained without the need for additional passes through the overlying structures and thereby minimizing patient discomfort and complications. This technique also allows continuous access to the target lesion while the initial samples are being analyzed by the cytopathologist, creating an easy path for obtaining new specimens and thus potentially increasing the diagnostic yield (**Fig. 1**). Fine-needle aspiration uses thin-walled 20- to 25-gauge needles that provide specimens suitable for cytologic and microhistologic evaluations[14,15] with minimal risk of complications compared with core-needle biopsies. Cutting needles (or core needles) provide core specimens for histologic evaluation and are available in various calibers. Modern small-caliber (18- to 20-gauge) cutting needles consistently provide high-quality specimens without increasing complication rates.[16,17] With this technique, the success rate of PIB is 70% to 95%, depending on the mix of organ systems, lesion size, and lesion location and the relative proportion of benign versus malignant lesions that are sampled.[11] Further understanding of the sample adequacy for PIB intended for molecular testing and genetic analysis is a subject of current investigations.

Portal Vein Embolization

The incidence of primary liver cancer has continued to rise over the past decade in the United States, and liver metastasis is still frequent.[18] In patients with primary tumors and metastases confined to the liver, liver resection remains the mainstay of curative

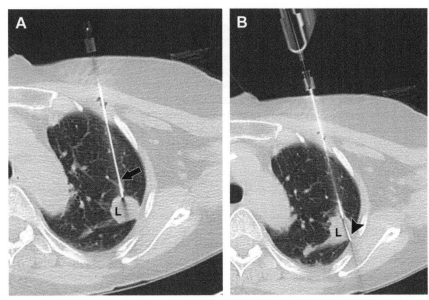

Fig. 1. Percutaneous CT-guided biopsy of a 2.0-cm lung lesion (L) using the coaxial technique. (*A*) A 19-gauge guide needle (*arrow*) placed at the vicinity of the lesion; (*B*) 20-gauge core needle (*arrowhead*) placed through the guide needle to obtain tissue samples. Pathology confirmed squamous cell carcinoma of the lung.

therapy. Despite technical advances in surgical technique and the care of postoperative patients, complications, such as fluid retention, cholestasis, and impaired synthetic function, still prolong recovery and hospital stays in patients who undergo hepatic resection. Among the elements associated with postoperative liver insufficiency, volume of the future liver remnant (FLR) is a strong and independent predictor of postsurgical hepatic dysfunction and complications.[19–21] The use of portal vein embolization (PVE) relies on the rationale of promoting preoperative increase in FLR by the hypertrophy caused by the redirection of blood flow to nonembolized liver segments, with the intent of reducing the incidence of postoperative liver insufficiency and increasing the number of patients eligible for major hepatic resection.[22,23]

The workup for PVE should begin with the calculation of total estimated liver volume (TELV) and the acquisition of volumetric CT images to calculate FLR volume. Among the ways of calculating TELV, some prefer the formula proposed by Vauthey and colleagues,[24] which was derived from the close relationship between body surface area and TELV (TELV = $-794.41 + 1267.28 \times$ body surface area). The FLR-TELV ratio is used as the standardized (preoperative) FLR that will be correlated with the surgical outcome. The FLR volume required to minimize the risk of hepatic failure after surgery is 20% and 30% in patients without cirrhosis who did and did not receive systemic chemotherapy, respectively, and 40% in patients with cirrhosis. Patients with an FLR volume below the appropriate threshold should be considered for PVE, considering individual factors on a case-by-case basis.[21,25–28] Contraindications for PVE include overt clinical portal hypertension, extensive portal vein tumor invasion, and complete lobar portal vein occlusion in view that the portal vein flow is already diverted in this situation.[29] Relative contraindications include partial tumor invasion of the portal vein, extrahepatic metastasis, tumor site precluding safe access to the portal vein, renal failure, and mild portal hypertension.

PVE is classically performed via 1 of the 3 different approaches: the percutaneous transhepatic, the percutaneous transjugular, or the intraoperative transileocolic venous approach. The most commonly used approach worldwide, the percutaneous transhepatic approach, can be categorized as contralateral or ipsilateral; the latter is gaining favor because it reduces the risk of injuring the FLR compared with the contralateral access (**Fig. 2**). A series of conventional angiographic catheters and guidewires are passed through the percutaneous vascular access to the portal vein system to perform portal vein venography, embolize the hepatic segments to be resected, and measure preembolization and postembolization pressures. Among the embolic materials preferred for PVE, we give preference to small (100-μm to 500-μm) calibrated particles and embolization coils within the secondary portal branches to further reduce the portal inflow that could lead to recanalization.[30] Patients who undergo PVE are discharged on the same day. A CT follow-up of 4 to 6 weeks is requested to assess the degree of hypertrophy of the FLR.

PVE provides high technical and clinical success rates, as indicated by hypertrophy of the FLR ranging from 28% to 46%. In a recent systematic review of 44 articles that included 1791 patients who underwent embolization, van Lienden and colleagues[31] calculated a mean hypertrophy rate of 37.9% ± 0.1%, a success rate of 99.3%, and a mortality rate of 0.1%. In a recent study of 358 patients from our institution, the median pre-PVE and post-PVE FLR volumes were 19.5% and 29.7%, respectively, and the rates of postoperative hepatic insufficiency and 90-day mortality were 8.3% and 3.8%, respectively.[32]

Cancer Treatment

Transarterial hepatic treatments

Transarterial interventional techniques used for palliation or bridge therapy of primary and secondary malignant hepatic tumors emerged due to the peculiarities of blood flow to primary and several secondary hepatic malignancies, which are preferentially supplied via the hepatic artery. Among these techniques, the most common are bland embolization of the arterial supply to the tumor to induce ischemia and tumor necrosis, regional intra-arterial infusion of cytotoxic or immunotherapeutic agents to enhance the tumoricidal effect, the combination of those techniques (chemoembolization), and transarterial delivery of yttrium-90 (^{90}Y)-coated microspheres (radioembolization).

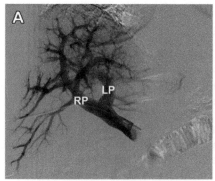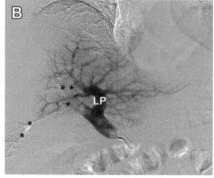

Fig. 2. Pre (A) and post (B) right portal (RP) vein embolization using the ipsilateral approach. Note the embolic material deposited on the right portal vein branches (*asterisks*) and patency of the left portal vein (LP) and its branches.

For transarterial chemoembolization (TACE), a chemotherapeutic drug or drugs are added to the embolic agent, on the basis of the theory that tumor ischemia caused by arterial embolization has a synergistic effect with the chemotherapeutic drugs. Several chemotherapeutic agents, most commonly doxorubicin and cisplatin, can be mixed with one or more embolic agents. Recently, the development of calibrated microparticles (DEB-TACE) has gained wide acceptance (**Fig. 3**). These drug-eluting microspheres allow more reliable distal occlusion of small vessels and delivery of high-dose chemotherapy to the tumor with a very low systemic circulation of the chemotherapeutic agent, thus reducing the associated systemic adverse effects when compared with other traditional forms of TACE.[33,34] Transarterial radioembolization (TARE) consists of the delivery of microspheres loaded with yttrium-90 (^{90}Y), a pure beta emitter. Like other transarterial therapies, ^{90}Y-loaded microspheres can deliver beta radiation preferentially to tumors following hepatic artery delivery via embolization of tumor-related arterioles. This approach potentially creates an intense local radiotherapeutic effect that is proportional to the density of the microsphere distribution. Compared with nonselective extracorporeal x-ray radiotherapy, TARE allows the particles to be deposited predominantly within the tumor vasculature, thereby leading to tumor damage while preserving the surrounding liver parenchyma. This feature allows the delivery of substantially higher radiation doses than those that can be safely delivered via external-beam radiotherapy.

TACE and TARE can be used as palliative treatment for patients who are not candidates for surgical resection or liver transplantation. They also can be used as neoadjuvant therapy with either the intent to prevent tumor progression or as a downstaging strategy for patients with a tumor burden beyond the acceptable inclusion criteria for liver transplantation. For patients with hepatocellular carcinoma (HCC) classified by the Barcelona Clinic Liver Cancer (BCLC) guidelines as intermediate stage (BCLC-B), transarterial chemoembolization is considered the standard of care.[35] In a recent study, a median survival of 42.8 months was achieved with the use of DEB-TACE loaded with doxorubicin in patients with BCLC-B.[36] For patients with unresectable metastatic colorectal disease to the liver, results of a recent phase I pilot study[37] and the final results of a phase III study,[38] respectively, demonstrated

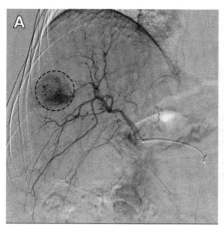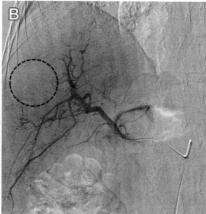

Fig. 3. Pre (*A*) and post (*B*) digital subtraction angiograms of the hepatic artery showing superselective drug-eluting beads transarterial chemoembolization of a 2.5-cm right hepatic hepatocellular carcinoma (*dotted black circle*).

that DEB-TACE loaded with irinotecan increased the 6-month overall response rate of hepatic lesions when compared with first-line systemic chemotherapy and increased overall survival, response rate, progression-free survival, and quality of life compared with second-line therapy. TARE has been investigated with patients with intermediate-stage or advanced-stage HCC. In a recent phase II trial, 17 patients with intermediate-stage HCC who did not have portal vein thrombosis were treated with TARE; disease control was achieved in 15 patients, time to progression was 13 months, and overall survival duration was 18 months (range, 12–38 months).[39] In a multicenter trial that assessed the use of radioembolization with ^{90}Y for patients with HCC, the 87 patients with BCLC-B HCC who were treated with ^{90}Y had a median survival of 16.9 months.[40] The result of the trial suggested that radioembolization with ^{90}Y may be particularly promising for patients with intermediate-stage HCC who are poor candidates for TACE as well for patients for whom prior TACE or bland embolization is ineffective, highlighting the possibility of using TARE as a complement to TACE.

Nonhepatic transarterial treatment

Intra-arterial procedures can be used to manage primary or secondary cancers, such as renal cell carcinoma (RCC) and pelvic and bone malignancies. These procedures can be used as a palliative stand-alone method, in combination with chemotherapy, ablative or surgical therapies, or as preoperative adjunct to facilitate surgical excision, reducing intraoperative blood loss and postoperative complications.

Renal artery embolization in the setting of RCC has been widely used since its introduction as a preoperative and palliative strategy.[41–48] Preoperative embolization can facilitate surgical excision by collapsing the tortuous veins covering the surface of the tumor and the renal hilum that can impede access to the renal artery during surgery. This technique also can reduce the size and extension of a tumor thrombus invading the renal vein or inferior vena cava, and it can reduce intraoperative blood loss and, although controversial, the operating time.[41,49] In general, nephrectomy is performed within 24 to 72 hours after embolization to take maximum advantage of the infarction-induced edematous rim around the kidney and to reduce distress from postembolization syndrome.[42] More recently, renal artery embolization has been used before thermal ablation for patients with RCC with the objective of reducing the heat-sink effect created by the vessels in the tumoral bed during ablation and potentially enhancing treatment efficacy by increasing the thermal ablated volume (Fig. 4).[50,51] Similarly, superselective tumor embolization has been used as an adjunct strategy to facilitate laparoscopic removal of tumors with a nephrometry score of 6 or higher to reduce blood loss and operating time while maintaining 5-year local recurrence rates similar to patients who undergo open partial nephrectomy.[52] Palliative embolization of RCC has been used with varying degrees of success for patients with unresectable RCC who are not candidates for surgical resection to control tumor-related symptoms, such as flank pain, hemorrhage, congestive heart failure due to large arteriovenous fistulas, hypercalcemia, hypertension, and polycythemia.[53–55] A review of all studies on arterial embolization for RCC published between 1973 and 1997 showed that only a small group of patients with massive hematuria, flank pain, or paraneoplastic syndrome may benefit from palliative embolization.[42] More recently, small case-series demonstrated successful control of hematuria and flank pain after renal embolization.[56,57] The effectiveness of this procedure in symptom palliation awaits further study and validation.

Regional intra-arterial chemotherapy and embolization can be used to treat pelvic malignancies. Intra-arterial chemotherapy, especially in combination with radical surgery, is useful in managing advanced uterine cervical carcinoma. In a study of

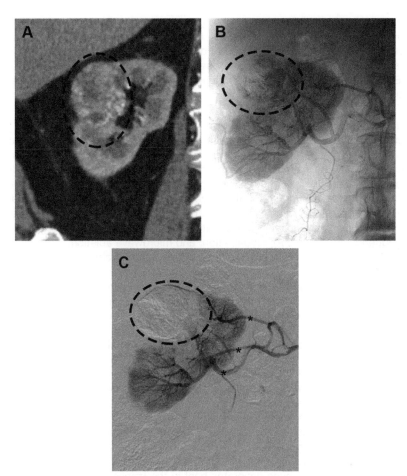

Fig. 4. A 79-year-old man with a right renal mass suspicious for renal cell carcinoma. (*A*) Coronal CT reconstruction showing the 3.5-cm lesion (*dotted circle*) in the midpole of the right kidney. Pre (*B*) and post (*C*) embolization of feeding vessels showing successful devascularization of the tumor (*dotted circles*) and patency of the branches supplying the kidney parenchyma (*asterisks*).

25 patients with stage IIB to IIIB uterine cervical carcinoma treated with pelvic intra-arterial cisplatin and bleomycin followed by surgery or radiotherapy, a clinical response rate of 80% and an operability rate of 72% was achieved.[58] Pelvic intra-arterial chemotherapy also can be followed by uterine artery embolization to enhance the local therapeutic effect.[59] The use of intra-arterial cisplatin administration in combination with radiotherapy for patients with muscle-invasive urinary bladder cancer has been investigated; the reported complete response rate ranged from 74% to 90%, the bladder preservation rate ranged from 75% to 100%, and the survival rate was similar to that achieved with cystectomy.[60–62]

Transcatheter arterial embolization for hypervascular primary and secondary bone tumors is generally performed preoperatively or for palliation. Hypervascular bone metastases, which are seen in 30% to 45% of patients with RCC and thyroid carcinoma,[63] are by far the most commonly embolized bone metastases. Owing to the hypervascular nature of these lesions, surgical intervention can be complicated by excessive, uncontrollable bleeding. The use of preoperative arterial embolization has been reported for bone metastases from renal, thyroid, breast, and lung malignancies and from melanoma, and has been shown to reduce intraoperative blood loss. Embolization also is used to inhibit tumor growth and to reduce pain or bleeding in patients with unresectable tumors.[63–66]

Percutaneous ablation therapy
Percutaneous therapy refers to the use of nonthermal and thermal percutaneous ablative technologies to treat cancer under imaging guidance. With this method, the target lesion is treated by the insertion of a needle or probe (or both) with subsequent delivery of energy or substance (or both) by imaging guidance. This technique is widely used for primary and metastatic tumors of the liver, lung, kidney, adrenal glands, and soft tissue. Nonthermal technology includes chemical ablation with ethanol or acetic acid instillation and irreversible electroporation. Thermal ablative technology includes radiofrequency ablation (RFA), cryoablation, and microwave ablation.

Percutaneous ethanol injection is the seminal percutaneous ablation technique. With a guiding needle, absolute ethanol is injected inside the tumor and around it, inducing coagulative necrosis as a result of cell dehydration, protein denaturation, and chemical occlusion of small vessels. This method is a well-established technique for treating nodular type HCCs. Although percutaneous ethanol injection is widely available and efficacious, the extent of necrosis obtained by this method is correlated with the size of the lesions: the complete response rate is higher in smaller HCCs than in large HCCs (90%, 70%, and 50% of tumors measuring <2, 2–3, and 3–5 cm, respectively).[67–69] Irreversible electroporation induces cell death by disrupting the electrical potential across cell membranes by creating permanent nanopores through the plasma membrane, which affects cell homeostasis.[70] Irreversible electroporation appears to be free from the heat-sink effect that affects other thermal ablative technologies and is safe for use with hepatic tumors adjacent to hepatic veins and portal pedicles.[71,72]

RFA involves delivering an alternating electrical current with a probe placed directly into the tumor. The resulting frictional heat and movement of electrons within the lesion and surrounding tissues generates heat in the immediate vicinity of the electrode. This heat is then conducted to the surrounding environment and results in coagulative necrosis of a finite volume of tissue. This technology has become the first-line modality for percutaneous hepatic ablation for patients with HCC and metastatic disease to the liver, mainly because it yields complete necrosis with fewer sessions than is required for percutaneous ethanol injection, thus leading to better local disease control.[73–77] The size and shape of the ablation zone varies depending on the amount of energy applied, type and number of electrodes, duration of ablation, and inherent tissue characteristics.[78] Because of its efficacy and safety profile, RFA is now offered to patients who are surgical candidates with comparable 5-year survival outcomes from resection.[79–82] The limitations of the technique include the heat-sink effect, whereby adjacent blood vessels produce perfusion-mediated attenuation of thermal energy deposition, potentially leading to incomplete ablation; large lesions (>5 cm); and proximity to thermally sensitive structures, such as the intestinal wall, gallbladder, diaphragm, and nerves, which can be damaged during the course of ablation.

Microwave (MW) ablation promotes tissue heating by causing polar water molecules to continuously realign with an oscillating electromagnetic field that emanates from the microwave antenna placed within the tumor. The continuous realignment creates heat by agitating water molecules in the surrounding tissue, thereby producing friction and heat and inducing cellular destruction via coagulative necrosis.[83] In contrast to RFA, microwave propagation is not affected by low electrical conductivity, high tissue impedance, or low thermal conductivity.[84] Compared with other available ablative technologies, MW creates larger tumor ablation volumes with consistently higher intratumoral temperatures, has faster ablation times, and an improved and a more favorable convection profile,[84] thus resulting in a reduction in the heat-sink effect created by vessels near to the ablated zone.[85] Recent improvements in MW engineering, along with expanded application of and experience with this technology, could create more effective ablation zones than RFA does (**Fig. 5**).[86–88]

Cryoablation, which causes rapid cooling of the targeted tissue, is performed by placing a cooling probe within the lesion, which promotes local ischemia and disrupts the cellular membrane. Ice crystals form within the cells and adjacent interstitium, causing cell dehydration and surrounding vascular thrombosis. Subsequently, when the tissues thaw, vascular occlusion leads to further ischemic injury, which initiates apoptosis.[89,90] Consistent tumor cell death is accomplished when the tissues are exposed to a temperature of −20°C or lower within an approximately 3-mm area inside the margins of the ice ball, which can be visualized under imaging guidance (**Fig. 6**). Treatment of large tumor volumes with cryoablation can, rarely, lead to the serious cytokine-mediated systemic inflammatory response associated with coagulopathy and multiorgan failure, myoglobinuria, and severe thrombocytopenia.[91–93]

Management of Cancer Complications

Biliary drainage

Patients with primary or secondary malignant biliary obstruction usually die due to liver insufficiency and cholangitis secondary to biliary obstruction.[94] For patients who failed to achieve biliary decompression via endoscopy, with high bile duct obstruction (above the cystic duct insertion[95]) or altered anatomy due to prior surgery, transhepatic percutaneous biliary drainage (PBD) can be used as an effective method for palliation.[95] PBD is usually performed in a staged approach until achievement of optimal drainage, but for most patients, liver function indices improve after the first session.[96]

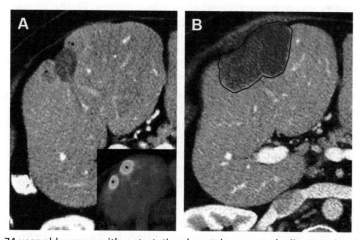

Fig. 5. A 74-year-old woman with metastatic colorectal cancer to the liver previously submitted to percutaneous RFA ablation. Six-month CT and positron emission tomography–CT (*inset*) follow-up (*A*) demonstrating recurrence at the ablated margins (*asterisks*) 6 months later around the previously ablated lesion. (*B*) Four-month CT follow-up after second session of percutaneous ablation with microwave showing adequate coverage of the recurrent tumor.

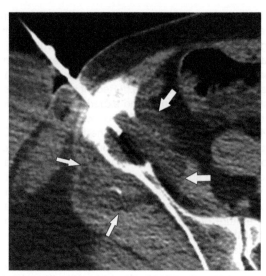

Fig. 6. Patient with metastatic RCC to the right iliac bone treated with cryoablation due to intractable pain. Note the ice-ball depicted during the ablation procedure (*arrows*). Patient had resolution of her pain following the procedure.

The initial biliary decompression can be achieved by placing a biliary drain either proximal (external) to or across the malignant obstruction (internal/external). External biliary drainage is associated with fluid and electrolyte imbalances due to loss of bile via the catheter to outside the body, malnutrition, and coagulopathy (due to the lack of bile aiding in the digestion of fat and fat-soluble minerals).[97,98] To address these issues, patients with an external biliary drain should have, whenever possible, their PBD converted to an internal/external drain with the aim of providing antegrade bile flow through the catheter lumen to the small bowel. Both external and external/internal biliary catheters should be exchanged every 2 to 3 months. Finally, for patients who are not candidates for surgery, internal biliary metallic internal stents can be used. A major advantage of using these stents is the absence of a catheter exiting the skin externally to the body, which improves the patient's comfort. Metallic stents are associated with a mean patency of 6 to 9 months and therefore should be used with patients with limited life expectancy.[99,100]

Regardless of the type of drainage chosen, patients who require biliary drainage must have a clearly defined goal and be aware of the maintenance requirements of external catheters and their impact on lifestyle.[101] In addition, the incidence of cholangitis among patients with cancer is higher than that in the general population, with an approximate incidence of 50% for those with external/internal drains, and the condition is more likely to develop the longer the catheter is used.[102,103] PBD can also be used in special situations, such as to optimize the drainage of intrahepatic bilomas (**Fig. 7**).

Urologic interventions

Malignant urinary obstruction is a common and threatening clinical picture due to the risk of developing renal function impairment, urinary tract sepsis, electrolyte disturbances, and metabolic acidosis. Ureteric obstruction is seen in a wide range of malignancies, most commonly those of gynecologic, gastrointestinal, urologic, and hematological origin. Its management requires urinary decompression, which is usually achieved by means of percutaneous nephrostomy. This procedure allows

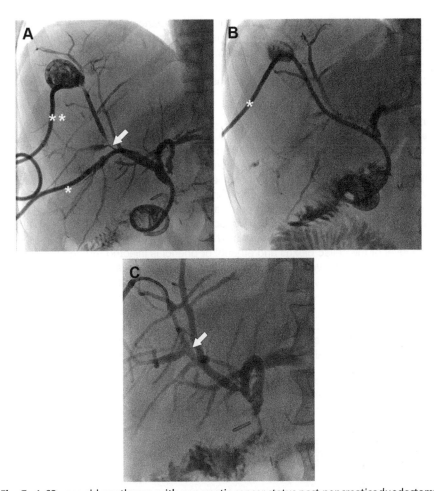

Fig. 7. A 62-year-old gentleman with pancreatic cancer status post pancreaticoduodectomy complicated with an intrahepatic infected biloma and hyperbilirubinemia. A percutaneous internal/external biliary drain (*asterisk*) along with an abscess drain (*double asterisk*) were placed under imaging guidance. (*A*) Follow-up cholangiogram and fistulogram demonstrated a stricture (*arrow*) between right anterior bile radicle communicating with the biloma and the main right bile duct. (*B*) Using the biloma percutaneous access, an internal/external biliary drain (*asterisk*) was placed through the focal stricture to address it, and the previous existing biliary drain was removed (not shown). (*C*) Two-month follow-up cholangiogram demonstrated resolution of the focal stricture (*arrow*). The biliary drain was removed and the patient remained asymptomatic with no evidence of biloma recurrence.

drainage of the urinary content, addresses the ominous consequences of urinary obstruction, and provides access for further urologic interventions. In cases of malignant or postoperative ureteric obstruction where retrograde stenting is unsuccessful or not feasible, antegrade percutaneous dilatation of the stricture can be performed, followed by placement of a nephroureteral stent across the stricture communicating the renal pelvis with the bladder. For patients who undergo radical cystectomy and ileal conduit, this stenting can be subsequently converted to an internal nephroureteral drain or to a retrograde nephroureteral catheter. Suprapubic catheters can be safely placed under fluoroscopy, ultrasonography, or CT guidance in patients with lower urinary tract obstruction with contraindications or inability to retain a transurethral drain catheter. Finally, patients with lower urinary tract fistulas who are poor candidates for surgery could benefit from percutaneous treatment by ureteral occlusion combined with insertion of a functioning percutaneous nephrostomy tube that allows diversion of urine from the fistula.[104]

Pain management

The prevalence of pain ranges from 40% to as high as 90% in patients with advanced cancer, making it a critical element of the care of patients with cancer. The mainstay therapy, opiates provide adequate pain control in 80% to 90% of these patients. For patients with localized pain who do not achieve adequate pain control or for whom the adverse effects of opiates are intolerable, image-guided procedures can be applied. Neuropathic pain associated with abdominal tumors, particularly gastric, esophageal, biliary, and pancreatic cancers, can be successfully managed with celiac plexus neurolysis. In this procedure, a fine needle is advanced under CT or fluoroscopy guidance at the level of the celiac plexus and ethanol or phenol is injected through the needle, causing irreversible nerve root destruction.[105,106] Percutaneous vertebroplasty can be performed for fractures secondary to neoplastic disease, thereby improving the patient's quality of life and reducing requirements for analgesia. Responses to this therapy are seen in 50% to 60% of oncologic patients who undergo vertebroplasty.[107] Percutaneous ablation can be used for patients with painful osseous metastasis who are not candidates for or who had a suboptimal response to radiotherapy with this technique, achieving pain control in more than 75% of patients.[108]

Treatment of vascular complications

Prehepatic portal vein obstruction in the oncologic population can occur as a consequence of direct tumor invasion to the portal vein, extrinsic compression, or periportal

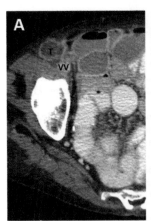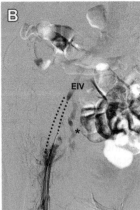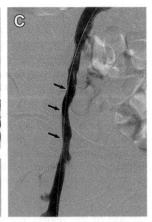

Fig. 8. (A) Abdominal CT demonstrating a metastatic colorectal tumor (T) to the abdominal wall invading the right external iliac/common femoral vessels (VV) complicated with venous thrombosis in an 80-year-old female patient. (B) Right femoral venography showing a filling defect and occlusion of the iliac vein (*dotted lines*) with collateral filling of the external iliac vein (EIV) (*asterisk*). (C) Catheter-direct thrombolysis was performed followed by mechanical thrombectomy and placement of stent-graft (*arrows*) with successful reperfusion of the affected segment. Patient maintained patency of the stent until her death, 1 year later after the intervention.

fibrosis after radiotherapy or surgery, or it can arise as a hypercoagulable state result-ing from malignancy. Placement of a percutaneous portal vein stent is a relatively safe and feasible alternative for these patients, providing marked relief from portal vein hypertension and improving liver function.[109,110] Patients presenting with malignant peripheral or central venous obstruction could benefit from percutaneous stent place-ment, which can occur before catheter-based thrombolysis and thrombectomy in patients presenting with acute thrombus (**Fig. 8**).[111] For patients with superior vena cava syndrome (SVCS), it is unclear whether a superior vena cava stent should be inserted before or after radiotherapy. The use of this stent as the primary therapy has been proposed for patients with life-threatening SCVS symptoms, such as signif-icant cerebral or laryngeal edema or hemodynamic compromise.[112] Primary and sec-ondary superior vena cava patency after stent placement in patients with malignant SVCS varies from 84% to 88% and 92% to 95%, respectively.[113,114]

SUMMARY

Cancer diagnosis and treatment comprises a number of diagnostic and therapeutic options performed by a wide range of medical specialists. Effective collaboration and precise understanding of the rationale of, levels of evidence of, and alternatives to the current standards of care should be acknowledged by all team members. Inter-ventional radiology provides minimally invasive procedures that play a critical role in the diagnosis, treatment, and management of cancer. The establishment of this spe-cialty as an integral part of the multidisciplinary oncologic team has brought clinical benefits for patients with cancer. Continuing support for translational and clinical investigation, clinical competence, and strong collaborative efforts between interven-tional radiologists and other medical specialists should be attained to improve the outcome of the treatment of this dreadful disease.

REFERENCES

1. Rosch J, Keller FS, Kaufman JA. The birth, early years, and future of interven-tional radiology. J Vasc Interv Radiol 2003;14(7):841–53.
2. Hickey R, Vouche M, Sze DY, et al. Cancer concepts and principles: primer for the interventional oncologist-part II. J Vasc Interv Radiol 2013;24(8):1167–88.
3. Hickey R, Vouche M, Sze DY, et al. Cancer concepts and principles: primer for the interventional oncologist-part I. J Vasc Interv Radiol 2013;24(8):1157–64.
4. Monfardini L, Della Vigna P, Bonomo G, et al. Interventional oncology in the elderly: complications and early response in liver and kidney malignancies. J Geriatr Oncol 2013;4(1):58–63.
5. Sheth RA, Hesketh R, Kong DS, et al. Barriers to drug delivery in interventional oncology. J Vasc Interv Radiol 2013;24(8):1201–7.
6. Wagner HN Jr, Conti PS. Advances in medical imaging for cancer diagnosis and treatment. Cancer 1991;67(Suppl 4):1121–8.
7. Schnall M, Rosen M. Primer on imaging technologies for cancer. J Clin Oncol 2006;24(20):3225–33.
8. Townsend DW, Carney JP, Yap JT, et al. PET/CT today and tomorrow. J Nucl Med 2004;45(Suppl 1):4S–14S.
9. Koh DM, Cook GJ, Husband JE. New horizons in oncologic imaging. N Engl J Med 2003;348(25):2487–8.
10. Kim ES, Herbst RS, Wistuba II, et al. The BATTLE trial: personalizing therapy for lung cancer. Cancer Discov 2011;1(1):44–53.

11. Gupta S, Wallace MJ, Cardella JF, et al. Quality improvement guidelines for percutaneous needle biopsy. J Vasc Interv Radiol 2010;21(7):969–75.

12. Liberman L. Centennial dissertation. Percutaneous imaging-guided core breast biopsy: state of the art at the millennium. AJR Am J Roentgenol 2000;174(5): 1191–9.

13. Gupta S, Madoff DC. Image-guided percutaneous needle biopsy in cancer diagnosis and staging. Tech Vasc Interv Radiol 2007;10(2):88–101.

14. Charboneau JW, Reading CC, Welch TJ. CT and sonographically guided needle biopsy: current techniques and new innovations. AJR Am J Roentgenol 1990; 154(1):1–10.

15. Reading CC, Charboneau JW, James EM, et al. Sonographically guided percutaneous biopsy of small (3 cm or less) masses. AJR Am J Roentgenol 1988; 151(1):189–92.

16. Hopper KD, Abendroth CS, Sturtz KW, et al. Blinded comparison of biopsy needles and automated devices in vitro: 2. Biopsy of medical renal disease. AJR Am J Roentgenol 1993;161(6):1299–301.

17. Hopper KD, Abendroth CS, Sturtz KW, et al. Blinded comparison of biopsy needles and automated devices in vitro: 1. Biopsy of diffuse hepatic disease. AJR Am J Roentgenol 1993;161(6):1293–7.

18. Simard EP, Ward EM, Siegel R, et al. Cancers with increasing incidence trends in the United States: 1999 through 2008. CA Cancer J Clin 2012; 62(2):124–5.

19. Shoup M, Gonen M, D'Angelica M, et al. Volumetric analysis predicts hepatic dysfunction in patients undergoing major liver resection. J Gastrointest Surg 2003;7(3):325–30.

20. Ribero D, Abdalla EK, Madoff DC, et al. Portal vein embolization before major hepatectomy and its effects on regeneration, resectability and outcome. Br J Surg 2007;94(11):1386–94.

21. de Meijer VE, Kalish BT, Puder M, et al. Systematic review and meta-analysis of steatosis as a risk factor in major hepatic resection. Br J Surg 2010;97(9): 1331–9.

22. Brouquet A, Andreou A, Shindoh J, et al. Methods to improve resectability of hepatocellular carcinoma. Recent Results Cancer Res 2013;190:57–67.

23. Rees M, John TG. Current status of surgery in colorectal metastases to the liver. Hepatogastroenterology 2001;48(38):341–4.

24. Vauthey JN, Abdalla EK, Doherty DA, et al. Body surface area and body weight predict total liver volume in Western adults. Liver Transpl 2002;8(3):233–40.

25. Pawlik TM, Olino K, Gleisner AL, et al. Preoperative chemotherapy for colorectal liver metastases: impact on hepatic histology and postoperative outcome. J Gastrointest Surg 2007;11(7):860–8.

26. Vauthey JN, Pawlik TM, Ribero D, et al. Chemotherapy regimen predicts steatohepatitis and an increase in 90-day mortality after surgery for hepatic colorectal metastases. J Clin Oncol 2006;24(13):2065–72.

27. Farges O, Belghiti J, Kianmanesh R, et al. Portal vein embolization before right hepatectomy: prospective clinical trial. Ann Surg 2003;237(2):208–17.

28. May BJ, Talenfeld AD, Madoff DC. Update on portal vein embolization: evidence-based outcomes, controversies, and novel strategies. J Vasc Interv Radiol 2013;24(2):241–54.

29. Madoff DC, Abdalla EK, Vauthey JN. Portal vein embolization in preparation for major hepatic resection: evolution of a new standard of care. J Vasc Interv Radiol 2005;16(6):779–90.

30. Avritscher R, de Baere T, Murthy R, et al. Percutaneous transhepatic portal vein embolization: rationale, technique, and outcomes. Semin Intervent Radiol 2008; 25(2):132–45.
31. van Lienden KP, van den Esschert JW, de Graaf W, et al. Portal vein embolization before liver resection: a systematic review. Cardiovasc Intervent Radiol 2013;36(1):25–34.
32. Shindoh J, Tzeng CW, Aloia TA, et al. Safety and efficacy of portal vein embolization before planned major or extended hepatectomy: an institutional experience of 358 patients. J Gastrointest Surg 2014;18(1):45–51.
33. Lammer J, Malagari K, Vogl T, et al. Prospective randomized study of doxorubicin-eluting-bead embolization in the treatment of hepatocellular carcinoma: results of the PRECISION V study. Cardiovasc Intervent Radiol 2010; 33(1):41–52.
34. Vogl TJ, Lammer J, Lencioni R, et al. Liver, gastrointestinal, and cardiac toxicity in intermediate hepatocellular carcinoma treated with PRECISION TACE with drug-eluting beads: results from the PRECISION V randomized trial. AJR Am J Roentgenol 2011;197(4):W562–70.
35. Llovet JM, Bruix J. Systematic review of randomized trials for unresectable hepatocellular carcinoma: chemoembolization improves survival. Hepatology 2003;37(2):429–42.
36. Burrel M, Reig M, Forner A, et al. Survival of patients with hepatocellular carcinoma treated by transarterial chemoembolisation (TACE) using drug eluting beads. Implications for clinical practice and trial design. J Hepatol 2012; 56(6):1330–5.
37. Martin RC 2nd, Scoggins CR, Tomalty D, et al. Irinotecan drug-eluting beads in the treatment of chemo-naive unresectable colorectal liver metastasis with concomitant systemic fluorouracil and oxaliplatin: results of pharmacokinetics and phase I trial. J Gastrointest Surg 2012;16(8):1531–8.
38. Fiorentini G, Aliberti C, Tilli M, et al. Intra-arterial infusion of irinotecan-loaded drug-eluting beads (DEBIRI) versus intravenous therapy (FOLFIRI) for hepatic metastases from colorectal cancer: final results of a phase III study. Anticancer Res 2012;32(4):1387–95.
39. Mazzaferro V, Sposito C, Bhoori S, et al. Yttrium(90) radioembolization for intermediate-advanced hepatocarcinoma: a phase II study. Hepatology 2013; 57(5):1826–37.
40. Sangro B, Carpanese L, Cianni R, et al. Survival after yttrium-90 resin microsphere radioembolization of hepatocellular carcinoma across Barcelona clinic liver cancer stages: a European evaluation. Hepatology 2011;54(3): 868–78.
41. Bakal CW, Cynamon J, Lakritz PS, et al. Value of preoperative renal artery embolization in reducing blood transfusion requirements during nephrectomy for renal cell carcinoma. J Vasc Interv Radiol 1993;4(6):727–31.
42. Kalman D, Varenhorst E. The role of arterial embolization in renal cell carcinoma. Scand J Urol Nephrol 1999;33(3):162–70.
43. Lanigan D, Jurriaans E, Hammonds JC, et al. The current status of embolization in renal cell carcinoma—a survey of local and national practice. Clin Radiol 1992;46(3):176–8.
44. Mebust WK, Weigel JW, Lee KR, et al. Renal cell carcinoma—angioinfarction. J Urol 1984;131(2):231–5.
45. Wallace S, Chuang VP, Swanson D, et al. Embolization of renal carcinoma. Radiology 1981;138(3):563–70.

46. Zielinski H, Szmigielski S, Petrovich Z. Comparison of preoperative embolization followed by radical nephrectomy with radical nephrectomy alone for renal cell carcinoma. Am J Clin Oncol 2000;23(1):6–12.

47. Wallace S, Carrasco H. Intra-arterial interventional therapy for malignant genitourinary neoplasms. Philadelphia: W B Saunders; 2000.

48. Subramanian VS, Stephenson AJ, Goldfarb DA, et al. Utility of preoperative renal artery embolization for management of renal tumors with inferior vena caval thrombi. Urology 2009;74(1):154–9.

49. Sweeney P, Wood CG, Pisters LL, et al. Surgical management of renal cell carcinoma associated with complex inferior vena caval thrombi. Urol Oncol 2003; 21(5):327–33.

50. Arima K, Yamakado K, Kinbara H, et al. Percutaneous radiofrequency ablation with transarterial embolization is useful for treatment of stage 1 renal cell carcinoma with surgical risk: results at 2-year mean follow up. Int J Urol 2007;14(7): 585–90 [discussion: 590].

51. Nakasone Y, Kawanaka K, Ikeda O, et al. Sequential combination treatment (arterial embolization and percutaneous radiofrequency ablation) of inoperable renal cell carcinoma: single-center pilot study. Acta Radiol 2012;53(4):410–4.

52. Simone G, Papalia R, Guaglianone S, et al. Zero ischemia laparoscopic partial nephrectomy after superselective transarterial tumor embolization for tumors with moderate nephrometry score: long-term results of a single-center experience. J Endourol 2011;25(9):1443–6.

53. Jacobs JA, Ring EJ, Wein AJ. New indications for renal infarction. J Urol 1981; 125(2):243–5.

54. Nurmi M, Satokari K, Puntala P. Renal artery embolization in the palliative treatment of renal adenocarcinoma. Scand J Urol Nephrol 1987;21(2):93–6.

55. Onishi T, Oishi Y, Suzuki Y, et al. Prognostic evaluation of transcatheter arterial embolization for unresectable renal cell carcinoma with distant metastasis. BJU Int 2001;87(4):312–5.

56. Munro NP, Woodhams S, Nawrocki JD, et al. The role of transarterial embolization in the treatment of renal cell carcinoma. BJU Int 2003;92(3):240–4.

57. Maxwell NJ, Saleem Amer N, Rogers E, et al. Renal artery embolisation in the palliative treatment of renal carcinoma. Br J Radiol 2007;80(950):96–102.

58. Kigawa J, Minagawa Y, Ishihara H, et al. The role of neoadjuvant intraarterial infusion chemotherapy with cisplatin and bleomycin for locally advanced cervical cancer. Am J Clin Oncol 1996;19(3):255–9.

59. Adachi S, Ogasawara T, Wakimoto E, et al. Phase I/II study of intravenous nedaplatin and intraarterial cisplatin with transcatheter arterial embolization for patients with locally advanced uterine cervical carcinoma. Cancer 2001;91(1): 74–9.

60. Eapen L, Stewart D, Collins J, et al. Effective bladder sparing therapy with intraarterial cisplatin and radiotherapy for localized bladder cancer. J Urol 2004; 172(4 Pt 1):1276–80.

61. Mokarim A, Uetani M, Hayashi N, et al. Combined intraarterial chemotherapy and radiotherapy in the treatment of bladder carcinoma. Cancer 1997;80(9): 1776–85.

62. Ikushima H, Iwamoto S, Osaki K, et al. Effective bladder preservation strategy with low-dose radiation therapy and concurrent intraarterial chemotherapy for muscle-invasive bladder cancer. Radiat Med 2008;26(3):156–63.

63. Barton PP, Waneck RE, Karnel FJ, et al. Embolization of bone metastases. J Vasc Interv Radiol 1996;7(1):81–8.

64. Gellad FE, Sadato N, Numaguchi Y, et al. Vascular metastatic lesions of the spine: preoperative embolization. Radiology 1990;176(3):683–6.
65. Chatziioannou AN, Johnson ME, Pneumaticos SG, et al. Preoperative embolization of bone metastases from renal cell carcinoma. Eur Radiol 2000;10(4): 593–6.
66. Smith TP, Gray L, Weinstein JN, et al. Preoperative transarterial embolization of spinal column neoplasms. J Vasc Interv Radiol 1995;6(6):863–9.
67. Lencioni R. Loco-regional treatment of hepatocellular carcinoma. Hepatology 2010;52(2):762–73.
68. Livraghi T, Bolondi L, Lazzaroni S, et al. Percutaneous ethanol injection in the treatment of hepatocellular carcinoma in cirrhosis. A study on 207 patients. Cancer 1992;69(4):925–9.
69. Sala M, Llovet JM, Vilana R, et al. Initial response to percutaneous ablation predicts survival in patients with hepatocellular carcinoma. Hepatology 2004;40(6): 1352–60.
70. Lee EW, Chen C, Prieto VE, et al. Advanced hepatic ablation technique for creating complete cell death: irreversible electroporation. Radiology 2010; 255(2):426–33.
71. Lencioni R, Crocetti L. Local-regional treatment of hepatocellular carcinoma. Radiology 2012;262(1):43–58.
72. Kingham TP, Karkar AM, D'Angelica MI, et al. Ablation of perivascular hepatic malignant tumors with irreversible electroporation. J Am Coll Surg 2012; 215(3):379–87.
73. Shiina S, Teratani T, Obi S, et al. A randomized controlled trial of radiofrequency ablation with ethanol injection for small hepatocellular carcinoma. Gastroenterology 2005;129(1):122–30.
74. Lin SM, Lin CJ, Lin CC, et al. Randomised controlled trial comparing percutaneous radiofrequency thermal ablation, percutaneous ethanol injection, and percutaneous acetic acid injection to treat hepatocellular carcinoma of 3 cm or less. Gut 2005;54(8):1151–6.
75. Brunello F, Veltri A, Carucci P, et al. Radiofrequency ablation versus ethanol injection for early hepatocellular carcinoma: a randomized controlled trial. Scand J Gastroenterol 2008;43(6):727–35.
76. Lencioni RA, Allgaier HP, Cioni D, et al. Small hepatocellular carcinoma in cirrhosis: randomized comparison of radio-frequency thermal ablation versus percutaneous ethanol injection. Radiology 2003;228(1):235–40.
77. Livraghi T, Meloni F, Di Stasi M, et al. Sustained complete response and complication rates after radiofrequency ablation of very early hepatocellular carcinoma in cirrhosis: is resection still the treatment of choice? Hepatology 2008;47(1): 82–9.
78. Ahrar K, Matin S, Wood CG, et al. Percutaneous radiofrequency ablation of renal tumors: technique, complications, and outcomes. J Vasc Interv Radiol 2005; 16(5):679–88.
79. Cho YK, Kim JK, Kim WT, et al. Hepatic resection versus radiofrequency ablation for very early stage hepatocellular carcinoma: a Markov model analysis. Hepatology 2010;51(4):1284–90.
80. Gillams AR, Lees WR. Five-year survival in 309 patients with colorectal liver metastases treated with radiofrequency ablation. Eur Radiol 2009;19(5):1206–13.
81. Gillams AR, Lees WR. Five-year survival following radiofrequency ablation of small, solitary, hepatic colorectal metastases. J Vasc Interv Radiol 2008;19(5): 712–7.

82. Oshowo A, Gillams A, Harrison E, et al. Comparison of resection and radiofrequency ablation for treatment of solitary colorectal liver metastases. Br J Surg 2003;90(10):1240–3.

83. Simon CJ, Dupuy DE, Mayo-Smith WW. Microwave ablation: principles and applications. Radiographics 2005;25(Suppl 1):S69–83.

84. Lubner MG, Brace CL, Hinshaw JL, et al. Microwave tumor ablation: mechanism of action, clinical results, and devices. J Vasc Interv Radiol 2010;21(Suppl 8): S192–203.

85. Yu NC, Raman SS, Kim YJ, et al. Microwave liver ablation: influence of hepatic vein size on heat-sink effect in a porcine model. J Vasc Interv Radiol 2008;19(7): 1087–92.

86. Shibata T, Iimuro Y, Yamamoto Y, et al. Small hepatocellular carcinoma: comparison of radio-frequency ablation and percutaneous microwave coagulation therapy. Radiology 2002;223(2):331–7.

87. Yu J, Liang P, Yu XL, et al. US-guided percutaneous microwave ablation versus open radical nephrectomy for small renal cell carcinoma: intermediate-term results. Radiology 2014;270(3):880–7.

88. Huang S, Yu J, Liang P, et al. Percutaneous microwave ablation for hepatocellular carcinoma adjacent to large vessels: a long-term follow-up. Eur J Radiol 2014;83(3):552–8.

89. Gage AA, Baust J. Mechanisms of tissue injury in cryosurgery. Cryobiology 1998;37(3):171–86.

90. Erinjeri JP, Clark TW. Cryoablation: mechanism of action and devices. J Vasc Interv Radiol 2010;21(Suppl 8):S187–91.

91. Bageacu S, Kaczmarek D, Lacroix M, et al. Cryosurgery for resectable and unresectable hepatic metastases from colorectal cancer. Eur J Surg Oncol 2007;33(5):590–6.

92. Seifert JK, France MP, Zhao J, et al. Large volume hepatic freezing: association with significant release of the cytokines interleukin-6 and tumor necrosis factor a in a rat model. World J Surg 2002;26(11):1333–41.

93. Sheen AJ, Poston GJ, Sherlock DJ. Cryotherapeutic ablation of liver tumours. Br J Surg 2002;89(11):1396–401.

94. Nordback IH, Pitt HA, Coleman J, et al. Unresectable hilar cholangiocarcinoma: percutaneous versus operative palliation. Surgery 1994;115(5):597–603.

95. Covey AM, Brown KT. Percutaneous transhepatic biliary drainage. Tech Vasc Interv Radiol 2008;11(1):14–20.

96. Saad WE, Wallace MJ, Wojak JC, et al. Quality improvement guidelines for percutaneous transhepatic cholangiography, biliary drainage, and percutaneous cholecystostomy. J Vasc Interv Radiol 2010;21(6):789–95.

97. Madoff DC, Wallace MJ. Palliative treatment of unresectable bile duct cancer: which stent? Which approach? Surg Oncol Clin N Am 2002;11(4):923–39.

98. Garcia MJ, Epstein DS, Dignazio MA. Percutaneous approach to the diagnosis and treatment of biliary tract malignancies. Surg Oncol Clin N Am 2009;18(2): 241–56, viii.

99. Wagner HJ, Knyrim K, Vakil N, et al. Plastic endoprostheses versus metal stents in the palliative treatment of malignant hilar biliary obstruction. A prospective and randomized trial. Endoscopy 1993;25(3):213–8.

100. Lee BH, Choe DH, Lee JH, et al. Metallic stents in malignant biliary obstruction: prospective long-term clinical results. AJR Am J Roentgenol 1997;168(3):741–5.

101. House MG, Choti MA. Palliative therapy for pancreatic/biliary cancer. Surg Oncol Clin N Am 2004;13(3):491–503, ix.

102. Nomura T, Shirai Y, Hatakeyama K. Bacteribilia and cholangitis after percutaneous transhepatic biliary drainage for malignant biliary obstruction. Dig Dis Sci 1999;44(3):542–6.
103. Carrasco CH, Zornoza J, Bechtel WJ. Malignant biliary obstruction: complications of percutaneous biliary drainage. Radiology 1984;152(2):343–6.
104. Avritscher R, Madoff DC, Ramirez PT, et al. Fistulas of the lower urinary tract: percutaneous approaches for the management of a difficult clinical entity. Radiographics 2004;24(Suppl 1):S217–36.
105. Titton RL, Gryzenia PC, Gervais DA, et al. Interventional radiology case conferences Massachusetts General Hospital. Continuous high-output drainage of hepatic abscess 3 months after radiofrequency ablation of hepatocellular carcinoma. AJR Am J Roentgenol 2003;180(4):1079–84.
106. Akhan O, Ozmen MN, Dincer A, et al. Liver hydatid disease: long-term results of percutaneous treatment. Radiology 1996;198(1):259–64.
107. McGraw JK, Lippert JA, Minkus KD, et al. Prospective evaluation of pain relief in 100 patients undergoing percutaneous vertebroplasty: results and follow-up. J Vasc Interv Radiol 2002;13(9 Pt 1):883–6.
108. Callstrom MR, Dupuy DE, Solomon SB, et al. Percutaneous image-guided cryoablation of painful metastases involving bone: multicenter trial. Cancer 2013; 119(5):1033–41.
109. Zhou ZQ, Lee JH, Song KB, et al. Clinical usefulness of portal venous stent in hepatobiliary pancreatic cancers. ANZ J Surg 2014;84(5):346–52.
110. Novellas S, Denys A, Bize P, et al. Palliative portal vein stent placement in malignant and symptomatic extrinsic portal vein stenosis or occlusion. Cardiovasc Intervent Radiol 2009;32(3):462–70.
111. Cheng S. Superior vena cava syndrome: a contemporary review of a historic disease. Cardiol Rev 2009;17(1):16–23.
112. Yu JB, Wilson LD, Detterbeck FC. Superior vena cava syndrome—a proposed classification system and algorithm for management. J Thorac Oncol 2008; 3(8):811–4.
113. Rowell NP, Gleeson FV. Steroids, radiotherapy, chemotherapy and stents for superior vena caval obstruction in carcinoma of the bronchus: a systematic review. Clin Oncol (R Coll Radiol) 2002;14(5):338–51.
114. Nagata T, Makutani S, Uchida H, et al. Follow-up results of 71 patients undergoing metallic stent placement for the treatment of a malignant obstruction of the superior vena cava. Cardiovasc Intervent Radiol 2007;30(5):959–67.

Index

Note: Page numbers of article titles are in **boldface** type.

Surg Oncol Clin N Am 23 (2014) 957–968
http://dx.doi.org/10.1016/S1055-3207(14)00072-6   **surgonc.theclinics.com**
1055-3207/14/$ – see front matter © 2014 Elsevier Inc. All rights reserved.

United States Postal Service

Statement of Ownership, Management, and Circulation
(All Periodicals Publications Except Requestor Publications)

1. Publication Title
Surgical Oncology Clinics of North America

2. Publication Number
0 1 2 - 5 6 5

3. Filing Date
9/14/14

4. Issue Frequency
Jan, Apr, Jul, Oct

5. Number of Issues Published Annually
4

6. Annual Subscription Price
$290.00

7. Complete Mailing Address of Known Office of Publication (Not printer) (Street, city, county, state, and ZIP+4®)

Elsevier Inc.
360 Park Avenue South
New York, NY 10010-1710

Contact Person
Stephen R. Bushing

Telephone (Include area code)
215-239-3688

8. Complete Mailing Address of Headquarters or General Business Office of Publisher (Not printer)

Elsevier Inc., 360 Park Avenue South, New York, NY 10010-1710

9. Full Names and Complete Mailing Addresses of Publisher, Editor, and Managing Editor (Do not leave blank)

Publisher (Name and complete mailing address)

Linda Belfus, Elsevier, Inc., 1600 John F. Kennedy Blvd. Suite 1800, Philadelphia, PA 19103-2899

Editor (Name and complete mailing address)

Jessica McCool, Elsevier, Inc., 1600 John F. Kennedy Blvd. Suite 1800, Philadelphia, PA 19103-2899

Managing Editor (Name and complete mailing address)

Adrianne Brigido, Inc., 1600 John F. Kennedy Blvd. Suite 1800, Philadelphia, PA 19103-2899

10. Owner (Do not leave blank. If the publication is owned by a corporation, give the name and address of the corporation immediately followed by the names and addresses of all stockholders owning or holding 1 percent or more of the total amount of stock. If not owned by a corporation, give the names and addresses of the individual owners. If owned by a partnership or other unincorporated firm, give its name and address as well as those of each individual owner. If the publication is published by a nonprofit organization, give its name and address.)

Full Name	Complete Mailing Address
Wholly owned subsidiary of	1600 John F. Kennedy Blvd. Ste. 1800
Reed/Elsevier, US holdings	Philadelphia, PA 19103-2899

11. Known Bondholders, Mortgagees, and Other Security Holders Owning or Holding 1 Percent or More of Total Amount of Bonds, Mortgages, or Other Securities. If none, check box ☒ None

Full Name	Complete Mailing Address
N/A	

12. Tax Status (For completion by nonprofit organizations authorized to mail at nonprofit rates) (Check one)
The purpose, function, and nonprofit status of this organization and the exempt status for federal income tax purposes:
☒ Has Not Changed During Preceding 12 Months
☐ Has Changed During Preceding 12 Months (Publisher must submit explanation of change with this statement)

PS Form 3526, August 2012 (Page 1 of 3 (Instructions Page 3)) PSN 7530-01-000-9931 PRIVACY NOTICE: See our Privacy policy in www.usps.com

---

13. Publication Title
Surgical Oncology Clinics of North America

14. Issue Date for Circulation Data Below
July 2014

15. Extent and Nature of Circulation

			Average No. Copies Each Issue During Preceding 12 Months	No. Copies of Single Issue Published Nearest to Filing Date
a. Total Number of Copies (Net press run)			454	482
b. Paid Circulation (By Mail and Outside the Mail)	(1)	Mailed Outside-County Paid Subscriptions Stated on PS Form 3541. (Include paid distribution above nominal rate, advertiser's proof copies, and exchange copies)	194	241
	(2)	Mailed In-County Paid Subscriptions Stated on PS Form 3541 (Include paid distribution above nominal rate, advertiser's proof copies, and exchange copies)		
	(3)	Paid Distribution Outside the Mails Including Sales Through Dealers and Carriers, Street Vendors, Counter Sales, and Other Paid Distribution Outside USPS®	73	85
	(4)	Paid Distribution by Other Classes Mailed Through the USPS (e.g. First-Class Mail®)		
c. Total Paid Distribution (Sum of 15b (1), (2), (3), and (4))			267	326
d. Free or Nominal Rate Distribution (By Mail and Outside the Mail)	(1)	Free or Nominal Rate Outside-County Copies Included on PS Form 3541	33	11
	(2)	Free or Nominal Rate In-County Copies Included on PS Form 3541		
	(3)	Free or Nominal Rate Copies Mailed at Other Classes Through the USPS (e.g. First-Class Mail)		
	(4)	Free or Nominal Rate Distribution Outside the Mail (Carriers or other means)		
e. Total Free or Nominal Rate Distribution (Sum of 15d (1), (2), (3) and (4))			33	11
f. Total Distribution (Sum of 15c and 15e)			300	337
g. Copies not Distributed (See instructions to publishers #4 (page #3))			154	145
h. Total (Sum of 15f and g)			454	482
i. Percent Paid (15c divided by 15f times 100)			89.00%	46.74%

16. Total circulation includes electronic copies. Report circulation on PS Form 3526-X worksheet.

17. Publication of Statement of Ownership
If the publication is a general publication, publication of this statement is required. Will be printed in the **October 2014** issue of this publication.

18. Signature and Title of Editor, Publisher, Business Manager, or Owner

Stephen R. Bushing – Inventory Distribution Coordinator

Date: September 14, 2014

I certify that all information furnished on this form is true and complete. I understand that anyone who furnishes false or misleading information on this form or who omits material or information requested on the form may be subject to criminal sanctions (including fines and imprisonment) and/or civil sanctions (including civil penalties).

PS Form 3526, August 2012 (Page 2 of 3)

Moving?

Make sure your subscription moves with you!

To notify us of your new address, find your **Clinics Account Number** (located on your mailing label above your name), and contact customer service at:

Email: journalscustomerservice-usa@elsevier.com

800-654-2452 (subscribers in the U.S. & Canada)
314-447-8871 (subscribers outside of the U.S. & Canada)

Fax number: 314-447-8029

Elsevier Health Sciences Division
Subscription Customer Service
3251 Riverport Lane
Maryland Heights, MO 63043

*To ensure uninterrupted delivery of your subscription,
please notify us at least 4 weeks in advance of move.

Printed and bound by CPI Group (UK) Ltd, Croydon, CR0 4YY

03/10/2024

01040488-0011